Advances in Blood Substitutes

Edited by

Robert M. Winslow Kim D. Vandegriff Marcos Intaglietta

University of California, San Diego

Volume 1	Blood Substitutes: Physiological Basis of Efficacy Winslow, Vandegriff, Intaglietta, editors ISBN 0-8176-3804-0
Volume 2	Blood Substitutes: New Challenges Winslow, Vandegriff, Intaglietta, editors ISBN 0-8176-3878-4
Volume 3	Advances in Blood Substitutes: Industrial Opportunities and Medical Challenges Winslow, Vandegriff, Intaglietta, editors ISBN 0-8176-3980-2

Advances in Blood Substitutes

From reviews of previous *Blood Substitutes* volumes--

"Overall, this volume offers concise and state-of-the-art overview of the subject, and as such the medical practitioner, hematologic specialist and investigator in blood substitutes will find it useful."

– The Quarterly Review of Biology, 1996

"This book is a good reference for all those who are interested in physiology of circulatory systems and the researchers and technologists who are interested in synthetic substitutes for biological materials."

– Journal of Cytology & Genetics, 1996

"There is now a concerted aim by both industry and academia to achieve the complete solution to the safe blood transfusion problem by the development of artificial blood substitutes. These efforts are summarized in this collection of essays edited by Winslow, Vandegriff and Intaglietta."

– European Review, 1996

Advances in Blood Substitutes

Industrial Opportunities and Medical Challenges

R. M. Winslow, M.D.
K.D. Vandegriff, Ph.D.
M. Intaglietta, Ph.D.
Editors

Birkhäuser
Boston • Basel • Berlin

Robert M. Winslow
School of Medicine
University of California
San Diego, CA 92161

Kim D. Vandegriff
School of Medicine
University of California
San Diego, CA 92161

Marcos Intaglietta
Dept. of Bioengineering
University of California
San Diego, CA 92161

Library of Congress Cataloging-in-Publication Data

Advances in blood substitutes : industrial opportunities and medical challenges / R.M. Winslow, K.D. Vandegriff, M. Intaglietta, editors.
p. cm.
Includes bibliographical references and index.
ISBN 0-8176-3980-2 (alk. paper). -- ISBN 3-7643-3980-2 (alk. paper)
1. Blood substitutes. I. Winslow, Robert M., 1941- . II. Vandegriff, Kim D. III. Intaglietta, Marcos.
[DNLM: 1. Blood Substitutes. 2. Hemoglobins--metabolism. 3. Fluorocarbons. 4. Polyethylene Glycols. 5. Oxygen--metabolism.
WH 450 A2441 1997]
RM171.7.A38 1997
615'.39--dc21
DNLM/DLC
for Library of Congress 97-22453
CIP

Printed on acid-free paper

Birkhäuser

ISBN 0-8176-3980-2
ISBN 3-7643-3980-2
Typeset by Renée Schad
Printed and bound by Quinn-Woodbine, Woodbine, NJ
Printed in the U.S.A.

9 8 7 6 5 4 3 2 1

Table of Contents

List of Contributors

Ann L. Baldwin, Ph.D.
Department of Physiology
College of Medicine
University of Arizona
Tucson, AZ 85724-5051

Pamela Bassett, D.M.D., M.B.A.
666 Fifth Avenue, 37th Floor
New York, NY 10103

Marvin L. Birnbaum, M.D., Ph.D.
Departments of Medicine & Physiology
University of Wisconsin — Madison
Madison, WI 53792

Elaine K. Daily, R.N., B.S., F.C.C.M.
Blood Substitutes
Baxter Healthcare
Route 120 & Wilson Road
Round Lake, IL 60073

John W. Eaton, Ph.D.
Baylor Medical College
Department of Pediatrics
One Baylor Plaza
Houston, TX 77030

Stephen F. Flaim, Ph.D.
Biological Sciences
Alliance Pharmaceutical Corp.
3040 Science Park Rd.
San Diego, CA 92121

Barbara Friensenecker, M.D.
Department of Bioengineering
University of California, San Diego
La Jolla,CA 92093-0412

Marcos Intaglietta, Ph.D.
Department of Bioengineering
University of California, San Diego
La Jolla,CA 92093-0412

Rakesh Jain, Ph.D.
Edwin L. Steele Laboratory
Massachusetts General Hospital *and*
Harvard Medical School
Boston, MA 02114

Heinz Kerger, M.D.
Department of Bioengineering
University of California, San Diego
La Jolla,CA 92093-0412

Kari L. Murad, Ph.D.
Department of Pathology (A-81)
Albany Medical College
47 New Scotland Avenue
Albany, NY 12208

Robert J. Przybelski, Ph.D.
Blood Substitutes
Baxter Healthcare
Route 120 & Wilson Road
Round Lake, IL 60073

Ronald J. Rohlfs, Ph.D.
Department of Medicine
School of Medicine
University of California, San Diego
Veterans Affairs Medical
Center (111-E)
3350 La Jolla Village Drive
San Diego, CA 92161

Hiromi Sakai, Ph.D.
Department of Polymer Chemistry
Advanced Research Institute for Science
and Engineering
Waseda University
Tokyo 169, Japan *and*
Department of Bioengineering (0412)
University of California, San Diego
Room 5608, Eng Bldg Unit 1
La Jolla, CA 92093-0412

Mark Scott, Ph.D.
Department of Pathology (A-81)
Albany Medical College
47 New Scotland Avenue
Albany, NY 12208

Vladimir P. Torchilin, Ph.D.
Department of Radiology
Harvard Medical School *and*
Chemistry Program, Center for Imaging and Pharmaceutical Research
Massachusetts General Hospital
149 13th Street
Charlestown, MA 02129-2060

Amy G. Tsai, Ph.D.
Department of Bioengineering
University of California, San Diego
La Jolla, CA 92093-0412

Sheung-Pun Tsai, Ph.D.
Department of Biochemistry
Hong Kong University of Science and Technology
Clear Water Bay
Kowloon, Hong Kong

Eishun Tsuchida, Ph.D.
Advanced Research Institute for Science and Engineering
Department of Polymer Chemistry
Waseda University
3-4 Ohkubo, Shinjuku-ku
Tokyo 169, Japan

Kim D. Vandegriff, Ph.D.
Department of Medicine
School of Medicine
University of California, San Diego
Veterans Affairs Medical Center (111-E)
3350 La Jolla Village Drive
San Diego, CA 92161

Robert M. Winslow, M.D.
Department of Medicine
School of Medicine
University of California, San Diego
Veterans Affairs Medical Center (111-E)
3350 La Jolla Village Drive
San Diego, California 92161

Jeffrey Tze-Fei Wong, Ph.D.
Department of Biochemistry
Hong Kong University of Science and Technology
Clear Water Bay
Kowloon, Hong Kong

List of Discussants

The following discussion participants are in addition to the Contributors. Numbers in parentheses are the Chapters in which Discussants participated.

Ruth Billings
Colorado State University
Fort Collins, CO (2)

Joeseppe Bonaventura
Duke University Medical Center
Durham, NC (4, 6, 11, 13, 14)

Giles R. Cokelet
University of Rochester
Rochester, NY (4, 6, 8, 12)

Maria Gawryl
Biopure Corporation
Cambridge, MA (2)

Armando Gonzales
Veterans Affairs Medical Center
San Francisco, CA (5, 14)

John Hearst
Cerus Corporation
Concord, CA (7, 9)

John Hess
U.S. Army
Bethesda, MD (7, 11, 12)

Rhoda E. Hirsch
Albert Einstein College of Medicine
Bronx, NY (2, 4)

Paul Johnson
University of California, San Diego
La Jolla, CA (4, 9, 10)

Peter Keipert
Alliance Pharmaceutical Corp.
San Diego, CA (4, 10, 14)

Jack Levin
University of California, San Francisco
San Francisco, CA (2, 4, 9)

Enzo Liguori
Army Hospital of Rome
Rome, ITALY (1)

Mark Lortie
University of California, San Diego
La Jolla, CA (2)

Dave Mailett
Rice University
Houston, TX (9)

Herbert J. Meiselman
University of Southern California
School of Medicine
Los Angeles, CA (1, 6, 7, 10, 11, 12)

William Phillips
University of Texas Health Science Center
San Antonio, TX (2, 8, 11, 13)

Vijay Sharma
University of California, San Diego
La Jolla, CA (14)

Lynn Ten Eyck
University of California, San Diego
La Jolla, CA (7)

Robert Woodson
University of Wisconsin
Madison, WI (6, 11)

Foreword

Each chapter of this volume is a contribution from an expert in the field, chosen by the editors to contribute to the 1997 "Current Issues in Blood Substitute Research and Development" course given in San Diego, March 17-19. The contributors were selected because of their expertise in areas which the editors believe to be critical to the advancement of the field, and which reflect activity in "hot" areas of relevant research.

While there is a continuity in style for the annual course, each year brings changes in emphasis and content. In previous years, we were often not able to provide time for participants to present their views and opinions. Consequently, this year we encouraged discussion after each presentation. These sessions were recorded, transcribed, and are printed with the chapters herein. We believe that the product is very close to the capturing this year's course in print, and trust readers will enjoy reading the always candid and often provocative remarks from the audience.

The price paid for inclusion of the discussion transcriptions was a delay in publication. Each author was allowed to edit his/her discussion section as well as the final version of the chapters prior to publication. The changes are mainly for grammar, and we tried, when possible, not to alter the conversational style of these interchanges.

While the discussions add an interesting component to the book, it also necessarily increased the amount of work required of the authors, editors, staff and assistants. The editors owe special thanks to Renée Schad, Program Manager for the Blood Substitutes research program at the University of California, San Diego, without whose assistance the creation of this book would not have been possible. We also wish to thank Dr. Ronald Rohlfs for his always enlightening comments and suggestions. We gratefully acknowledge Shirley Kolkey and her assistants at Complete Conference Management for their skillful organization of the course. We also wish to acknowledge the continued support of the National Institutes of Health (NHLBI), in particular, Dr. George Nemo and his staff.

Finally, we wish to thank all the authors and participants of the course. Without their continued efforts, there would be no current issues in research and development of blood substitutes for us to update.

Robert M. Winslow

Kim D. Vandegriff

Marcos Intaglietta

Preface

During the initial planning stages for this volume, our working subtitle was "New Directions", because we have become extremely excited over the past several years about how studying cell-free oxygen carriers has changed the fundamental way in which we think about oxygen transport. However commercialization of these products has accelerated also (two products are in Phase III clinical trials), and, we believe, the prospect of clinically available solutions is at least as exciting as the scientific advances. Hence, our hybrid subtitle is "Industrial Opportunities and Medical Challenges"

We believe that the scientific advances discussed in this volume will contribute significantly to future generations of products, and that these new thoughts and theories will become increasingly important as first-generation products are replaced by more sophisticated and cost-effective ones. This book, thus, represents new advances both in commercialization and in our understanding of the basic workings of blood substitutes as medical products.

A new feature added to this year's book is a discussion section at the end of each chapter. These discussions followed the presentations of these chapters at the 1997 "Current Issues in Blood Substitute Research and Development" course given in San Diego in 1997. Exciting new ideas arose out of these exchanges, and we hope that this addition to the book will stimulate new ideas in the readers as well.

The review of the 1996 literature by Winslow (Chapter 1) has become a staple of the course, providing a path to steer through the abounding literature on blood substitutes and related fields. The literature is broken into a number of useful categories that outrange the review from previous years, reflecting both the increasing interest in the field and the expanding indications and scientific evaluations under study.

Advances in product development are covered in diverse chapters ranging from pharmacoeconomics of blood substitutes by Bassett (Chapter 3) to the efficacy of a perfluorocarbon-based oxygen carriers by Flaim (Chapter 6) to strategies employed in developing a hemoglobin-based product for its pressor effect by Przybelski, Daily and Birnbaum (Chapter 5).

New technologies are introduced in chapters by Sakai *et al.* (Chapter 8) on encapsulated hemoglobin using polyethylene glycol modified liposomes and by Scott, Murad and Eaton (Chapter 7) on polyethylene glycol modified red blood cells. The use of poly ethylene glycol modification became a "hot topic" this year due to its inert and highly interesting chemical properties. This is advanced in more detail by Torchilin (Chapter 13) in the chapter on the chemistry of modification of molecules and particles using polyethylene glycol. An older, and somewhat related technology, that still looks very promising is revisited by Tsai and Wong (Chapter 12) in their chapter on dextran conjugated hemoglobin.

A new indication for tumor oxygenation is reviewed by Jain (Chapter 4), providing an in-depth and fascinating overview of tumor microcirculation and new developments in cancer therapy. The microcirculation is explored further in a chapter by Baldwin (Chapter 2) in which ultrastructural inflammatory effects and extravasation are addressed. These two chapters lead to new experimental approaches and reveal new avenues that are just under exploration in this field.

Several paradigms are reevaluated in this volume. A new theory on the oxygen delivery by hemoglobin-based oxygen carriers is developed in a mathematical model presented by Winslow and Vandegriff (Chapter 9). Rohlfs, Vandegriff and Winslow (Chapter 14) provide a chapter on nitric oxide binding to hemoglobin-based oxygen carriers and its physiologic implication. Tsai *et al.* (Chapter 10) challenge assumptions about viscosity in the efficacy of blood substitutes. Finally, Vandegriff, Rohlfs and Winslow (Chapter 11) challenge assumptions about colloid osmotic properties in the design of blood substitutes. All of these chapters develop new ideas that are aimed to help the field continue to grow in the coming years.

As in each of the two previous years, this book is dedicated to updating the current state of the art in blood substitute research and development. The recent success of moving products into advanced clinical trials has come out of years of rigorous work toward this end. We feel that this book reflects the excitement in the field as hard work is finally being realized in tangible goals.

This book is the result of the effort of an entire generation of blood substitute scientists. However, selection of authors and subjects for the current volume is our responsibility alone. We have tried to provide an interesting and exciting volume this year. We always look forward to the response the book receives.

Robert M. Winslow

Kim D. Vandegriff

Marcos Intaglietta

Chapter 1

Blood Substitutes: 1996 in the Literature

Robert M. Winslow, M.D.

1.1 Introduction

The year 1996 in the "blood substitute" literature continued to follow the trends set in 1994 and 1995. That is, there appears to be less emphasis on specific biochemical modifications of hemoglobin and perfluorocarbon chemistry, and more on clinical trials and related issues. There was an ever larger number of meetings and symposia on the subject, and even more appear to be slated for 1997, as products near the market and clinic.

The term "blood substitutes" is falling out of favor in many circles because it carries the connotation of over-promise and failure. Instead, we are seeing terms such as HBOC (hemoglobin-based oxygen carrier), therapeutic oxygen carrier, cell-free oxygen carrier and hemodiluent used. These terms more accurately reflect the fact that none of the products being developed today is a true blood substitute. Rather, each fulfills some function of blood, like oxygen transport or volume expansion.

Whether we like it or not, however, "blood substitute" is an index term for much of the current literature having to do with oxygen carriers. Thus a Medline search for blood substitutes will yield citations for coagulation factors and platelets, for example, which are not of immediate interest for our forum on oxygen carriers. However, citations for plasma expanders such as starches, albumin and gelatin also are uncovered, and many of these are of great interest to us. This year's search, as in the past, is for the index term "blood substitute" and I have culled the result to eliminate those citations which I believe are of little or no relevance to the development of oxygen carriers. Searches for terms such as "hemoglobin", "perfluorocarbons", "polyethylene glycol", for example, would yield many citations, some of which might also be of interest. This strategy is dangerous, of course, since our audience is diverse, and each of us has our own special set of interests. Finally, I have included some references that do not appear in a standard Medline search but which have been brought to my attention during the year by colleagues or by reading related literature.

During the past year, a number of colleagues have sent me reprints of their work, with the suggestion that they be included in the next review. This carries the strong inference that I have offended some of my colleagues in the past, and to them I apologize. If I have overlooked significant contributions to the literature in 1996 it is totally out of ignorance: no effort has been made to judge quality or relevance in this summary, with the exception that I have marked with an asterisk (*) the articles that I believe are worth special attention.

1.2 News, Reviews and Editorials

Progress in 1996 was marked by the approval by the FDA of Phase III clinical trials for Baxter's product, HemeAssist (known as DCLHb), which is being developed based on a strategy to exploit the product's vasoactivity (Gibbs, Hensley, Fricker). Reviews and editorials in 1996, however, were mixed. These ranged from the optimistic documentation of the progress of clinical development to pessimistic reviews of older published literature (Eaton, Hess, Hess and Reiss). The articles by Hess and by Hess and Riess cite some of the same properties as preventing blood substitutes from fulfilling their promise as resuscitation solutions as Baxter exploits in their clinical trials. Perhaps this contradiction will be resolved in the near future as new data come to light; the Hess and Hess and Riess reviews deal with outdated data which do not adequately reflect the current state of the "blood substitute" field.

Thoughtful reviews of the emerging products and their potential impact on clinical practice are provided by Dietz *et al.*, Joyner and Faust, and Mallick and Bodenham. The review by Gould and Moss summarizes the experience of these two pioneers in development of one product, glutaraldehyde-polymerized human hemoglobin. Thomas presents a summary of an important conference held in Edinburgh in the fall of 1995 in which alternatives to transfusion were discussed at length. Although autologous transfusion, rather than blood substitutes, was the primary focus of that conference, the discussion points out that not every system of medical practice has the same requirements for transfusion services.

1. **Ben-Hur, E., and B. Horowitz**. Virus inactivation in blood [editorial]. *AIDS* 10: 1183-1190, 1996.

2. **Dietz, N.M., M.J. Joyner, and M.A. Warner**. Blood substitutes: fluids, drugs, or miracle solutions? *Anesth. Analg.* 82: 390-405, 1996.

3. **Eaton, J.W.** Hemoglobin-based blood substitutes: a dream-like trade of blood and guile? *J. Lab. Clin. Med.* 127: 416-417, 1996.

4. **Fricker, J.** Artificial blood--bad news for vampires? *Lancet* 347: 1322, 1996.

5. **Gibbs, W.W.** Artificial blood quickens. Several short-term substitutes approach final clinical trials. *Sci. Am*er. 275: 44-48, 1996.

6. **Gould, S.A., and G.S. Moss.** Clinical development of human polymerized hemoglobin as a blood substitute. *World J. Surg.* 20: 1200-1207, 1996.

7. **Hensley, S.** Baxter's blood substitute OK'd for trauma testing. Mod. Healthcare 26: 16, 1996.

8. **Hess, J.R.** Blood Substitutes. *Semin. Hematol.* 33: 369-378, 1996.

9. **Hess, J.R., and Reiss, R.F.** Resuscitation and the limited utility of the present generation of blood substitutes. *Trans. Med. Rev.* X: 276-285, 1996.

10. **Joyner, M.J., and R.J. Faust.** Blood Substitutes: What is the target? In *Blood Substitutes: New Challenges* (R.M. Winslow, K.D. Vandegriff, and M. Intaglietta, eds). Boston: Birkhäuser, 1996, pp. 15-33.

11. **Mallick, A., and A.R. Bodenham.** Modified haemoglobins as oxygen-transporting blood substitutes. *Br. J. Hosp. Med.* 55: 443-448, 1996.

12. **Sekiguchi, S., and K. Ikebuchi.** [Present status and future of blood management in Japan]. *Nippon Naika Gakkai Zasshi* 85: 862-870, 1996.

*13. **Thomas, M.J.** Royal College of Physicians, Edinburgh: final consensus statement. Consensus Conference on Autologous Transfusion, 4-6 October, 1995. *Vox Sang.* 70: 183-184, 1996.

1.3 Products

The commercial products in development as of approximately September, 1996, are summarized in a review by Winslow (26), in which multiple databases were searched, including those for patents and news announcements as well as the scientific literature.

A very careful description of a hemoglobin modification process was provided by Bucci *et al.* This article is detailed enough so that most standard biochemical laboratories should be capable of producing cross-linked hemoglobin if the procedures are followed in detail. As pointed out in the accompanying editorial by Winslow (1996a), this type of communication has been lacking in the field in general, and has led to controversies over whether products from one laboratory are comparable to those from others. For example, whether or not the Baxter DCLHb and the Army's αα-Hb are, in fact, the same product is still not resolved. It is hoped that more generic products, such as the one described by Bucci *et al.*, will be described in the future so that academic work on blood substitutes need not be impeded by such controversies. Other hemoglobin products and methods are described in the articles by Greenwald *et al.* and Pavlik *et al.*

Engineering recombinant hemoglobin has become the focus of many groups after the pioneering work at Somatogen showed that large-scale production is a realistic goal. Articles by Manning and Sanders *et al.* delve into associated issues and discuss in detail the various properties of hemoglobin that may be of importance in the design of a blood substitute: subunit interaction, oxidation, free-radical formation, and oxygen affinity.

Liposome-encapsulated hemoglobin (LEH) is discussed in several articles. Biological effects of LEH in the U.S. Navy's program are presented by Rollwagen *et al.*, while Tsuchida's group in Japan characterizes its liposomes in the article by Sakai *et al.* In spite of the complexity of production techniques, LEH is showing promise in its biological effects. The article by Rohlfs and Vandegriff suggests that production might be simplified in the future.

*14. **Bucci, E., A. Razynska, H. Kwansa, B. Matheson-Urbaitis, M. O'Hearne, J.A. Ulatowski, and R. C. Koehler.** Production and characteristics of an infusible oxygen-carrying fluid based on hemoglobin intramolecularly cross-linked with sebacic acid. *J. Lab. Clin. Med.* 128: 146-153, 1996.

15. **Greenwald, R.B., A. Pendri, A. Martinez, C. Gilbert, and P. Bradley.** PEG thiazolidine-2-thione, a novel regent for facile protein modification: Conjugation of bovine hemoglobin. *Bioconjug. Chem.* 7: 638-641, 1996.

16. **Ivanitski, G.R., and S.I. Vorob'ev.** [Organization of mobile structures in the blood stream--basis for the function of perfluorocarbon "artificial blood"]. *Biofizika* 41: 178-190, 1996.

17. **Leslie, S.B., S. Puvvada, B.R. Ratna, and A.S. Rudolph.** Encapsulation of hemoglobin in a bicontinuous cubic phase lipid. *Biochemica Biophysica Acta* 1285: 246-254, 1996.

*18. **Manning, J.M.** Examples of chemical modification and recombinant DNA approaches with hemoglobin. *Transfus. Clin. Biol.* 3: 109-111, 1996.

19. **Pavlik, P.A., M.K. Boyd, and K.W. Olsen.** Molecular dynamics of a hemoglobin crosslinking reaction. *Biopolymers* 39: 615-618, 1996.

20. **Rohlfs, R.J., and K.D. Vandegriff.** Non-phospholipid liposomes: A novel method for the preparation of hemoglobin-containing lipid vesicles. In *Blood Substitutes: New Challenges* (R.M. Winslow, K.D. Vandegriff, and M. Intaglietta, eds.). Boston: Birkhäuser, 1996, pp. 163-184.

*21. **Rollwagen, F.M., W.C. Gafney, N.D. Pacheco, T.A. Davis, T.M. Hickey, T.B. Nielsen, and A.S. Rudolph.** Multiple responses to administration of liposome-encapsulated hemoglobin (LEH): Effects on hematopoiesis and serum IL-6 levels. *Exp. Hematol.* 24: 429-436, 1996.

*22. **Sakai, H., K. Hamada, S. Takeoka, H. Nishide, and E. Tsuchida.** Physical properties of hemoglobin vesicles as red cell substitutes. *Biotechnol. Prog.* 12: 119-125, 1996.

*23. **Sanders, K.E., G. Ackers, and S. Sligar.** Engineering and design of blood substitutes. *Curr. Opinion Struct. Biol.* 6: 534-540, 1996.

24. **Szebeni, J., N.M. Wassef, A.S. Rudolph, and C.R. Alving.** Complement activation in human serum by liposome-encapsulated hemoglobin: the role of natural anti-phospholipid antibodies. *Biochem. Biophys. Acta* 1285: 127-130, 1996.

25. **Winslow, R.M.** Blood substitutes: science or business? *J. Lab. Clin. Med.* 128: 126-127, 1996.

*26. **Winslow, R.M.** Blood substitutes in development. *Exp. Opin. Invest. Drugs* 5: 1443-1452, 1996.

1.4 Effects

More products are now available to investigators than have been in previous years, but still the literature on biological effects is heavily weighted toward industrial research using proprietary products.

1.4.1 Hemodynamic effects

Although the hemodynamic effects of perfluorocarbon emulsions are fairly straightforward, the vasoactivity of hemoglobin solutions is still not completely understood. Gulati *et al.* show that endothelin probably plays some role in this activity. The Amend *et al.* paper studies the hemodynamic response of bled dogs to resuscitation with cell-free (unmodified) hemoglobin compared to shed blood and confirms that blood is the superior product. But the studies underline the effects of cell-free hemoglobin that seem to be characteristic of many products: reduced cardiac output, hypertension, and bradycardia. Excretion of N-acetyl-beta-D-glucosaminidase (NAG) was significantly elevated in the hemoglobin animals, reflecting renal damage produced by that solution. Traditionally, it has been assumed that most of these unfavorable side-effects could be eliminated by purification and cross-linking of hemoglobin.

Such a product is the object of the paper by Kasper *et al.*, which reports a study of a purified, cross-linked bovine hemoglobin (HBOC-201) in a human study of perioperative hemodilution. These authors report that as a result of a hemodilution of 3 ml/kg, surgical patients demonstrate an increase of mean arterial pressure of 140% over control, an increase of systemic vascular resistance to 169% and reduction of cardiac index to 75% of control. They conclude that HBOC-201, at a dose of 3 ml/kg, impairs oxygen delivery because of adverse effects on cardiac output.

The study by Jia *et al.* was one of the most important hemoglobin papers of the year. In it, the authors find a significant difference between arterial and venous S-nitrosohemoglobin (SNO-hemoglobin). They proposed a transport function for the β93 cysteine residue, whereby hemoglobin is S-nitrosylated in the lung and the NO group is released in tissue, helping to maintain capillary flow. These findings spawned considerable speculation about the role of hemoglobin in regulation of vessel tone and blood pressure, and will surely lead to further exploration of these phenomena in the coming years. The general roles of the mediators NO and CO were reviewed by Motterlini in 1996.

27. **Amend, J., C. Ou, C. Ryan-MacFarlane, P.J. Anderson, N. Amend, and G.P. Biro.** Systemic responses to SFHS-infusion in hemorrhaged dogs. *Artif. Cells Blood Substit. Immobil. Biotechnol.* 24: 19-34, 1996.

28. **Gulati, A., A.C. Sharma, and G. Singh.** Role of endothelin in the cardiovascular effects of diaspirin crosslinked and stroma reduced hemoglobin. *Crit. Care Med.* 24: 137-147, 1996.

*29. **Jia, L., J. Bonaventura, and J.S. Stamler.** S-nitrosohaemoglobin: a dynamic activity of blood involved in vascular control. *Nature* 380: 221-226, 1996.

*30. **Kasper, S.M., M. Walter, F. Grune, A. Bischoff, H. Erasmi, and W. Buzello.** Effects of a hemoglobin-based oxygen carrier (HBOC-201) on hemodynamics and oxygen transport in patients undergoing preoperative hemodilution for elective abdominal aortic surgery. *Anesth. Analg.* 83: 921-927, 1996.

*31. **Ulatowski, J.A., T. Nishikawa, B. Matheson-Urbaitis, Bucci, E., Traystman, R.J., and R.C. Koehler.** Regional blood flow alterations after bovine fumaryl ββ-crosslinked hemoglobin transfusion and nitric oxide synthase inhibition. *Crit. Care Med.* 24: 558-565, 1996.

1.4.2 Volume and oncotic effects

As the unique effects of hemoglobin are understood better, attention is directed to volume effects, since hemoglobin is oncotically active. Furthermore, the amount of oncotic pressure exerted by hemoglobin depends to a strong degree on the type of chemical modification to which it has been subjected. An excellent overview of oncotic forces and fluid shifts in the body is presented in the article by Michel. In it, the author traces the development in concepts of the various fluid spaces and their regulation from Starling up to the present.

Further insight into oncotic and volume effects is gained from the increasing interest in the starches. These products are synthetic, inexpensive, and have fewer side-effects than traditional plasma-expanders. Therefore, they are being used more in clinical settings around the world and may represent a commercial target for hemoglobin or perfluorocarbon-based products in the future. Oncotic effects have not been the primary target of blood-substitute research, because it has always been assumed that the optimal product should have the same oncotic activity as blood. However, interesting insights are provided by oncotic effects with regard to the blood-brain barrier (Chi *et al.*), brain injury (Cole *et al.*), endothelin levels (Garcia-Sepulcre *et al.*) and brainstem evoked potentials (Detsch *et al.*), all of which are relevant to blood-substitute development. Burg *et al.* even show that osmotic forces may influence gene expression.

32. **Burg, M.B., E.D. Kwon, and D. Kultz.** Osmotic regulation of gene expression. *FASEB J.* 10: 1598-1606, 1996.

33. **Chi, O.Z., X. Lu, H.M. Wei, J.A. Williams, and H.R. Weiss.** Hydroxyethyl starch solution attenuates blood-brain barrier disruption caused by intracarotid injection of hyperosmolar mannitol in rats. *Anesth. Analg.* 83: 336-341, 1996.

34. **Cole, D.J., J.C. Drummond, P.M. Patel, J.C. Nary, and R.L. Applegate.** Effect of oncotic pressure of diaspirin cross-linked hemoglobin (DCLHb) on brain injury after temporary focal cerebral ischemia in rats. *Anesth. Analg.* 83: 342-347, 1996.

35. **Detsch, O., M. Heesen, J. Muhling, A. Thiel, B. Bachmann-Mennenga, and G. Hempelmann.** Isovolaemic haemodilution with hydroxyethylstarch has no effect on somatosensory evoked potentials in healthy volunteers. *Acta Anaesthesiol. Scand.* 40: 665-670, 1996.

36. **Garcia-Sepulcre, M.E., F. Carnicer, M. Mauri, A. Prieto, and M. Perez-Mateo.** Increased plasma endothelin in liver cirrhosis and response to plasma volume expansion [letter]. *Am. J. Gastroenterol.* 91: 2452-2453, 1996.

*37. **Michel, C.C.** One hundred years of Starling's hypothesis. *News Physiol. Sci.* 11: 229-237, 1996.

1.4.3 Perfusion and regional blood flow

Understanding of the local effects of either hemoglobin solutions or perfluorocarbons may not be complete for some time because of the array of macromolecules that mediate microvascular effects. These include substances that act either as vasodilators or vasoconstrictors, those which promote neovascularization, and the myriad adhesion molecules that are being described. The paper by Gennaro *et al.* studies eicoasanoid release in skeletal muscle after ischemia and reperfusion, for example.

38. **Gennaro, M., C. Mohan, and E. Ascer**. Perfluorocarbon emulsion prevents eicoasanoid release in skeletal muscle ischemia and reperfusion. *Cardiovasc. Surg.* 4: 399-404, 1996.

39. **Golubev, A.M., M.A. Magomedov, T.A. Leont'eva, and T.S. Guseinov**. [The biomicroscopic evaluation of the blood microcirculatory bed in the mesentery of the small intestine during experimental perftoran infusion under normovolemia]. *Morfologiia* 109: 36-40, 1996.

40. **Traylor, R.J., and R.G. Pearl**. Crystalloid *versus* colloid versus colloid: all colloids are not created equal. *Anesth. Analg.* 83: 209-212, 1996.

1.4.4 Gas transport

In theory, exchange of oxygen should be facilitated by the presence of cell-free oxygen carriers, as shown by a number of models such as the one discussed by Shah and Mehra and Page *et al.* In practice, this has been difficult to demonstrate, either because of vasoactive effects in the case of hemoglobins, or because so little of the product can be administered in the case of the perfluorocarbon emulsions. Nevertheless, Keipert *et al.* continue to show beneficial effects of perfluorocarbon emulsions.

The paper by Hughes *et al.* (41) is of interest because it studies gas exchange in humans hemodiluted with up to 40 g of polymerized bovine hemoglobin. They found that although peak plasma concentrations did not exceed 2 g/dl, the pulmonary diffusing capacity increased up to 20% above baseline in the highest dose groups, compared to controls who demonstrated reduced diffusing capacity. The diffusing capacity paralleled plasma hemoglobin, suggesting a cause and effect relationship.

The overlooked property of hemoglobin, CO_2 transport, was reviewed by Winslow with a view toward implications for blood substitutes.

*41. **Hughes, G.S., Jr., E.J. Antal, P.K. Locker, S.F. Francom, W.J. Adams, and E.E. Jacobs.** Physiology and pharmacokinetics of a novel hemoglobin-based oxygen carrier in humans. *Crit. Care Med.* 24: 756-764, 1996.

42. **Hughes, G.S., Jr., S.F. Francom, E.J. Antal, W.J. Adams, P.K. Locker, E.P. Yancey, and E.E. Jacobs.** Effects of a novel hemoglobin-based oxygen carrier on percent oxygen saturation as determined with arterial blood gas analysis and pulse oximetry. *Ann. Emerg. Med.* 27: 164-169, 1996.

43. **Keipert, P.E., N.S. Faithfull, D.J. Roth, J.D. Bradley, S. Batra, P. Jochelson, and K.E. Flaim.** Supporting tissue oxygenation

during acute surgical bleeding using a perfluorochemical-based oxygen carrier. *Adv. Exp. Med. Biol.* 388: 603-609, 1996.

44. **Page, T.C., C.B. McKay, W.R. Light, and J.D. Hellums.** Experimental simulation of oxygen transport in microvessels. In *Blood Substitutes: New Challenges* (R.M. Winslow, K.D. Vandegriff, and M. Intaglietta, eds). Boston: Birkhäuser, 1996, pp. 132-145.

45. **Shah, N., and A. Mehra.** Modeling of oxygen uptake in perfluorocarbon emulsions. Some comparisons with uptake by blood. *ASAIO J.* 42: 181-189, 1996.

1.4.5 Endothelium and microvascular effects

Microcirculation studies are among the most exciting to be carried out with cell-free oxygen carriers. The papers by Tsai *et al.* and Intaglietta *et al.* present an entirely new theoretical analysis which points to the importance of blood viscosity in oxygen transport. This analysis would not have been possible without data from studies with "blood substitutes" because they offer the possibility to dissociate blood viscosity, oncotic pressure, oxygen affinity, and oxygen capacity in order to study the separate effects of these variables. Essentially, Intaglietta proposes that a link between blood viscosity and microvascular flow may enable cell-free oxygen carriers to realize their full potential. The relationship between viscosity and vasoconstriction, which are reciprocal in hemorrhage, may be explained by the growing knowledge about transduction of shear stress into chemically-mediated vasoactivity in the studies of Frangos, including the paper by Gudi *et al.* Similar lines of research are represented by the papers of Boldt *et al.* and Karmaker and Dhar.

46. **Boldt, J., M. Heesen, W. Padberg, K. Martin, and G. Hempelmann.** The influence of volume therapy and pentoxifylline infusion on circulating adhesion molecules in trauma patients. Anesthesia 51: 529-535, 1996.

*47. **Gudi, S.R.P., C.B. Clark, and J.A. Frangos.** Fluid flow rapidly activates G proteins in human endothelial cells. Involvement of G proteins in mechanicochemical signal transduction. *Circ. Res.* 79: 834-839, 1996.

*48. **Intaglietta, M., P.C. Johnson, and R.M. Winslow.** Microvascular and tissue oxygen distribution. *Cardiovasc. Res.* 32: 632-643, 1996.

49. **Karmakar, N., and P. Dhar.** Effect of steady shear stress on fluid filtration through the rabbit arterial wall in the presence of macromolecules. *Clin. Exp. Pharmacol. Physiol.* 23: 299-304, 1996.

50. **Tsai, A.G., H. Kerger, and M. Intaglietta.** Microvascular oxygen distribution: Effects due to free hemoglobin in plasma. In *Blood Sub-*

stitutes: New Challenges (R.M. Winslow, K.D. Vandegriff, and M. Intaglietta, eds.). Boston: Birkhäuser, 1996, pp. 124-131.

1.5 Efficacy

Efficacy of blood-substitute solutions has always been assumed, and efforts are now underway in large-scale clinical trials to provide proof. However since the details of the activity of the materials are still under study, animal research continues. A part of the problem in studying efficacy is that no end point is universally accepted. Subcutaneous oxygen tension and gastrointestinal PO_2 are used in the studies of Drucker *et al.* and Frankel *et al.*, respectively. Biochemical and acid-base effects are studied in the papers by Conover *et al.* and Leppaniemi *et al.*, while survival and gas transport are the end points in the abstract by Winslow *et al.* The hemodilution model (Conover *et al.*) suggests that polyethylene glycol bovine hemoglobin (PEG-Hb) could be useful in this procedure, which is gaining in popularity.

*51. **Conover, C.D., P. Malatesta, L. Lejeune, C.L. Chang, and R.G. Shorr.** The effects of hemodilution with polyethylene glycol bovine hemoglobin (PEG-Hb) in a conscious porcine model. *J. Invest. Med.* 44: 238-246, 1996.

*52. **Drucker, W., F. Pearce, L. Glass-Heidenreich, H. Hopf, C. Powell, M.G. Ochsner, H. Frankel, D. Murray, M. Nelson, H. Champion, G. Rozycki, J. Silva, D. Malcolm, J. DeNobile, D. Harviel, and N. Rich.** Subcutaneous tissue oxygen pressure: a reliable index of peripheral perfusion in humans after injury. *J. Trauma* 40: S116-S122, 1996.

*53. **Frankel, H.L., H.B. Nguyen, T. Shea-Donohue, L.A. Aiton, J. Ratigan, and D.S. Malcolm.** Diaspirin cross-linked hemoglobin is efficacious in gut resuscitation as measured by a GI tract optode. *J. Trauma* 40: 231-240; discussion, 241, 1996.

54. **Leppaniemi, A., R. Soltero, D. Burris, E. Pikoulis, J. Ratigan, C. Waasdorp, H. Hufnagel, and D. Malcolm.** Early resuscitation with low-volume PolyDCLHb is effective in the treatment of shock induced by penetrating vascular injury. *J. Trauma* 40: 242-248, 1996.

55. **Winslow, R.M., A. Gonzales, and M. Gonzales.** Physiologic effects of hemoglobin-based oxygen carriers compared to red blood cells in acute hemorrhage. [abstract] *Blood* 88: 626a, 1996.

1.6 Toxicity

Toxicity remains an important subject as clinical applications for blood substitutes broaden. Many academic laboratories focus on adverse effects of blood substitutes as industry focuses on clinical applications. The traditional toxicities of hemoglobin solutions include vasoactivity and renal damage, while perfluorocarbon toxicities involve inflammatory responses and thrombocytopenia.

1.6.1 Coagulation and liver function

In 1996 there were a number of studies of coagulation. Dilution of coagulation factors has long been recognized to occur with aggressive hemodilution with dextrans, starches, and even in patients receiving massive amounts of plasma or other blood products, including red cells. This must be kept in mind in consideration of future clinical applications, since neither hemoglobin solutions nor perfluorocarbon emulsions contain coagulation factors, and platelets will be diluted by simple mathematical relationships.

Bleeker and coworkers reported morphologic findings in the gastrointestinal mucosa of animals which had received glutaraldehyde polymerized hemoglobin. They concluded that this abnormality could be corrected by alteration of the conditions of polymerization. Coagulation abnormalities, including deficits of factor VIII, are well known to follow administration of gelatins and some starches, but so far have not been reported with hemoglobin or perfluorocarbon solutions.

*56. **Bleeker, W., J. Agterberg, E. La Hey, G. Rigter, L. Zappeij, and J. Bakker.** Hemorrhagic disorders after administration of glutaraldehyde-polymerized hemoglobin. In *Blood Substitutes: New Challenges* (R.M. Winslow, K.D. Vandegriff, and M. Intaglietta, eds.). Boston: Birkhäuser, 1996, pp. 112-123.

57. **Mardel, S.N., F. Saunders, L. Ollerenshaw, C. Edwards, and D. Baddeley.** Reduced quality of *in-vitro* clot formation with gelatin-based plasma substitutes [letter]. *Lancet* 347: 825, 1996.

58. **Heath, M.L.** Clot formation and gelatin-based plasma substitutes [letter]. *Lancet* 347: 1336, 1996.

59. **Mardel, S.N., F.M. Saunders, L.D. Ollerenshaw, and D.T. Buddeley.** Haemodilution induces a hypercoagulable state [letter]. *Br. J. Anaesth.* 77: 700-701, 1996.

1.6.2 Liver function

There have been few studies of specific abnormalities of liver function in recent years. The group represented by the paper by Eldridge *et al.* has conducted histological studies for many years with polyoxyethylene-modified hemoglobin and report specific lesions.

60. **Eldridge, J., R. Russell, R. Christenson, R. Sakamoto, J. Williams, M. Parr, B. Trump, P. Delaney, and C.F. Mackenzie.** Liver function and morphology after resuscitation from severe hemor-

rhagic shock with hemoglobin solutions or autologous blood. *Crit. Care Med.* 24: 663-671, 1996.

1.6.3 Infection and endotoxin

A major fear has been that cell-free hemoglobin might either promote bacterial growth or it might diminish the ability of the reticuloendothelial system to remove blood-borne bacteria. One potential mechanism for hemoglobin toxicity of this type is interference with platelet and phagocyte function, resulting from scavenging of NO by hemoglobin, as reviewed by Krishnamurti and Alving. A second possible difficulty, raised by the Levin group, is a specific binding mechanism for hemoglobin and endotoxin. In spite of these two concerns, studies such as the one by Langermans *et al.* have failed to show significantly increased mortality when bacteria and hemoglobin are administered together.

*61. **Krishnamurti, C., and B. Alving.** Biological consequences of cross-linked hemoglobin in animal models of surgery and endotoxemia. In *Blood Substitutes: New Challenges* (R.M. Winslow, K.D. Vandegriff, and M. Intaglietta, eds.). Boston: Birkhäuser, 1996, pp. 99-111.

*62. **Langermans, J.A., M. van Vuren-van der Hulst, and W.K. Bleeker.** Safety evaluation of a polymerized hemoglobin solution in a murine infection model. *J. Lab. Clin. Med.* 127: 428-434, 1996.

*63. **Levin, J., R.I. Roth, W. Kaca, M. Yoshida, and D. Su.** Hemoglobin-endotoxin interactions. In *Blood Substitutes: New Challenges* (R.M. Winslow, K.D. Vandegriff, and M. Intaglietta, eds.). Boston: Birkhäuser, 1996, pp. 185-202.

1.6.4 Neurologic injury

Hemoglobin has been shown to be toxic to isolated neurons in the past, but the paper by Reasoner raises the additional issue that the degree of volume expansion (or contraction) prior to experimental central nervous system infarction has important consequences for the extent of infarct. This type of study underscores the importance of a thorough understanding of the oncotic effects of plasma expanders and blood substitutes and the specific implications for clinical applications such as neurological disease and stroke.

64. **Reasoner, D.K., K.H. Ryu, B.J. Hindman, J. Cutkomp and T. Smith.** Marked hemodilution increases neurologic injury after focal cerebral ischemia in rabbits. *Anesth. Analg.* 82: 61-67, 1996.

1.7 Clinical Applications

As more products enter clinical trials, attention is focused on clinical applications. This is to be expected because companies are making marketing plans, and strategies are being formulated for achieving regulatory approval. The chapter by Winslow discusses the many different properties of the current crop of potential blood substitutes and explores how these properties make them more or less attractive for specific applications. Blood substitutes are being viewed less as blood substitutes and more as therapeutic agents to be used in well-defined clinical situations.

65. **Winslow, R.M.** Blood substitute oxygen carriers designed for clinical applications. In *Blood Substitutes: New Challenges* (R.M. Winslow, K.D. Vandegriff, and M. Intaglietta, eds.). Boston: Birkhäuser, 1996, pp. 60-73.

1.7.1 Shock, trauma and hemorrhage

Blood has been used to treat hemorrhagic shock by the inescapable logic that what's lost should be replaced. It is not that simple, of course, because of the numerous physiologic and biochemical adaptations that come into play when significant volume is lost. Essential to the clinical management of patients in shock is the assessment of the severity of the shock state, so that the therapy can be tuned to the requirement. Baron and Scalea discuss the physiology of shock and suggest that simple measurements like blood pressure, heart rate and hematocrit may not be the best indices to follow. Instead, they propose more attention be paid to acid-base balance, lactic acid, central venous oxygen tension and oxygen transport parameters.

The two papers by Mackay *et al.* and Nho *et al.* propose that transfusion of whole blood in shock may not be the most efficacious approach to therapy and instead hemodilution, either with polyglycine or PEG-hemoglobin, may be better.

*66. **Baron, B.J., and T.M. Scalea.** Acute blood loss. *Emerg. Med. Clin. North Amer.* 14: 35-55, 1996.

67. **Mackay, Z., Q. Shugufta, M. Din, and A.A. Guru.** Hemodilution in complicated high velocity vascular injuries of limbs. *J. Cardiovasc. Surg. (Torino)* 37: 217-221, 1996.

68. **Nho, K., R. Linberg, M. Johnson, C. Gilbert, and R. Shorr.** PEG-hemoglobin: An efficient oxygen-delivery system in the rat exchange transfusion and hypovolemic shock models. *Art. Cells, Blood Substit., and Immobil. Biotech.* 22: 795-803, 1996.

1.7.2 Perioperative hemodilution

After sustained popularity in Europe, perioperative hemodilution is gaining a foothold in North America as well, as reviewed in the article by Kreimeier and Messmer. There are a number of reasons for this, including the fear of transfusion of infected blood and blood conservation, but the physiological benefits now seem to be appreciated also. New, more highly purified hydroxyethyl starches are now available, and some of the preparations (for example, Pentastarch) have higher oncotic pressure than the older preparations. It appears that albumin is being replaced by the starches as the first choice of many physicians because of the high cost of albumin, primarily, but also because the effects of starches may be more sustained. The properties of alternatives, including dextran-40, dextran-60, hydroxyethylstarch-200, gelatin and albumin are compared in the paper by Freyburger *et al.*

69. **Blanloeil, Y., and Y. Leteurnier.** [Indications and role of albumin for vascular loading during postoperative intensive care]. *Ann. Fr. Anesth. Reanim.* 15: 497-506, 1996.

70. **Brutocao, D., S.L. Bratton, J.R. Thomas, P.F. Schrader, P.G. Coles, and A.M. Lynn.** Comparison of hetastarch with albumin for postoperative volume expansion in children after cardiopulmonary bypass. *J. Cardiothorac. Vasc. Anesth.* 10: 348-351, 1996.

71. **Carli, P.** [Indications and role of albumin for vascular loading during prehospital care]. *Ann. Fr. Anesth. Reanim.* 15: 470-472, 1996.

72. **Fosse, E., and H.E. Heier.** [Changing the use of albumin at the Oslo hospital]. *Tidsskr Nor Laegeforen* 116: 54-57, 1996.

*73. **Freyburger, G., M. Dubreuil, M.R. Boisseau, and G. Janvier.** Rheological properties of commonly used plasma substitutes during preoperative normovolaemic acute haemodilution. *Br. J. Anaesth.* 76: 519-525, 1996.

74. **Gerard, J.L., and H. Bricard.** [Indications and role of albumin for vascular loading in the operating room]. *Ann. Fr. Anesth. Reanim.* 15: 481-490, 1996.

75. **Grathwohl, K.W., B.J. Bruns, C.J. LeBrun, A.K. Ohno, T.A. Dillard.** Does hemodilution exist? Effects of saline infusion on hematologic parameters in euvolemic subjects. *South Med. J.* 89: 51-5, 1996.

*76. **Kreimeier, U., and K. Messmer.** Hemodilution in clinical surgery: state of the art 1996. *World J. Surg.* 20: 1208-1217, 1996.

77. **McCall, W.G.** Physiological and practical considerations of fluid management. *CRNA* 7: 62-70, 1996.

1.7.3 Transfusion therapy

The HIV epidemic has forever changed transfusion practices worldwide, as demonstrated in the review by Frey and Messmer. However, blood is safer now than it ever has been. The aggregate risk of viral transmission from transfused blood is estimated by Schreiber *et al.* as 1/34,000 units, a figure which makes blood transfusion of less risk than that of the underlying disease or clinical indication, as pointed out in the accompanying editorial by Paul Holland.

Nevertheless, strategies are now in place to minimize blood transfusions, such as perioperative hemodilution and autologous transfusion. The latter technique seems to have reached its maximum in terms of number of patients who are eligible or units of blood saved.

*78. **Frey, L., and K. Messmer.** Transfusion therapy. *Current Opin. Anaesthesiol.* 9: 183-187, 1996.

79. **Holland, P.V.** Viral infections and the blood supply. *N. Engl. J. Med.* 334: 1734-1735, 1996.

80. **Oberhauser, M., H.J. Bardenheuer, H. Bernasconi, T. Genz, and U. Kreimeier.** [Isovolemic hemodilution for avoiding homologous blood transfusion effectiveness in large gynecologic interventions]. *Infusionsther. Transfusionsmed.* 23: 15-23, 1996.

*81. **Schreiber, G.B., M.P. Busch, S.H. Kleinman, and J.J. Korelitz.** The risk of transfusion of transmitted viral infections. *N. Engl. J. Med.* 334: 1685-1690, 1006.

1.7.4 Burn

Burn injury is a new section in this year's literature review. This unique injury involves massive fluid shifts from the intravascular to the interstitial spaces, and issues of oncotic pressure become very important. The paper by Guha *et al.*, points out that a scald injury in sheep reduced the cardiac output by 30%, the mean arterial pressure by 20%, and the systemic hematocrit increased by 10 to 15%. They found that therapy with hypertonic saline dextran or hetastarch reduced the volume of fluid needed, and therefore edema, significantly.

*82. **Guha, S.C., M.P. Kinsky, B. Button, D.N. Herndon, L.D. Traber, D.L. Traber, and G.C. Kramer.** Burn resuscitation: crystalloid *versus* colloid versus hypertonic saline hyperoncotic colloid in sheep. *Crit. Care Med.* 24: 1849-1857, 1996.

1.7.5 Liquid ventilation

Although not a "blood substitute" application, liquid breathing is a "spin-off" of blood substitute research. The paper by Leach *et al.* describes the use of perflubron in premature infants with respiratory distress syndrome, with impressive results.

*83. **Leach, C.L., J.S. Greenspan, D.S. Rubenstein, T.H. Shaffer, M.R. Wolfson, J.C. Jackson, R. DeLemos, and B.P. Fuhrman.** Partial liquid ventilation with perflubron in premature infants with severe respiratory distress syndrome. *New Eng. J. Med.* 335: 761-767, 1996.

1.8 Discussion

Meiselman: As a newcomer to this field, I am reminded of the work in the early sixties on hemodilution with rheomacrodex, which is 40,000 molecular weight dextran, and macrodex which is a 70,000 molecular weight dextran. The extensive literature at that time argued the pros and cons of hemodilution. It seems like we need to look at that experience and incorporate it with the new concepts that are being developed in terms of recombinant or PEG-hemoglobin. There was an enormous amount of both animal and theoretical work done with *in vivo* observations of microcirculatory blood flow in burn and other conditions.

Winslow: It is an excellent comment. The products we have to study now are so much better: they don't interact with factor VIII, allergic and anaphylactic reactions are fewer, and now we have solutions that carry oxygen.

Intaglietta: You have made a very impressive review of the literature, and at least to me, it has been obvious for quite some time, whenever there is a question about blood substitutes or this field, one should actually come to you and short circuit the whole investigative process. I was wondering whether in your view of this year's literature, you have found work in the development of blood substitutes or similar materials in countries outside of the United States, Europe and Japan. We have two distinguished visitors from Brazil, two from Mexico, one from Italy, and one from Hong Kong, in addition to the group from Waseda University in Tokyo. Maybe you have seen some other activities that we are unaware of by just looking at the literature.

Winslow: I should have stated in my introduction that the review is not representative of the non-English literature. There were, however, a number of very interesting related articles from foreign countries that I didn't mention. For example, I have been very impressed at the level of Russian science in spite of the abysmal level of support from the Russian government. Relevant work in Russia seems to be focused in two areas, perfluorocarbons and polyethylene glycol (PEG). There have been reports of PEG-modified materials, not hemoglobin necessarily, but other molecules that have very significant volume expansion properties. The Japanese literature is also under-represented, again because very often we can only get titles. But we are going to have a presentation by Dr. Sakai, and we have quite a number of visitors this year from Japan, so I am hoping we will get more insight as we go. Italy has a long tradition of work in hemoglobin, but there was apparently little activity in this field. France, Germany, the Netherlands and U.K. have all contributed significantly in past years.

Intaglietta: I wonder if Dr. Ligouri who I see here in the audience, might comment on what it happening in Italy in the development of blood substitutes.

Ligouri: I don't know exactly the proceedings in Italy for blood substitutes because I am a cardiovascular surgeon. But just yesterday Dr. Winslow said to me that in Italy a group in Milan has some experience in blood substitutes like the San Diego group.

Bonaventura: With respect to the Italian situation, I worked for three years in the Rome lab of Antonini, Brunori and Jeffries Wyman, and I gave a lecture on blood substitutes there just three months ago. The biggest problem is the lack of support from the Italian government for research in this area. Enrico Bucci and Clara Fronticelli have their origins in that group, and they are, of course, carrying out Italian-style research in the United States. But what I would like to point out is that much of the fundamental work, which provides the hemoglobin biochemistry groundwork for what is being done in hemoglobin-based oxygen carriers, came from that group in Rome. In fact there is a lot of overlooked, old literature concerning modified hemoglobin and glutaraldehyde cross-linked erythrocytes. Maurizio Brunori and Bruno Giardina have done a number of very interesting experiments with these "red cell rocks", which can be washed with deionized water— they don't break, and they still bind oxygen reversibly.

Chapter 2

Blood Substitutes and the Intestinal Microcirculation: Extravasation and Ultrastructural Alterations

Ann Baldwin, Ph.D.

2.1 Introduction

Three necessary requirements for hemoglobin (Hb)-based blood substitutes are (i) that they remain in the circulation for an appropriate time period, (ii) that they do not alter the mechanisms of macromolecular exchange between blood and tissue, and (iii) that they do not cause tissue damage. A problem with hemoglobin-based blood substitutes is that they may leave the circulation and produce cytotoxic side effects. One vital organ which is particularly adversely affected during hemorrhagic shock is the intestine. Shock results in loss of gut mucosal integrity, allowing translocation of bacteria and endotoxins into the circulation, resulting in a systemic inflammatory response. The intestine is also important with respect to the immune system because the mucosa contains Peyer's patches, or organized aggregates of lymphoid tissue in between the villi. Peyer's patches play a key role in the initiation and expression of mucosal immunity. For these reasons we decided to focus on the intestine with respect to its responses to blood substitutes.

Previous studies have shown that commercially available hemoglobin extravasates from fenestrated intestinal mucosal capillaries only 30 seconds after injection (Milici and Bankston 1982). One approach that is being taken to reduce extravasation is to bind Hb to a larger molecule, such as polyethylene glycol-conjugated (PEG) hemoglobin (PEG-Hb). This procedure increases the molecular Stokes Einstein radius from 5 nm to 25 nm. However, we have shown that PEG-Hb extravasates rapidly from intestinal mucosal capillaries and causes epithelial detachment in villi near Peyer's patches. In this chapter studies are described in which the time course of extravasation of PEG-Hb from the intestinal microcirculation is determined using epifluorescence microscopy in combination with video imaging and analysis. Further studies are described in which electron microscopy is used to determine the transendothelial pathways followed by PEG-Hb and to characterize the ultrastructural changes caused by microvascular infusion of PEG-Hb.

Finally, the possible mechanisms responsible for tissue damage are described and possible protocols to ameliorate such damage are discussed.

2.2 Extravasation of PEG-Hb

2.2.1 Methods

PEG-Hb was labeled with fluoroisothiocyanate (FITC) using a protocol supplied by "Molecular Probes". Briefly, a sample of PEG-Hb was degassed and dissolved in 0.15 M sodium bicarbonate, and FITC in dimethyl sulfoxide was added dropwise. The reaction was incubated at room temperature with continuous stirring. After one hour, the reaction was stopped by adding freshly prepared 1.5 M hydroxylamine, pH 8.0. The reaction product was incubated for an additional 30 minutes, and then the unbound FITC was removed by passing the product through a gel filtration column at 10°C. The bound FITC-PEG-Hb was filtered just before use.

Male Sprague-Dawley rats (350-450 g) were anesthetized with sodium pentobarbitone (6 mg/100g wt., i.p.). FITC-PEG-Hb (2 mg/ml) was injected into the rats via the superior mesenteric artery or femoral vein. A timer was started on injection of the tracer, and the mucosa was scanned using a light microscope with epifluorescence while videotaping the image. Preliminary experiments were performed in which the whole field of view was scanned to determine whether there were any sites of preferential extravasation. Extravasation occurred preferentially within villi adjacent to Peyer's patches. In each subsequent experiment, two adjacent Peyer's patches were selected and surrounding villi scanned at various times after injection. In order to observe exactly the same villi at different time points throughout the experiment, the following protocol was developed. Each Peyer's patch was treated as a clock face, and the villi located at the noon, 3-pm, 6-pm and 9-pm positions were focused on in turn and the exact time of observation noted.

Extravasation caused villi to become bright in contrast to the surrounding epithelium. In order to quantitate the degree of brightness at a given time-point, the following method was used. The videotape of each experiment was played back using a recorder connected to a TV monitor and to a computer equipped with a video acquisition card. The image of each focused villus was grabbed so that it could be analyzed using an analog to digital (A-to-D) converter and computer software (NIH-Image). The average intensity of each villus minus the background was determined at each time-point.

A villus was considered "bright" if its intensity, measured using the A-to-D converter, exceeded 45 pixels. This was the value that correlated best with the intensity of villi that were "brighter than control", as judged by eye. The percentage of bright villi was counted at various time points after injection. Average villus intensities (including villi that were not "bright") were measured for each experiment. In addition, the distribution of extravasated PEG-Hb within each villus was recorded by obtaining a concentration profile across the villus at different times after injection.

2.2.2 Results

Preliminary experiments showed that extravasation of FITC-Hb, unlike that of FITC-albumin, initially occurred only at villi surrounding Peyer's patches, suggesting that activation of cells which normally reside within Peyer's patches may be involved. Villi surrounding a Peyer's patch are shown in Figure 2.1. Extravasation near Peyer's patches started at 2 minutes. At this point, the PEG-Hb was just beginning to leave the microcirculation and fluorescence was just detectable within the villi. By 5 minutes, fluorescence had accumulated within villi adjacent to Peyer's patches. By 8 minutes, about 20% of selected villi, (but few away from Peyer's patches), were bright and some tracer was observed between occasional Peyer's patch villi; this was accompanied by epithelial sloughing.

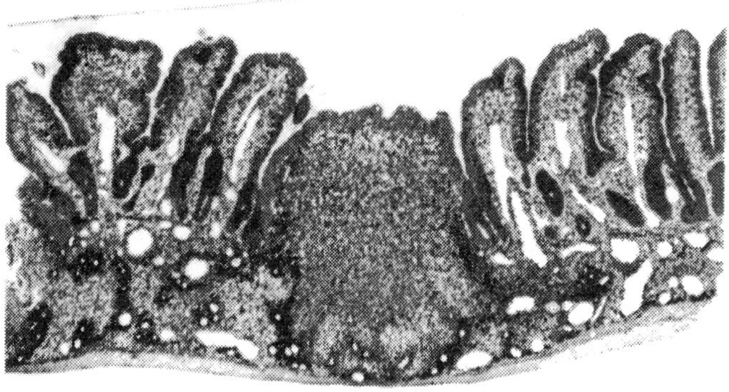

Figure 2.1.

By 10 minutes, the intensity within villi adjacent to Peyer's patches started to fall as the FITC-PEG-Hb leaked out through the villus epithelium (Figure 2.2). By this time, the borders around the villi became less defined as the epithelial layer fragmented. Extravasation away from

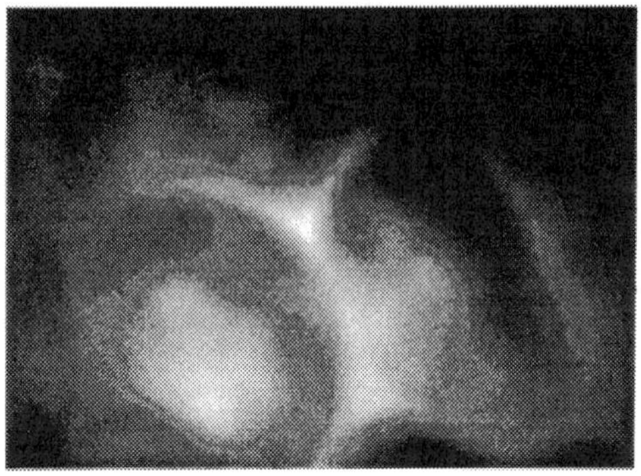

Figure 2.2.

Peyer's patches was delayed by about 10 minutes. The time course of extravasation, evaluated in terms of percentage of bright Peyer's patch villi and in terms of the mean intensity of Peyer's patch villus interstitium, respectively, are shown in Figures 2.3 and 2.4. The results

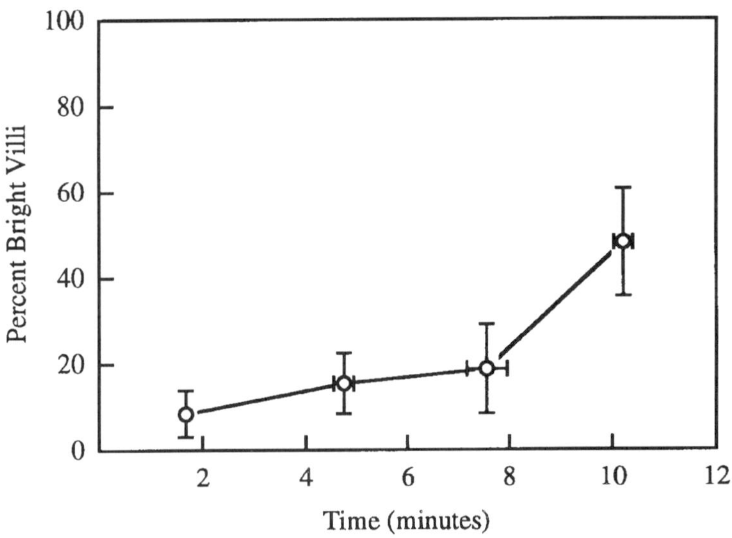

Figure 2.3. Percentage of bright villi after FITC-PEG-Hb injections.

were averaged over 8 experiments. In both cases, extravasation after 10 minutes was significantly greater than at 2 minutes. Figure 2.5 shows typical concentration profiles through a villus at two different time points (2 minutes and 10 minutes) after injection. These two profiles through the single villus reflect similar results to those seen when results are averaged.

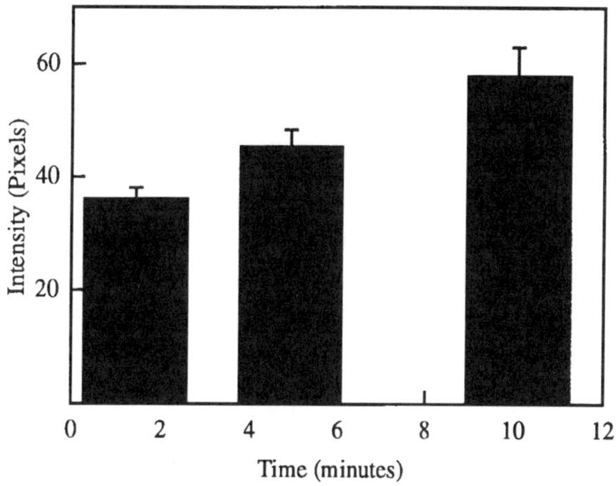

Figure 2.4. Mean fluorescence intensity of villus interstitium after FITC-PEG-Hb injection.

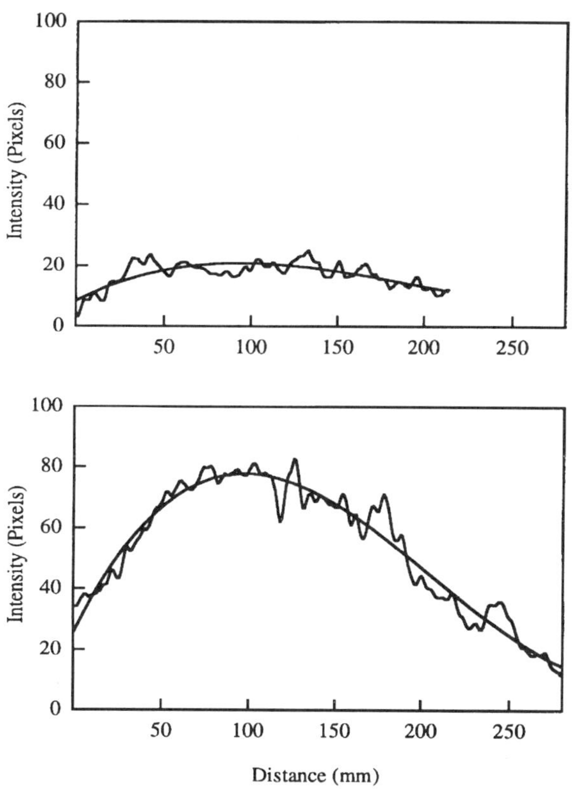

Figure 2.5. Concentration profiles of extravasated PEG-Hb in a villus, at 2 minutes (top) and 10 minutes (bottom), after injection.

2.3 Ultrastructural Effects of PEG-Hb

2.3.1 Methods

The following study was performed to determine the transendothelial pathways followed by PEG-Hb and to characterize tissue damage. Male Sprague-Dawley rats (350 g - 450 g) were anesthetized with pentobarbitone (6 mg/100g wt., i.p.). A cannula was placed retrograde in the abdominal aorta distal to the superior mesenteric artery. Ten mg of PEG-Hb (2 mg/ml) in Hepes buffered saline (HBS) was injected through a 0.2-micron filter via the cannula and allowed to circulate for 2, 8, 15, 30, 60 or 90 minutes. In control rats, HBS replaced PEG-Hb. Three animals were used for each group. The intestine was perfusion-fixed, stained with diaminobenzidine (DAB) and prepared for electron microscopy. The DAB was used as a stain for hemoglobin in order to determine the pathways taken by PEG-Hb as it extravasates. Although DAB also stains specific granules in immune cells, this property does not compromise its effectiveness as a label for Hb in our experiments.

2.3.2 Results - pathways of transendothelial passage

Staining with diaminobenzidine showed that after 2 minutes, Hb filled endothelial vesicles, both attached to, and apparently separate from, the luminal membrane. Endothelial cell junctions, open to the basement membrane, also contained Hb (Figure 2.6).

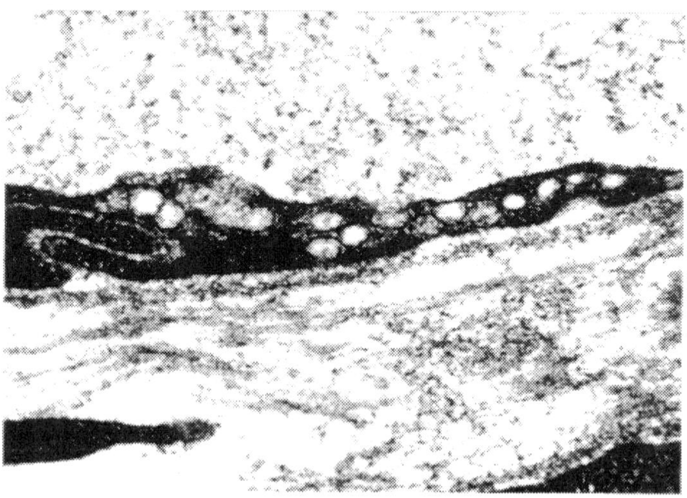

Figure 2.6.

Since this type of junction (zonnula adherens) is too narrow (3 nm) to permit passage of a molecule as large as PEG-Hb (25 nm), this indicates that the junctions are becoming widened as a result of PEG-Hb perfusion. It is possible that PEG-Hb may penetrate the junctions and then gain access to endothelial vesicles which are open to the abluminal endothelial surface.

Alternatively, extravasation of PEG-Hb may occur both via leaky junctions and by pinocytosis. Fenestrae are unlikely to be pathways for extravasation because our electron microscopy studies show that PEG-Hb actually reduces the number of single diaphragmed fenestrae per endothelial cell (Figure 2.7). However, the number of "transitional" fenestrae, or those which possess a double or triple diaphragm, is increased by PEG-Hb. Control preparations showed endothelial junctions which contained "tight" regions, and thus were not open to the basement membrane. These experiments indicate that PEG-Hb, or a breakdown product, such as Hb or heme, causes endothelial junctions to widen and then serve as a transport pathway. Thus, binding Hb to PEG does not prevent its extravasation across intestinal mucosal capillaries.

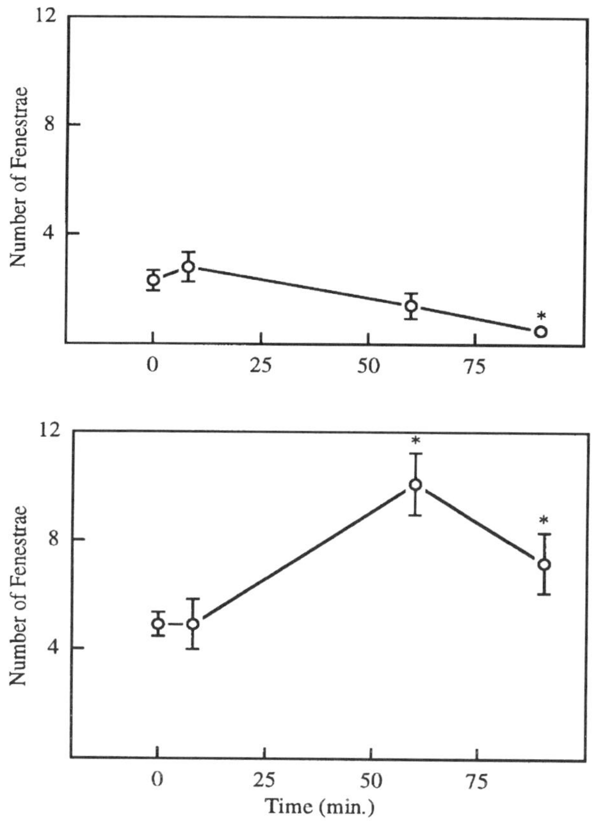

Figure 2.7. Mean number of fenestrae (single diaphragm (top)), double or triple (bottom) per intestinal mucosal capillary section. *Indicates significant difference from control.

2.3.3 Other Ultrastructural Effects

In control preparations, epithelial cells adhered closely to each other and to the basement membrane. Some lymphocytes (L) were seen between epithelial cells (E) close to the basement membrane and adjacent to capillaries (C), (Figure 2.8). Two minutes after PEG-Hb injection, at villi close to Peyer's patches, epithelial cells started to separate from each other and show long finger-like cytoplasmic projections. At 8 minutes after injection, epithelial cells were detaching from basement membrane, the cytoplasmic projections were more pronounced and the subepithelial tissue was edematous. Mast cells (MC) were present beneath the epithelium and were often in the process of degranulating, and thus releasing histamine (Figure 2.9). Lymphocytes, which were normally wedged tightly between pairs of epithelial cells at their basal aspect, had moved up closer to the lumen. This change was probably due to passive migration of the lymphocytes (*i.e.*, space filling). It is unlikely that lymphocytes play an active role so soon after PEG-Hb injection. Eosinophils (EO) could be seen beneath the epithelium (Figure 2.10). Compared with neutrophils, it is doubtful that eosinophils are of significant importance in protection against the usual types of infection. However, eosinophils have a special propensity to collect in tissues in which allergic reactions have occurred.

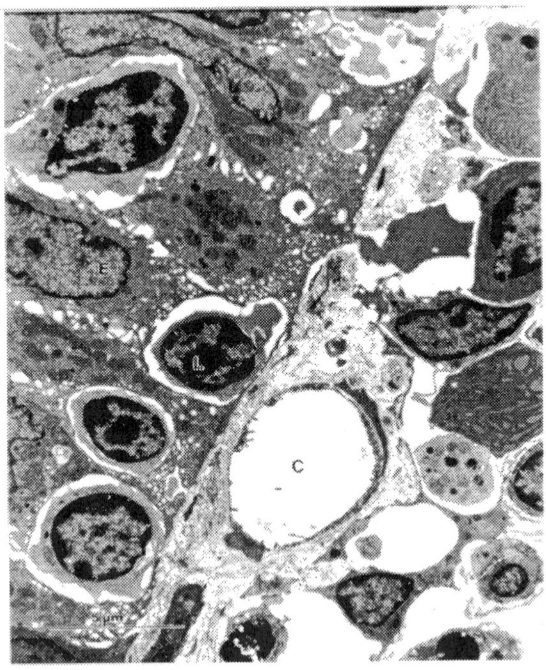

Figure 2.8.

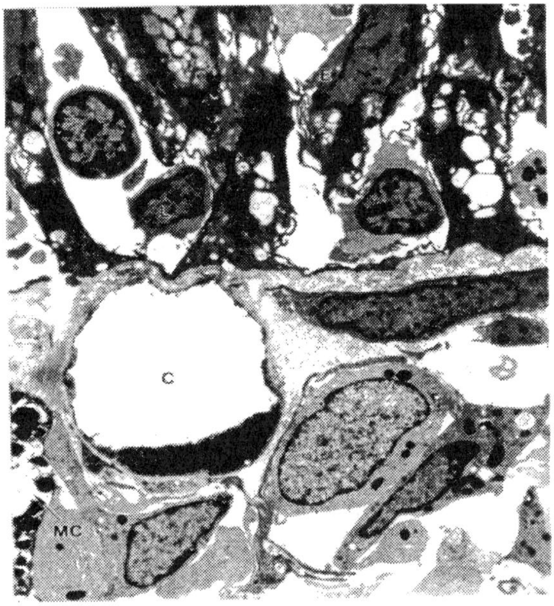

Figure 2.9.

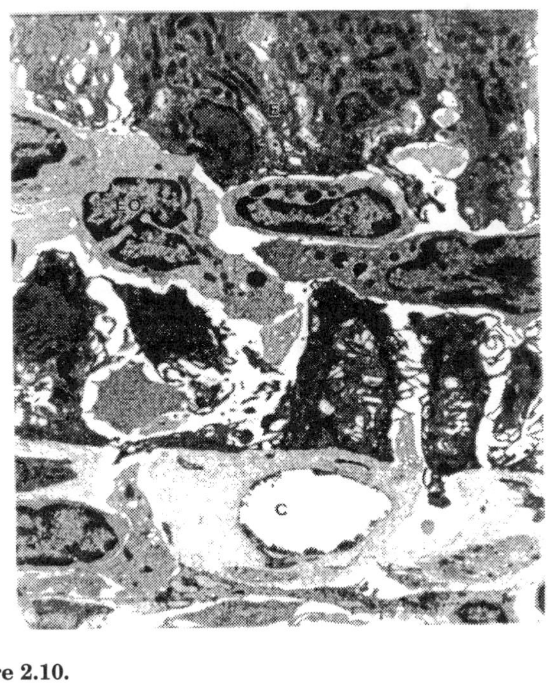

Figure 2.10.

These cells were normally not seen in controls. Often, collagen fibers were observed arranged circumferentially around the capillaries in a highly organized fashion. This abundance and organization of collagen fibers was not seen in control preparations. Previous authors (Moore *et al.* 1992) have suggested that collagen-epithelial interactions are important in restitution after injury, and that collagen can be produced locally and rapidly (within 60 minutes) at the site of injury to allow restitution of the villus tip epithelium to proceed. After 15-minutes circulation time of PEG-Hb, there appeared to be some recovery. There was less epithelial sloughing, subepithelial edema was reduced, and the lymphocyte arrangement was more organized (Figure 2.11). Specimens which were fixed 60 and 90 minutes after injection of PEG-Hb showed improved recovery. In villi away from Peyer's patches similar changes occurred, except their time course was delayed by 6-7 minutes.

To summarize, interstitial damage is caused by the extravasating Hb, either *per se* or in conjunction with activated resident immune cells. The appearance of degranulating mast cells and eosinophils in the villus interstitium following PEG-Hb injection indicates an inflammatory or allergic response to PEG-Hb, which appears to be transient.

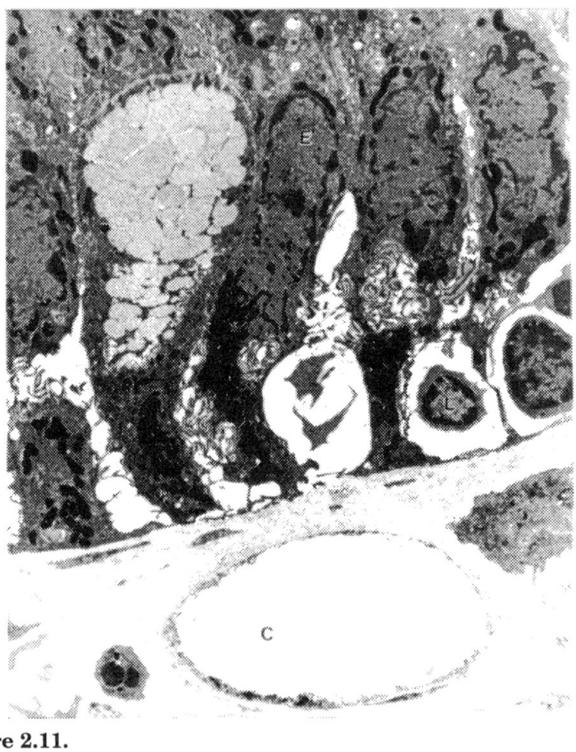

Figure 2.11.

The ultrastructural changes produced by circulation of PEG-Hb follow a time course that is consistent with the passage of fluorescently-labeled PEG-Hb from the blood stream, through the villus interstitium and into the intestinal lumen, both close to and away from Peyer's patches. Extravasation near Peyer's patches starts within 2 minutes. By 10 minutes most selected villi (but none away from Peyer's patches) are usually bright, and some tracer is observed between occasional Peyer's patch villi; this is accompanied by epithelial sloughing. The epithelial damage near Peyer's patches has been confirmed using transmission electron microscopy. Thus the PEG-Hb is not only crossing the microvascular walls, it is also damaging the epithelium and entering the intestinal lumen.

Previous studies, involving exchange transfusion with cross-linked Hb, have demonstrated hepatic injury with acute inflammatory cell infiltration by days 1 and 4, which was resolved by day 15. Also, Hb positive material has been seen in capillary endothelial cells (Smith *et al.* 1990). In the same study, degeneration and regeneration of kidney epithelial cells was observed. The epithelial damage, inflammatory cell infiltration, and the transient nature of these responses are similar to our observations in the intestine in response to PEG-Hb.

2.4 Conclusions

Our most significant finding so far is that the potential hemoglobin-based oxygen carrier, PEG-Hb, causes a transient inflammatory or allergic response in the intestine. This response, which lasts for at least one hour, enhances extravasation of the PEG-Hb, and also increases transport of plasma proteins from the blood stream into the intestinal lumen. Thus, transport of nutrients and drugs between blood and tissue will also be compromised during this time period. Since the damage is resolved in a few hours, it may easily remain undetected in routine preclinical safety studies. However, the interaction of PEG-Hb with pathologic states, such as prolonged ischemia and hemorrhagic or septic shock, is unknown. Such pathologic states will often be evident in patients in need of transfusions. Therefore, it is vital to develop protocols to reduce intestinal extravasation and subsequent inflammation.

Two possible causes for the damaging effects of PEG-Hb on the intestine are: (i) complement activation and/or (ii) generation of oxygen-free radicals.

2.4.1 Complement activation

The complement system provides the first line of defense against foreign cells or particles, ensuring their cytolytic and phagocytic removal. A survey of the literature reveals that injected hemoglobins cause complement activation only if they contain impurities, such as endotoxins or stromal phospholipids (Feola *et al.* 1988). Hemoglobins encapsulated using liposomes have also been shown to activate complement, while the free Hb did not in this case (Szebeni *et al.* 1994). Impurities have been shown to cause complement activation by the alternative pathway (Szebeni *et al.* 1994). Human Hb transfusates may also contain trace membrane fragments with blood group antigens which activate complement by the classical pathway if injected into humans (Chang and Lister 1992).

When complement C3a is formed, it equilibrates rapidly across capillaries due to its low molecular weight (9000). The peak concentration in blood is reached in 15 minutes, and then it rapidly declines to normal in 60 minutes. This time course is similar to that of the intestinal ultrastructural response to PEG-Hb. It has been shown that infusion of bacterial endotoxin (lipopolysaccharide, LPS) and Hb results in synergistic toxicity (Chang and Lister 1992, Kaca and Roth 1995). Physiologically significant levels of LPS are present in circulating blood in a variety of clinical conditions, such as shock and hypoxia, which lead to deterioration of mucosal barriers. Thus, the use of "toxin-free" Hb may still result in deleterious effects due to complement activation.

2.4.2 Generation of oxygen-free radicals

Autoxidation of oxyhemoglobin, in which the iron is in the Fe^{II} form, to methemoglobin, in which the iron is in the Fe^{III} form, results in generation of superoxide radicals (Misra and Fridovich 1972; Wever, Oudega and Van Gelder 1973). This autoxidation occurs in the presence of hydrogen peroxide, H_2O_2. One example of a circumstance under which H_2O_2 is produced is during tissue reperfusion with oxygenated media after hypoxia. The superoxide radicals which form during autoxidation lead to lipid peroxidation damage of membrane components and are thought to play an important role in increasing capillary permeability (Granger, Rutili and McCord 1991). In addition, H_2O_2 and oxyHb or metHb can produce ferryl heme, Fe^{IV}, a highly reactive species that can peroxidize lipids, degrade carbohydrates and cross-link proteins (Giulivi and Davies 1990):

$$HbFe^{II}\,O_2 + H_2O_2 \rightarrow HbFe^{IV}\,OH + OH^- + O_2$$

$$HbFe^{III} + H_2O_2 + H^+ \rightarrow HbFe^{IV}\,OH + H_2O$$

Superoxide radical and H_2O_2 can also cause hemoglobin to release free iron, which can then catalyze production of hydroxyl radical, $^{\bullet}OH$, by the Fenton reaction (Misra and Fridovich 1972):

$$Fe^{II} + H_2O_2 \rightarrow Fe^{III} + {}^{\bullet}OH + OH^-$$

Intact Hb does not catalyze $^{\bullet}OH$ production (Halliwell and Gutteridge 1986). The hydroxyl radical has been shown to cause physical disruption of the intestinal mucosal epithelium. Bacteria can then cross the gastrointestinal mucosal barrier and spread systemically (Deitch *et al.* 1990).

The Fe^{III} which is formed can react with superoxide radicals to produce more Fe^{II}:

$$Fe^{III} + O_2^- \rightarrow Fe^{II} + O_2$$

The Fe^{II} then undergoes the Fenton reaction to produce more $^{\bullet}OH$. Thus, the combination of H_2O_2 and Fe^{2+} represents a highly toxic potential.

In normal blood, the reservoir of heme iron is compartmentalized within the erythrocyte, which limits its ability to act as a catalyst. Erythrocytes are rich in antioxidant enzymes, such as superoxide dismutase (SOD) and catalase, which inactivate the superoxide radical and H_2O_2, respectively (Wever, Oudega and Van Gelder, 1973). These enzymes are in close proximity to Hb within the erythrocytes, and although Hb can release catalytic iron when exposed to oxidant stress, injury is limited because the enzymes react with the resultant oxygen-free radicals before they reach the red cell membrane.

There are many examples of hemoglobin-induced tissue damage that have been shown to result, at least partially, from action of oxygen-free radicals produced by free iron. When the free radicals are inactivated with SOD and/or catalase or the free iron is chelated with deferoxamine, the damage is reduced. For example, Paller (1988) showed that deferoxamine reduced renal dysfunction and accompanying free radical-mediated lipid peroxidation during heme-protein-induced acute renal failure. Deferoxamine also prevents oxyHb-induced endothelial and smooth muscle cell cytoskeletal injury (Comair, Schipper and Brem 1993). Hemoglobin has been shown to potentiate oxidant injury, and resultant increased capillary permeability, in isolated rat lungs (Seibert *et al.* 1991). Significantly more free Fe^{II} was present when hemoglobin was added to perfusates, and it was concluded that the Fe^{II} was producing hydroxyl radicals via the Fenton reaction.

2.4.3 Implications for blood substitute design

The studies described above indicate that hemoglobin-based blood substitutes may intensify the effects of ischemia in patients with hemorrhage or trauma, who receive Hb for red blood cell replacement. Therefore, efforts must be made to reduce the damaging effects of complement activation and oxygen-free radical generation. As indicated previously, the way to reduce complement activation is to eliminate impurities from hemoglobin. With regard to reducing the generation of free radicals, little progress has been made. However, several methods are currently being developed to effectively scavenge oxygen-free radicals.

Firstly, one approach is to incorporate SOD and catalase into cross-linked hemoglobin (D'Agnillo and Chang 1993). This technique ensures that the free-radical scavengers are in close contact with the source of the oxygen-free radicals, the hemoglobin, and also effectively addresses the problem that free SOD has a short half-life in blood (10 - 40 minutes). Secondly, another way of increasing the half-lives of SOD and catalase is to bind them to PEG. Polyethylene glycol-SOD has a half-life of several days, and PEG linkage increases the half-life of catalase from 2 to 50 hours (Burnham 1994). Thirdly, the protective effect of selenium on Hb-mediated lipid peroxidation is being investigated (Simoni *et al.* 1995). The rational for using selenium is that it has very powerful antioxidant properties. Hemoglobin's oxidative reactions are very complex, and so total protection cannot be achieved using hydroxyl radical scavengers exclusively. The real test for these new developments is whether they can be incorporated into transfusion strategems in such a way that sensitive tissues, such as the intestine, are not subjected to damage, even transient, in conditions of ischemia.

2.5 Acknowledgments

The experimental work was supported by NIH grant HL 93018. I would like to thank Ms. Lisa Wilson and Mr. Dirk Hamlyn who assisted in the experiments described in this study, specifically with regard to surgical procedures and data acquisition, respectively.

2.6 References

Burnham, N.L. Polymers for delivering peptides and proteins. *Am. J. Hosp. Pharm.* 51: 210-218, 1994.

Chang, T.M.S., and C. Lister. A preclinical screening test for modified hemoglobin to bridge the gap between safety studies and use in humans. *Biomat., Artif. Cells, Immobil. Biotech.* 20: 565-573, 1992.

Comair, Y.G., H.M. Schipper, and S. Brem. The prevention of oxyhemoglobin-induced endothelial and smooth muscle cytoskeletal injury by deferoxamine. *Neurosurgery* 32: 58-64, 1993.

D'Agnillo, F., and T.M. Chang. Cross-linked hemoglobin-superoxide dismutase-catalase scavenges oxygen-derived free-radicals and prevents methemoglobin formation and iron release. *Biomat., Artif. Cells, Immobil. Biotech.* 21(5): 609-621, 1993.

Deitch, E.A., W. Bridges, L. Ma, R. Berg, R.D. Specian, and D.N. Granger. Hemorrhagic shock-induced bacterial translocation: the role of neutrophils and hydroxyl radicals. *J. Trauma* 30: 942-952, 1990.

Feola, M., J. Simoni, M. Dobke, and P.C. Canizaro. Complement activation and the toxicity of stroma-free hemoglobin solutions in primates. *Circ. Shock* 25: 275-290, 1988.

Giulivi, C., and K.J.A. Davies. A novel antioxidant role for hemoglobin: the comproportionation of ferryl hemoglobin with oxyhemoglobin. *J. Biol. Chem.* 265: 19453-19460, 1990.

Granger, D.N., G. Rutili, and J.M. McCord. Superoxide radicals in feline intestinal ischemia. *Gastroenterology* 81: 22-29, 1981.

Halliwell, B., and J.M.C. Gutteridge. Oxygen free radicals and iron in relation to biology and medicine: some problems and concepts. *Arch. Biochem. Biophys.* 246: 501-514, 1986.

Kaca, W., and R. Roth. Activation of complement by human hemoglobin and by mixtures of hemoglobin and bacterial endotoxin. *Biochim. Biophys. Acta.* 1245: 49-56, 1995.

Milici, A.J., and P.W. Bankston. Fetal and neonatal rat intestinal capillaries: permeability to carbon, ferritin, hemoglobin, and myoglobin. *Am. J. Anat.* 165: 165-186, 1982.

Misra, H.P., and I. Fridovich. The generation of superoxide radical during the autoxidation of hemoglobin. *J. Biol. Chem.* 247: 6960-6962, 1972.

Moore, R., J. Madri, S. Carlson, and J.L. Madara. Collagens facilitate epithelial migration in restitution of native guinea pig intestinal epithelium. *Gastroenterology* 102: 119-130, 1992.

Paller, M.S. Hemoglobin- and myoglobin-induced acute renal failure in rats: role of iron in nephrotoxicity. *Am. J. Physiol.* 255(Renal Fluid Electrolyte Physiol. 24): F539-F544, 1988.

Seibert, A.F., A.E. Taylor, J.B. Bass, and J. Haynes, Jr., Hemoglobin potentiates oxidant injury in isolated rat lungs. *Am. J. Physiol.* 260 (Heart Circ. Physiol. 29): H1980-H1984, 1991.

Simoni, J., G. Simoni, E.L. Garcia, S.D. Prien, R.M. Tran, M. Feola, and G.T. Shires. Protective effect of selenium on hemoglobin mediated lipid peroxidation *in vivo*. *Art. Cells, Blood Substit., Immobil. Biotech.* 23: 469-486, 1995.

Smith, C.D., S.T. Schuschereba, J.R. Hess, L. McKinney, D. Bunch, and P.D. Bowman. Liver and kidney injury after administration of hemoglobin cross-linked with bis(3,5-dibromosalicyl) fumarate. *Biomat., Artif. Cells, Artif. Org.* 18: 251-261, 1990.

Szebeni J., N.M. Wassef, H. Spielberg, A.S. Rudolph, and C.R. Alving. Complement activation in rats by liposomes and liposome-encapsulated hemoglobin: evidence for anti-lipid antibodies and alternative pathways activation. *Biochem. Biophys. Res. Comm.* 205: 255-263, 1994.

Wever, R., B. Oudega, and B.F. Van Gelder. Generation of superoxide radicals during the autoxidation of mammalian oxyhemoglobin. *Biochem. Biophys. Acta.* 302: 475-478, 1973.

2.7 Discussion

Levin: You've alluded to other cross-linked hemoglobins that produce the same effect. Would you specify which two you're talking about?

Baldwin: One is the alpha-alpha cross-linked from the U.S Army, and the other one, I can't tell you.

Levin: Secondly, your structural changes are quite striking. Do you have any evidence that the villi are sloughing, are actually being lost?

Baldwin: The villi themselves don't slough; it's just the epithelial cells which slough, but the villi themselves stay intact under our conditions, in our preparation.

Levin: And finally, I'd just like to suggest that by using radio-labeled preparations, you might get some interesting quantification of the actual loss you are seeing, and that could be very informative.

Baldwin: Yes, I think so.

Gawryl: Did you characterize your labeled pegylated hemoglobin? Specifically, do you know what the concentration of endotoxin was in that solution?

Baldwin: Yes, we had it measured after we had labeled, and it was 0.6 EUs, and I think that is probably the maximal dose for humans, but we did some ultrastructural experiments where we injected that same dose of endotoxin by itself, and we saw some difference compared to controls, but nothing on this scale.

Gawryl: Secondly, did that labeling procedure cause any denaturation of that hemoglobin?

Baldwin: No, it didn't.

Gawryl: And how did you measure that?

Baldwin: One thing, we worried in case we might convert the oxyhemoglobin to methemoglobin, so we checked by spectrophotometry, and we had the same Soret absorption peak.

Gawryl: Did you look for a free heme in that solution?

Baldwin: No we didn't.

Rohlfs: Very nice talk. How much of your effect can be explained by fluid shifts?

Baldwin: Well, as far as ultrastructural studies are concerned, we have injected the same volume, 5 ml, of substance which is isotonic with plasma, and we don't get anything like these ultrastructural differences. We've also done experiments where we've injected 5 ml which is not isosmotic with plasma, just without any albumin in it, and we don't find any differences between those two.

Rohlfs: We've found that the pegylated hemoglobin brings a lot of water with it. If it's in the vascular space, it draws a lot of water in there, so perhaps it's carrying water with it into the villi.

Baldwin: That's possible, but also, as I mentioned before, we found exactly the same things going on with hemoglobin with no PEG, so that wouldn't totally explain it.

Billings: Ann, as you know, we've done a lot of work looking for inflammatory reactions and oxidative reactions in the liver, and the alpha-alpha cross-linked hemoglobin which we get from the U.S. Army is remarkably unreactive in our system. So, I'm prompted to ask one question. Have you confirmed any of your morphological observations with any biochemical and molecular measurements? Have you measured that there are mediators being released from mast cells, for example, or anything else on a biochemical level that would confirm that this is significant?

Baldwin: No, we haven't, but that would definitely be a good thing to do. With regard to your comment that the alpha-alpha cross-linked from the U.S. Army was unreactive, we have found so far that it produces the least damage of all of them that we've used in our system.

Billings: I think the possibility that you're looking at some heme-mediated reactions is very real, particularly with the labeled material, so I am prompted to ask where is the label? Is it on the heme? Is it on the protein, or where is it?

Baldwin: Well, we have got the protocol from Molecular Probes. I know that you can link FITC to the heme and also you can link it to the globins, but you use different procedures, and I would have to check with them to see exactly where our FITC is. But one thing we could do is look at both.

Lortie: I found the demonstration of the rapid change in the number of fenestra very elegant, and I wasn't aware that this could happen so quickly. So perhaps you could tell me if that is a first-time demonstration, and what mediators might be regulating this rapid change? I know you've published on the role of nitric oxide via the intravascular side of things. Do you think this is a nitric oxide mediated phenomenon?

Baldwin: Well, this is the first time. I haven't seen anyone else publish this kind of work. As far as nitric oxide, that's a good point. We did do some studies where we used nitric oxide inhibitors, and we looked at the same thing, and we did find a change in the fenestrae when we inhibited nitric oxide, they did seem to disappear.

Lortie: And just a quick technical question. Is this an *in situ* isolated perfused model you are using? When you give the hemoglobin, is the hemoglobin circulating and loaded with oxygen?

Baldwin: I should have made it clearer. We injected the hemoglobin. We tried various, different ways; we tried through the femoral artery, the femoral vein, the tail vein, and the superior mesenteric artery, and all four gave the same results. This is circulation through the whole body.

Lortie: Okay, so you do have circulating white blood cells on board.

Baldwin: Yes.

Hirsch: With respect to where you infused the material, I was wondering if you had a chance to look at the histology of other tissues. Is the hemoglobin sequestered at other sites, and how is it broken down? Do you see the same type of changes in the junctions in other tissues?

Baldwin: The only other microcirculation we looked at was the mesentery, and we did see the same thing in the junctions there, but we haven't looked at other organs.

Hirsch: And have you see any macrophage activity?

Baldwin: Yes, we do.

Hirsch: So, do you think there is an immediate reaction in terms of particle-type recognition, or is it too small?

Baldwin: I would think that particle-type recognition would take longer than the time course that we see these changes taking place.

Hirsch: And a technical question. In terms of your measuring fluorescent brightness, would you be able to have an assessment if the total FITC-labeled hemoglobin permeates the tissue? Can you use that as, let's say, 100% extravasation and then use your brightnesses to give you a percent measurement or a relative percent measurement?

Baldwin: Yes, that would be possible. We haven't done that yet. We've done that with the studies on FITC albumin.

Hirsch: And, the last question. I've labeled hemoglobin with fluorescent probes and often you see changes in oxygen affinity which would indicate conformational changes also. Did you measure the oxygen affinity change of the FITC-labeled hemoglobin?

Baldwin: No, we didn't.

Phillips: Have you looked at the effect of PEG by itself or else PEG linked to other protein molecules, and have you seen these effects with any other kind of proteins?

Baldwin: PEG by itself, we keep meaning to do it, but we haven't done it yet, and the reason is that it's low on my list of priorities is because we think this seems to be a heme mediated response, because we see it with hemoglobins that don't have PEG on them, but, yes, we ought to look at PEG alone.

Winslow: Do you filter the solutions as they go into the animal through a submicron filter?

Baldwin: Yes, we do.

Winslow: I also want to follow up on Ron Rohlf's point about the oncotic pressure. There is a tremendous difference in oncotic pressure between these hemoglobins, and Ron raised a very good question. It seems to me that the appropriate control would be Pentastarch which has the same oncotic pressure as PEG hemoglobin, but of course, is a totally different molecule. I think that might be worth trying.

Baldwin: Yes, we would like to try that.

Chapter 3

A Discussion of Pharmacoeconomics Applied to Blood Substitutes

Pamela Bassett, D.M.D., M.B.A.

3.1 Introduction

Pharmacoeconomics examines the costs and the consequences of health interventions. The results of pharmacoeconomic studies provide the economic reasons to use a particular product based on direct comparisons of costs and outcomes of competing products or interventions. In today's healthcare marketplace, providers, and specifically managed care organizations (MCOs), are forced to make difficult choices about which products will be made available for use in their organizations. It is now imperative to make pharmacoeconomic study results available to decision makers for review in order to achieve product acceptance for use in most organizations (Clifton and Blumenschein 1995). Without the results of a pharmacoeconomic study at product launch, the likelihood of product use and acceptance in today's market is extremely low. Therefore, implementing pharmacoeconomic studies during clinical trials is recommended.

If properly planned, the results of pharmacoeconomic studies will elucidate the true value of the product. In the case of blood substitutes, there may be cost-savings, such as lower inventory costs, fewer diagnostic tests or even improved outcomes in certain indications, which lower the overall costs of treatment. These cost-savings are the components for developing a pricing strategy of blood substitutes. It may be a fallacy to assume that blood substitutes must be priced in the same range as a unit of red blood cells. Pricing blood substitutes as equivalent to donor red blood cells may not take into account the costs and consequences of blood substitute use and may result in minimizing their real value. For at least two decades, health care delivery discussions have focused on cost-reductions. In fact, health policy is about achieving economic efficiency, not, as often stated, cost-reduction. Although the blood banking system has begun to react to cost pressures, the competitive nature of the market has not yet had an impact in this segment. However, as competing products, such as blood substitutes, become available, this will no longer be true. Ultimately, the competitive market process may determine where blood goes: for clinical use and/or for further processing as a blood substitute. A key part of this determination will be how blood and other competing products contribute to economic efficiency. In the process of making this set of determinations towards creating efficiency, the value of the outcomes may determine how nations ultimately utilize their blood supplies; and where and how it should be directed.

3.2 The Role of Pharmacoeconomics

In a healthcare environment with unlimited resources, pharmacoeconomic studies are unnecessary. However, in the U.S. and globally, healthcare resources are restricted. The restriction of resources fuels competitive market forces, particularly in the U.S. In contrast to competitive markets in many industries, decisions in the healthcare market are not made exclusively at the consumer level. The healthcare market is a non-traditional competitive market with multi-point decision-making, where neither the decision-maker nor the user are directly faced with the price of the product. Pharmacoeconomic studies can explain the true impact of using any particular therapeutic agent; in terms of both cost consequences and clinical outcomes. These studies are therefore necessary to inform decision-making (Torrance *et al.* 1996). Beyond using pharmacoeconomic study results for purchasing decisions, these data may be used by regulators, hospitals, MCOs and other insurers as important input to the development of clinical guide-lines. Manufacturers may use results to decide whether development should move forward or be halted during Phase II clinical trials. If development continues into Phase III clinical trials, pharmacoeconomic data can be used to develop pricing strategies and be incorporated into the product marketing plans.

3.3 Overview of Pharmacoeconomic Study Design

The field of pharmacoeconomics has grown tremendously in the past ten years and encompasses a wide body of knowledge. There are numerous detailed reviews of the subject in both journals and textbooks (Clemens *et al.* 1995, Coyle 1996, Drummond and Davies 1991, Drummond and Stoddart 1984, Eisenberg *et al.* 1994, Feeny *et al.* 1996, Hillman and Kim 1995, Mauskopf *et al.* 1996, Rutten-van Molken, van Doorslaer and van Vliet 1994, Task Force on Principles for Economic Analysis of Health Care Technology 1995, Torrance *et al.* 1996, Torrance *et al.* 1995). Below, the pharmacoeconomic study design is very briefly highlighted.

The economic analysis of a new therapeutic agent will ideally cover three areas. First, the impact of health-services resources must be examined, including the costs associated with the new therapeutic as well as the savings of resources that may result from discontinued therapies as a result of using the new agent. Both monetary (costs of products, diagnostics, labor and services) and non-monetary (changes in blood pressure, rates of infection, quality of life, morbidity and mortality) measurement of costs, benefits and the outputs of health services are useful in representing the overall value of the therapeutic agent. Second, the impact on the resources of the community must be considered as inputs to the analysis as well. These include inputs from patients, families and agencies that may become involved with the treatment or be affected by use of the therapeutic indirectly: for example, the patient's time in obtaining treatment or the involvement of social services support. A community viewpoint and societal perspective should be used. Finally, and most importantly, the new therapeutic's impact on health status must be examined (Drummond and Stoddart 1984).

If, by way of medical evaluation, the new agent is deemed equivalent to an existing therapy in terms of outcomes, and the outcome is "worth having", then an economic study can compare the two ways of achieving the effect, oftentimes using a Cost-Minimization Analysis (CMA). If different outcomes are achieved, then the extra benefits, savings of resources or quality of life changes must be examined, often using a Cost-Consequence Analysis (CCA), Cost-Effectiveness Analysis (CEA) and/or Cost-Benefit Analysis (CBA). There is overlap among the techniques, and the use of one does not preclude the use of another. In fact, a natural hierarchy suggests that data flow from cost-consequence to cost-effectiveness analysis to cost-benefit. Most often, the marginal effort required to add techniques is small.

Economic analyses must clearly specify the target population for the therapeutic agent: that is, what types of patients, with what disease, of what severity, with or without what other co-morbidities, what age group, and so on. Because the therapeutic agent may be cost effective for some subgroups of patients and not for others, it will be important to identify the groups under study and, when appropriate, to undertake separate analyses for different groups. Patient groups that differ on effectiveness, cost or preferences may therefore differ on cost effectiveness and should be studied separately, data permitting.

The relevant comparators may be other drugs, other medical care such as surgery, or even no treatment. The use of existing practice as a comparator may be the single most prevalent clinical practice or it could be current practice(s) weighted by market share.

The cost measurements for resources used in treatment must first be described in natural, non-monetary units. The cost valuation or unit prices must also be considered. Economic definitions of costs should be used and the concept of opportunity cost recognized. When possible, standard cost values should be used in costing out resource utilization. Alternative values should be presented as sensitivity analyses.

Costs and effects should be reported as incremental, that is, as differences between two alternatives. It is also useful to report total costs and total outcomes for each of the alternatives - the drug and each of the comparator treatments. The totals enable users to better appreciate the magnitudes involved, as well as allowing future users to make comparisons with new or different comparator treatments, as part of bringing studies up to date or transferring study results across geographic or practice boundaries.

3.4 Planning for Pharmacoeconomic Studies

3.4.1 When to incorporate pharmacoeconomic study into clinical trials

Decision criteria for the inclusion of economic analysis into clinical trials can be based upon what happens to resources at the healthcare delivery level. Issues including whether the therapeutic agent will alter the use of resources, whether there are potentially large-resource consequences, and the priority decision makers place on the use of the resource are at stake. These criteria are highlighted in Table 3.1.

Table 3.1 When to incorporate pharmacoeconomic studies into clinical trials.

Altering Use of Resources	• When results of clinical trials are likely to be influential in deciding future patterns of care • Pressure to adopt or not adopt the therapy means this could be the last trial
Resource Consequences are Large	• Potentially significant unit cost difference between alternatives • Radically different alternatives • Very large patient population affected
Importance of Resource Use to Decision Makers	• When questions of resource use are a priority • Changes in the allocation of resources and subsequent costs

Source: Drummond and Stoddart 1984

When facing a decision to build economic analysis into the clinical trials, in addition to examining the use of resources, the status of alternative therapies and the market outlook are also a consideration. To ensure value of the economic analysis itself, sizable amounts of scarce resources should be at stake prior to undertaking the study. When the technology underlying each alternative is well understood or when the alternative therapies are of a radically different nature, economic analysis should be incorporated into trials. Finally, when decision-making responsibility, with respect to product use, is fragmented, and, when the parties involved in the decision-making process may be at odds, it is important to conduct economic studies in conjunction with trials. In the case of blood substitutes, these criteria for including economic analysis into clinical trials are met.

3.4.2 Timing of studies

The methods, means and timing of the information collected during pharmacoeconomic studies are as important as the information itself (Bloom and Fendrick 1996). Theoretically, pharmacoeconomic studies may be conducted at any time during a product's life cycle. The timing of the studies largely depends upon the needs of the recipients of the study results. For example, studies conducted during early clinical trials may guide the development process, including market plans. Studies conducted during Phase III may be used for pricing and formulary decisions and may form the basis for initial clinical and prescribing guidelines. Effectiveness data, *versus* original efficacy data, collected during Phase IV clinical trials, may be used to update prior study results.

The advantages of implementing pharmacoeconomic studies during clinical trials are significant. First, the marginal cost of collecting additional data during the trial period is small and will decrease expenditures *versus* conducting separate pharmacoeconomic studies. Second, given the importance of having pharmacoeconomic data available prior to product launch, not moving forward with studies during the trial phases may stall market acceptance. Finally, the results of the pharmacoeconomic study will "explain" the implications of the new therapeutic agent, creating a framework for decision-making, both clinical and administrative.

3.5 Discussion

To date, pharmacoeconomic regulations are in place in Australia and Canada to aid in the reimbursement decisions for drugs. In Australia, manufacturers have been required to submit pharmacoeconomic data in support of drug applications for inclusion in the national reimbursement scheme since January, 1993. The requirement to submit pharmacoeconomic data to participate in government controlled reimbursement systems is a trend that is expected to grow. According to a recent survey of health economists in Europe, economic evaluations are currently used in a number of European countries as an input into decisions about drug reimbursement (Johannesson 1995).

The importance of pharmacoeconomics in the U.S. is underscored by the Pharmaceutical Research and Manufacturers of America (PhRMA) having adopted a voluntary set of principles to provide guidance for its member companies on the conduct and evaluation of pharmacoeconomic research in January, 1995. The principles were prepared by a working group of pharmacoeconomic scientists from the PhRMA Task Force on the Economic Evaluation of Pharmaceuticals. The Task Force has made recommendations to guide the selection of methodology and reporting of research. These recommendations were reviewed by a panel of academic experts and outside reviewers. The PhRMA approach is meant to ensure soundness of the research methods used, full disclosure and transparency of all methods, analyses and results (Clemens *et al.* 1995).

The current focus on economic analysis is a result of the demand to demonstrate value for money spent. The need to demonstrate value is escalating as the healthcare provider market continues to mature, and the resources of MCOs and other healthcare decision makers shrink further (Wanke and Ryan 1996). At the current annual escalation rate, as much as 90% of the U.S. population may be participating in MCOs by 1998, the first year when blood-substitute products may become available. The integration of federal programs with new private sector initiatives will result in more than 95% of the U.S. population receiving health care from some type of managed care system by the end of the century (Santell 1996). The implications of an MCO-controlled marketplace for blood substitutes are that presenting results from pharmacoeconomic studies could make the difference between quick market diffusion with significant market share and lackluster market acceptance, since product prices and value received will require justification.

The issue of pricing and value are ordinarily settled in the operation of a free-market economy, where industry customarily sets the price of a new product close to the price of an already marketed product in order to compete effectively. However, the healthcare market is not a free market economy. To set an appropriate price requires an understanding of the value of blood substitutes and involves examining how their use can alter the course of treatment and associated costs in specific settings. Further, blood substitutes may or may not be competing with red blood cells. The price targets for a commercially available blood substitute are quoted with some frequency, usually in a range from \$300 to \$600 per unit. However, these potential prices are not presented with supporting data based on the results of pharmacoeconomic studies. A simplistic unit-to-unit pricing strategy, *e.g.*, a unit of red blood cells is \$350, therefore, a unit of a blood substitute should be \$350, may be misleading by not taking into account the potential contribution of blood substitutes to overall cost reductions and economic efficiency. If prices for blood substitutes incorporate pharmacoeconomic data, the resulting pricing strategies may or may not be equivalent to a unit of red blood cells, and the value of any particular blood substitute can be substantiated based upon data derived from use in the clinical setting. Clinical trials incorporating pharmacoeconomic studies comparing various treatment approaches, *e.g.*, blood substitute use *versus* red blood cell use, interventions such as acute normovolemic hemodilution (ANH), *etc.*, may elucidate both the better treatment choices and the better economic choices, on a specific indication by indication basis.

3.6 References

Bloom, B.S., and A.M. Fendrick. Timing and timeliness in medical care evaluation. *PharmacoEconomics* 9: 183-187, 1996.

Clemens, K., R. Townsend, F. Luscombe, J. Mauskopf, J. Osterhaus, and J. Bobula. Methodological and conduct principles for pharmacoeconomic research. *PharmacoEconomics* 8: 169-174, 1995.

Clifton, G.D., and K. Blumenschein. The use of pharmaceuticals in critical care, the importance of outcome prediction models. *PharmacoEconomics* 7: 388-392, 1995.

Coyle, D. Statistical analysis in pharmacoeconomic studies. *PharmacoEconomics* 9: 506-516, 1996.

Drummond, M., and L. Davies. Economic analysis alongside clinical trials: revisiting the methodological issues. *International Journal of Technology Assessment in Health Care* 7: 561-573, 1991.

Drummond, M.F., and G.L. Stoddart. Economic analysis and clinical trials. *Controlled Clinical Trials* 5: 115-128, 1984.

Eisenberg, J., H. Glick, K. Schulman, *et al.* Pharmacoeconomics: economic evaluation of pharmaceuticals. In: *Pharmcoepidemiology, 2nd ed.* (B. Strom, ed.). Chichester: John Wiley and Sons Ltd., 1994.

Feeny, D., W. Furlong, M. Boyle, and G.W. Torrance. Multiattribute health status classification systems, health utilities index. *PharmacoEconomics* 7: 490-502, 1996.

Hillman, A.L., and M.S. Kim. Economic decision making in healthcare, a standard approach to discounting health outcomes. *PharmacoEconomics* 7: 198-205, 1995.

Johannesson, M. Economic evaluation of drugs and its potential uses in policy making. *PharmacoEconomics* 8: 190-198, 1995.

Mauskopf, J., K. Schulman, L. Bell, and H. Glick. A strategy for collecting pharmacoeconomic data during Phase II/III clinical trials. *PharmacoEconomics* 9: 264-277, 1996.

Rutten-van Molken, M., E. van Doorslaer, and R. van Vliet. Statistical analysis of cost outcomes in a randomized controlled clinical trial. *Health Economics* 3: 333-345, 1994.

Santell, J.P. Projecting future drug expenditures - 1996. *American Journal of Health-System Pharmacists* 53: 139-150, 1996.

Task Force on Principles for Economic Analysis of Health Care Technology. Economic analysis of health care technology: a report on principles. *Annals of Internal Medicine* 122: 61-70, 1995.

Torrance, G.W., D. Blaker, A. Detsky, W. Kennedy, F. Schubert, D. Menon, P. Tugwell, R. Konchak, E. Hubbard, and T. Firestone. Canadian guidelines for economic evaluation of pharmaceuticals. *PharmacoEconomics* 9: 535-559, 1996.

Torrance, G.W., W. Furlong, D. Feeny, and M. Boyle. Multi-attribute preference functions, health utilities index. *PharmacoEconomics* 7: 503-520, 1995.

Wanke, L.A., and G.M. Ryan. Strategic planning for applied pharmacoeconomics programs. *Pharmacy Practice Management Quarterly* 15: 64-74, 1996.

Chapter 4

Tumor Microcirculation: Role in Drug and Nutrient Delivery

Rakesh K. Jain, Ph.D.

ABSTRACT

To reach cancer cells in a tumor, a blood-borne molecule must make its way into the blood vessels of the tumor and across the vessel wall into the interstitium, and finally migrate through the interstitium. Unfortunately, tumors often develop in ways that hinder each of these steps. Our research goals are to analyze each of these steps experimentally and theoretically, and then integrate the resulting information in a unified theoretical framework. Oxygen, one of the smallest blood-borne molecular species, is potentially the most important enhancer of cancer radiation treatment. Its arrival to the needed sites potentially is determined by the unique transport characteristics of the tumor microcirculation. Thus, our analysis and synthesis approach allows us to obtain a better understanding of physiological barriers in solid tumors and to develop novel strategies to exploit and/or overcome these barriers for improved cancer treatment.

4.1 Introduction

Cancer is the second leading cause of death in the United States and in many industrialized countries (Beardsley 1994). After the primary tumor has been surgically removed and/or sterilized by radiation, the residual disease is usually managed with a variety of systemic therapies. For these therapies to be successful, they must satisfy two requirements: (1) the relevant agent must be effective in the *in vivo* orthotopic microenvironment of tumors; and, (2) this agent must reach the target cells *in vivo* in optimal quantities. Our research is aimed at examining the latter issue — the delivery of therapeutic agents to solid tumors and normal host tissues.

All therapeutic agents can be divided into three categories: molecules, particles and cells. Blood-borne molecules or particles that enter the tumor vasculature reach cancer cells via distribution through the vascular compartment, transport across the microvascular wall, and transport through the interstitial compartment. For a molecule of given size, charge, and configuration, each of these transport processes may involve diffusion and convection. In addition, during the journey, the molecule may bind nonspecifically to proteins or other tissue components, bind specifically to the target(s), or be metabolized (Jain 1994a). Some of these physiological parameters are also important for heat transfer in normal and tumor tissues during hyperthermic treatment of cancer (Jain 1994b).

The delivery of small molecules to a tumor is critically dependent on the quantitative understanding of transport phenomena in the microcirculation. More specifically, we need information on: (1) how angiogenesis takes place and what determines blood flow heterogeneities in tumors; (2) how blood flow influences the metabolic microenvironment in tumors and how the microenvironment affects the biological properties of tumors (*e.g.*, vascular permeability, cell adhesion); (3) how material moves across the microvascular wall; and, (4) how it moves through the interstitial compartment and the lymphatics. Analysis of these processes is made for molecules, particles and cells, and the information is integrated in a unified framework for scale-up from mice to humans.

4.2 Experimental and Theoretical Approaches

We have utilized five approaches to gain insight into the pathophysiology of solid tumors:

(1) A tissue-isolated tumor which is connected to the host's circulation by a single artery and a single vein (Sevick and Jain 1988). This technique was originally developed by P.M. Gullino at the National Cancer Institute in 1961 for rats (Gullino 1970); we have recently adapted it to mice (Kristjansen *et al.* 1994).

(2) A modified Sandison rabbit ear chamber (Zawicki *et al.* 1981), a modified Algire mouse dorsal chamber (Leunig *et al.* 1994b), and a cranial window in mice and rats (Yuan et al. 1994b). The ear chamber has the advantage of superior optical quality, and the mice of working with immunodeficient and genetically engineered animals (Milstone *et al.* 1996, Yamada *et al.* 1995). Recently, we have developed a quantitative angiogenesis assay using these windows to study the physiology of vessels induced by individual growth factors (Dellian *et al.* 1996b). We also perfuse single vessels of tumors in these windows (Lichtenbeld *et al.* 1996) and utilize two acute preparations: liver and mesentery.

(3) *In vitro* methods to assess the deformability, adhesion and permeability of normal and neoplastic cells (Melder *et al.* 1996, Munn, Melder

and Jain 1996, Traykov and Jain 1987), as well as measurements of adhesion molecules' expression in intact monolayers (Munn *et al.* 1995).

(4) Routine molecular biology techniques (e.g., *in situ* hybridization, Southern, Northern and Western blotting) (Yuan *et al.* 1996).

(5) Mathematical models to describe and integrate the data obtained from the above four approaches to scale up biodistribution data from mice to humans and to design future experiments (Baxter and Jain 1989, Baxter and Jain 1990, Baxter and Jain 1991a, Baxter and Jain 1991b, Baxter *et al.* 1994, Baxter *et al.* 1995, Eskey *et al.* 1994, Jain and Baxter 1988, Jain and Wei 1977, Netti *et al.* 1995, Netti *et al.* 1996, Yuan, Baxter and Jain 1991).

While each of these approaches has its limitations, it is their combination that has led to the development of the framework for tumor microcirculation and drug delivery described in this article.

4.2.1 Distribution through vascular space

The tumor vasculature consists of both vessels recruited from the preexisting network of the host vasculature and vessels resulting from the angiogenic response of host vessels to cancer cells (Folkman 1995, Jain 1988). Movement of molecules through the vasculature is governed by the vascular morphology (*i.e.*, the number, length, diameter, and geometric arrangement of various blood vessels) and the blood flow rate (Baish *et al.* 1996, Gazit *et al.* 1995, Less *et al.* 1991).

Although the tumor vasculature originates from the host vasculature, and the mechanisms of angiogenesis are similar (Folkman 1995, Patan, Munn and Jain 1996), its organization may be completely different depending on the tumor type, its growth rate, and its location (Less *et al.* 1991). The architecture and blood flow are different not only among various tumor types but also between a spontaneous tumor and its transplants (Jain 1988). For example, unlike normal tissue, where red blood cell (RBC) velocity is dependent on vessel diameter, there is no such dependence in tumors (Leunig *et al.* 1992b, Yuan *et al.* 1994b). Furthermore, RBC velocity may be an order of magnitude lower in tumors compared to the host vessels. The temporal and spatial heterogeneity in tumor blood flow (Figure 4.1) may, in part, be a result of elevated geometric and viscous resistance in tumor vessels (Less *et al.* 1997, Sevick and Jain 1989a, Sevick and Jain 1989b, Sevick and Jain 1991a), coupling between high vascular permeability and elevated interstitial fluid pressure (Netti *et al.* 1996), and vascular remodeling by intussusception (Patan, Munn and Jain 1996).

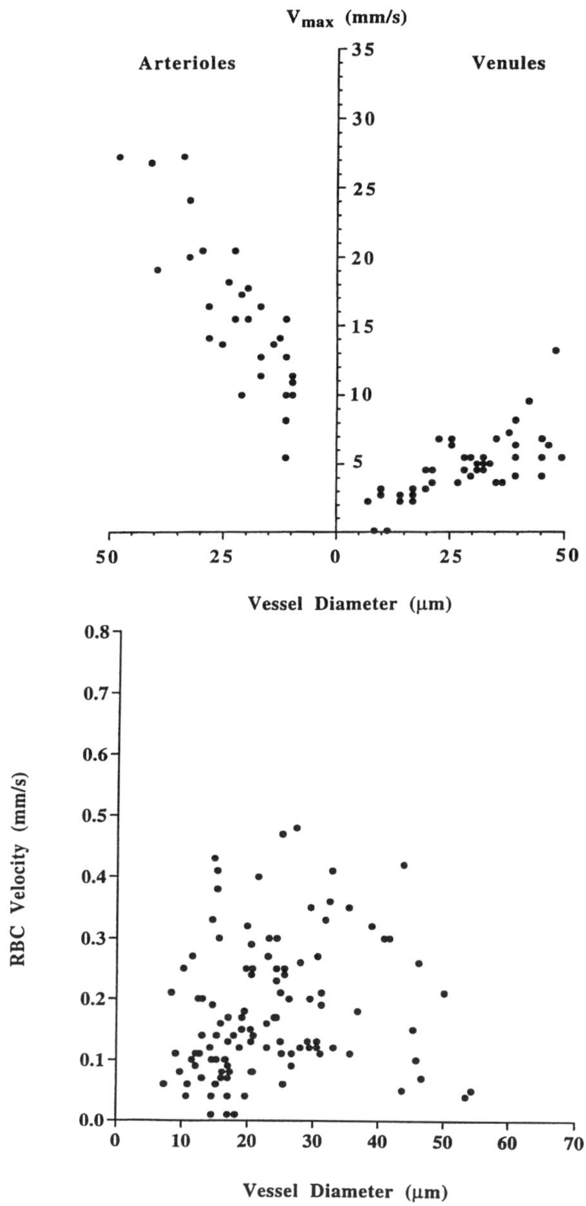

Figure 4.1. Blood velocity as a function of vessel diameter in normal pial vessels (top panel) and a human glioma (U87) xenograft on the pial surface (bottom panel). Note that in normal microcirculation, blood velocity is dependent on vessel diameter, whereas in tumors, there is no such dependence. Furthermore, the blood velocity in tumor vessels is about an order of magnitude lower than in host vessels (Adapted from Yuan *et al.* 1994b).

Based on perfusion rates, four regions can be recognized in a tumor: an avascular, necrotic region, a semi-necrotic region, a stabilized microcirculation region, and an advancing front (Endrich *et al.* 1979). Intra-tumor blood flow distributions in spontaneous animal and human tumors are now being investigated using nuclear magnetic resonance, positron emission tomography (Melder *et al.* 1993), and functional computed tomography (Eskey *et al.* 1992, Eskey *et al.* 1994, Hamberg *et al.* 1994). While limited, these results are in concert with the transplanted tumor studies: blood flow rates in necrotic and semi-necrotic regions of tumors are low (Figure 4.2), while those in non-necrotic regions are vari-

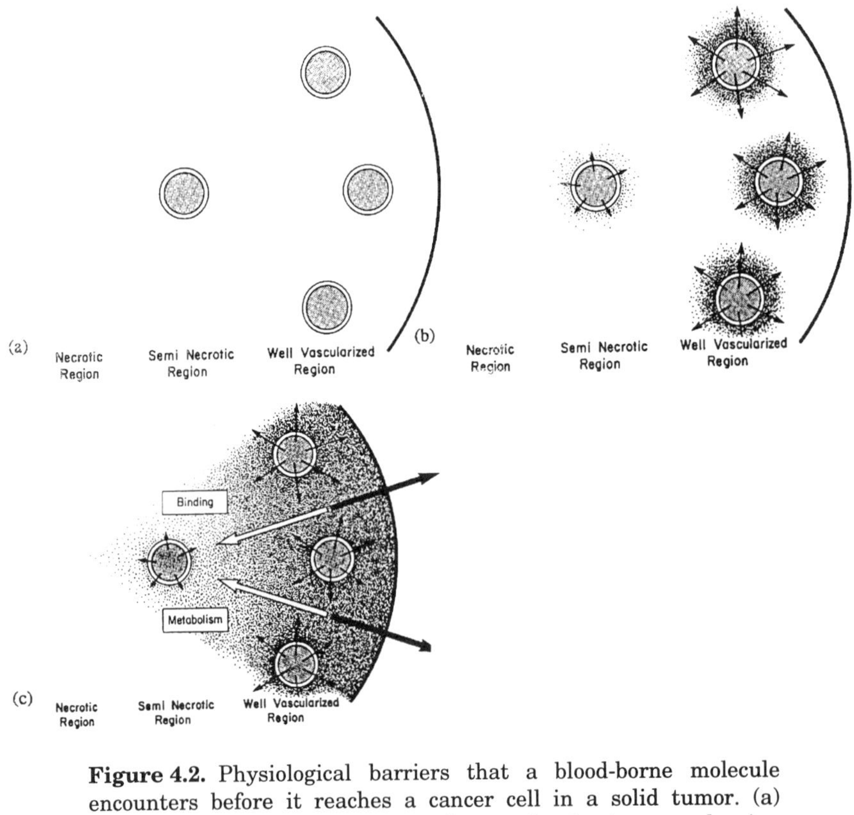

Figure 4.2. Physiological barriers that a blood-borne molecule encounters before it reaches a cancer cell in a solid tumor. (a) Schematic of a heterogeneously perfused tumor showing well-vascularized periphery, a semi-necrotic, intermediate zone, and an avascular, necrotic central region. Note: Immediately after i.v. injection, the molecules are delivered to perfused regions only. (b) Low interstitial pressure in the periphery permits adequate extravasation of fluid and macromolecules. (c) These macromolecules move toward the center by the slow process of diffusion. In addition, interstitial fluid oozing from tumor carries macromolecules with it by convection into the normal tissue. Note: Interstitial movement may be further retarded by binding. Products of metabolism may be cleared rapidly by blood. (Reproduced from Jain 1989).

able and can be substantially higher than in surrounding (contralateral) host normal tissues (Vaupel and Jain 1991). Considering these spatial and temporal heterogeneities in blood supply, coupled with variations in the vascular morphology at both microscopic and macroscopic levels, it is not surprising that the spatial distribution of nutrients and therapeutic agents in tumors is heterogeneous and that the average uptake decreases, in general, with an increase in tumor weight. This perfusion heterogeneity also makes it difficult to heat the tumor periphery during hyperthermia (Jain 1994b).

4.2.2 Metabolic microenvironment

The temporal and spatial heterogeneities in blood flow are expected to lead to a compromised metabolic microenvironment in tumors. To quantify the spatial gradients of key metabolites, we have recently adapted two optical techniques: fluorescence ratio-imaging microscopy (FRIM) and phosphorescence quenching microscopy (PQM) (Dellian *et al.* 1996a, Helmlinger *et al.* 1997, Martin and Jain 1994, Torres-Filho *et al.* 1994). As shown in Figure 4.3, both pH and pO_2 decrease as one moves away from tumor vessels, leading to acidic and hypoxic regions in tumors. While low pO_2 and pH are detrimental to some therapies (*e.g.*, radiation), they might enhance the effect of certain drugs, if the drug could be delivered in adequate quantities in those regions (Jain, Shah and Finney 1984, Nozue *et al.* 1996, Ward and Jain 1988).

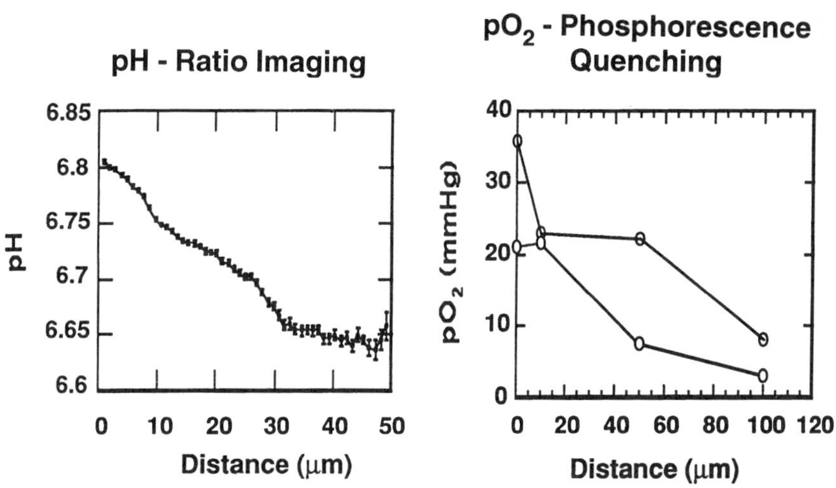

Figure 4.3. Spatial gradients of metabolites in tumors. Left panel: pH gradients measured using fluorescence ratio imaging microscopy (Adapted from Martin and Jain 1994). Right panel: pO_2 gradients measured using phosphorescence quenching (Adapted from Torres-Filho *et al.* 1994). Distance from the vessel wall, in microns, is shown on the x-axis, with zero being the vessel wall.

To gain further insight into tumor metabolism, we combined two powerful approaches: magnetic resonance spectroscopy and tissue-isolated tumors. The former allows us to measure the energy level in tumors, while the latter allows us to control the supply of individual substrates (*e.g.*, glucose, oxygen) to the tumor. Using this approach, we have recently shown that solid tumors depend more on glucose than on oxygen to maintain their ATP level (Eskey *et al.* 1993).

4.2.3 Transport across the microvascular wall

Once a blood-borne molecule reaches an exchange vessel, its extravasation occurs by diffusion and convection and, to some extent, presumably by transcytosis (Jain 1987a). Diffusive flux is proportional to the exchange vessel's surface area, S (cm^2), and the difference between the plasma and interstitial concentrations, C_p - C_i (g/m). Convection is proportional to the rate of fluid leakage, J_f (m/s), from the vessel. J_f, in turn, is proportional to S and the difference between the vascular and interstitial hydrostatic pressures, p_v - p_i (mm Hg), minus the osmotic reflection coefficient (σ) times the difference between the vascular and interstitial osmotic pressures π_v - π_i (mm Hg). The proportionality constant that relates transluminal diffusion flux to concentration gradients, (C_p - C_i), is referred to as the vascular permeability coefficient, P (cm/s), and the constant that relates fluid leakage to pressure gradients is referred to as the hydraulic conductivity, L_p (cm/mm Hg · s). The effectiveness of the transluminal osmotic pressure difference in producing fluid movement across a vessel wall is characterized by σ, which is close to 1 for a macromolecule and close to zero for a small molecule. Thus, the transport of a molecule across normal or tumor vessels is governed by three transport parameters (P, L_p, and σ), the surface area for exchange, and the transvascular concentration and pressure gradients.

Vascular permeability and hydraulic conductivity of tumors, in general, is significantly higher than that of normal tissues (Dvorak *et al.* 1995, Gerlowski and Jain 1986, Jain 1987a, Sevick and Jain 1991b, Yuan *et al.* 1993, Yuan *et al.* 1994a, Yuan *et al.* 1994b), and hence, these vessels may lack permselectivity (Yuan *et al.* 1995). Positively charged molecules have a higher permeability (Dellian *et al.* 1996c). Despite increased overall permeability, not all blood vessels of a tumor are leaky, and even leaky vessels have a finite pore size (Hobbs *et al.* 1996). Our hypothesis is that the large pore size in tumors represents wide inter-endothelial junctions (Roberts and Palade 1997).

Not only does the vascular permeability vary from one tumor to the next, but within the same tumor it varies both spatially and temporally (Jain 1987a). The local microenvironment plays an important role in controlling vascular permeability. For example, a human glioma (HGL21) is fairly leaky when grown subcutaneously in immunodeficient mice, but it exhibits blood-brain barrier properties in the cranial window. We have not seen such site-dependent differences for other tumors. Our working hypothesis is that the host-tumor interactions control the production and secretion of cytokines associated with permeability changes (*e.g.*, VPF/VEGF and its inhibitors). A better understanding of the molecular mechanisms of permeability-regulation in tumors is likely to yield strategies for improved drug delivery (Yuan *et al.* 1996).

If tumor vessels are indeed "leaky" to fluid and macromolecules, then what leads to the poor extravasation of these agents in various regions of tumors? As shown by us and others (Arbit, Lee and DiResta 1994, Boucher, Baxter and Jain 1990, Boucher and Jain 1992, Curti *et al.* 1993, Jain 1987b, Less *et al.* 1992), experimental and human tumors exhibit high interstitial fluid pressure. Furthermore, the uniformly high pressure drops precipitously to normal values in the tumor's periphery or in the peritumor region (Baxter and Jain 1989, Boucher, Baxter and Jain 1990, Jain and Baxter 1988). This may lower fluid extravasation in the high pressure regions, especially because the oncotic and hydrostatic pressures are also equal between the intravascular and extravascular space (Boucher and Jain 1992). Because the transvascular transport of macromolecules in normal tissues occurs primarily by convection (Jain 1987a, Rippe and Haraldsson 1987), convective transport of macromolecules in the center of tumors may be less than in the tumor periphery (Baxter and Jain 1989, Jain and Baxter 1988, Lichtenbeld *et al.* 1996). Additionally, the average vascular surface area per unit tissue weight decreases with tumor growth, hence reduced transvascular exchange would be expected in large tumors compared with small tumors (Baxter and Jain 1989, Baxter and Jain 1990).

4.2.4 Transport through interstitial space and lymphatics

Once a molecule has extravasated, its movement through the interstitial space occurs by diffusion and convection (Jain 1987b). Diffusion is proportional to the concentration gradient in the interstitium, and convection is proportional to the interstitial fluid velocity, u_i (cm/s). The latter, in turn, is proportional to the pressure gradient in the interstitium. Just as the interstitial diffusion coefficient, D (cm^2/s), relates the diffusive flux to the concentration gradient, the interstitial hydraulic conductivity, K (cm^2/mm Hg $\cdot$ s), relates the interstitial velocity to the pressure gradient (Jain 1987b). Values of these transport coefficients are determined by the structure and composition of the interstitial compartment as well as the physicochemical properties of the solute molecule (Berk *et al.* 1997, Chary and Jain 1989, Johnson *et al.* 1995, Nugent and Jain 1984, Swabb, Wei and Guillino 1974).

Using fluorescence recovery after photobleaching (FRAP), we found D of various molecules to be about one-third that in water and similar to that in the host tissue (Chary and Jain 1989). Similarly, the value of K for a human colon carcinoma xenograft (LS174T) measured using two different methods was higher than that of a hepatoma (Swabb, Wei and Guillino 1974), which in turn was higher than that of the liver. Given these relatively high values of D and K, why do exogenously injected macromolecules not distribute uniformly in tumors? As discussed next, there are two reasons for this apparent paradox.

The time constant for a molecule with diffusion coefficient D to diffuse across distance L is approximately $L^2/4D$. For diffusion of IgG in tumors, this time constant is on the order of one hour for a 100-μm distance, days for a 1-mm distance, and months for a 1-cm distance. So for a 1-mm tumor, diffusional transport would take days, and for a 1-cm tumor, it would take months. If the central vessels have collapsed completely due to cellular proliferation and interstitial matrix rearrangement, there would be no delivery of macromolecules by blood flow to this necrotic center. Binding may further retard the transport in tumors (Baxter and Jain 1991a, Baxter and Jain 1991b, Berk *et al.* 1993, Kaufman and Jain 1990, Kaufman and Jain 1991).

As mentioned earlier, interstitial fluid pressure is high in the center of tumors and low in the periphery and surrounding tissue (Baxter and Jain 1989, Boucher, Baxter and Jain 1990, Jain and Baxter 1988). Therefore, one would expect interstitial fluid motion from the tumor's periphery into the surrounding normal tissue. In various animal and human (xenograft) tumors studied to date, 6% to 14% of plasma entering the tumor has been found to leave from the tumor periphery (Jain 1987a, Jain 1989). This fluid leakage leads to a radially outward interstitial fluid velocity of 0.1 to 0.2 μm/s at the periphery of 1-cm tissue-isolated tumor (Jain 1987a). A macromolecule at the tumor periphery has to overcome this outward convection to diffuse into the tumor. The relative contribution of this mechanism of heterogeneous distribution of antibodies in tumors may be smaller than the contribution of heterogeneous extravasation due to elevated pressure and necrosis (Baxter and Jain 1989).

In most normal tissues, extravasated macromolecules are taken up by the lymphatics and brought back to the central circulation. Because of the lack of functional lymphatics within the tumor, the fluid and macromolecules oozing from the tumor surface must be picked by the peritumor host lymphatics (Baxter and Jain 1990). To characterize the transport into and within the lymphatic capillaries, we have recently developed a mouse tail model (Leu *et al.* 1994). Our current efforts are directed towards understanding changes in lymphatic transport in the presence of a tumor.

The parameters discussed govern the transport of molecules in tumors. An equally significant and necessary component in the understanding of tumor transport properties involves the mechanisms associated with the transport of cells. These mechanisms are governed by both local hydrodynamic forces and adhesive forces, however they are not germane to the transport of small molecular species in the context of oxygen carrying plasma expanders that may be used to enhance radiation therapy, and will not be reviewed here (Melder *et al.* 1996, Munn, Melder and Jain 1996).

4.2.5 Pharmacokinetic modeling: Scale-up from mouse to human

So far we have analyzed each of the steps in the delivery of molecules to and within solid tumors. Can we take this information and integrate it in a unified framework? We have been successful to some extent in this endeavor, using physiologically-based pharmacokinetic modeling. This approach, pioneered by two chemical engineers K. Bischoff and R.L. Dedrick in the 1960's, has been applied successfully to describe and scale-up the biodistribution of low molecular weight agents (for a review, see Dedrick 1973, Gerlowski and Jain 1983, Jain 1994b). We have extended this approach to macromolecules and cells (Baxter *et al.* 1995).

In this approach, a mammalian body is represented by a number of physiological compartments interconnected anatomically. The volume and blood flow rate to each of these compartments/organs are known or can be measured. The parameters that characterize transport across the sub-compartments (*i.e.*, vascular, interstitial and cellular) and the metabolism of various agents are not generally known and cannot be easily measured. Our philosophy has been to use as many measured parameters as possible and estimate the remaining parameters by fitting the model to the murine biodistribution data. By scaling-up the parameters using well-defined scale-up laws (Dedrick 1973), we then predict the biodistribution in human patients and compare with clinical data. Discrepancies between predictions and actual data help us in identifying inter-species differences, and force us to question our model assumptions. This is an evolutionary process - as our understanding of underlying physiology and biochemistry improves, the relevant parameters are modified and the model is refined further. The model is useful not only for designing murine experiments and/or clinical trials, but also in identifying the sensitive parameters that need careful measurement and analysis. If we need detailed spatial information about a tissue/organ, then we develop a distributed parameter model for that organ, *e.g.*, tumor (Baxter and Jain 1989, Baxter and Jain 1990, Baxter and Jain 1991a, Baxter and Jain 1991b, Baxter *et al.* 1995, Jain and Wei 1977). While simple in principle, this cyclic approach of analysis and synthesis has served as a useful paradigm for developing a deeper understanding of drug and cell distribution in normal and malignant tissues. The level of sophistication of these models is likely to improve with our understanding of underlying principles (Baish *et al.* 1996).

4.3 Bench to Bedside

The physiologic factors that contribute to the poor delivery of therapeutic agents to tumors include heterogeneous blood supply, interstitial hypertension, relatively long transport distances in the interstitium, and cellular heterogeneities (Figure 4.2). How can these physiologic barriers be exploited or overcome?

Several physical (*e.g.*, radiation, heat) and chemical (*e.g.*, vasoactive drugs) agents may lead to an increase in tumor blood flow or vascular permeability (Dudar and Jain 1984, Fukumura *et al.* 1995, Jain 1987a, Jain and Ward-Hartley 1984, Kristensen *et al.* 1996), lower pH (Jain, Shah and Finney 1984, Ward and Jain 1988) or increase in pO_2 (Nozue *et al.* 1996). Another approach may be based on increasing the interstitial transport rate of molecules by increasing K or D enzymatically (Boucher, Leunig and Jain 1996, Jain 1989, Swabb, Wei and Guillino 1974) or using multi-step approaches (Baxter and Jain 1996, Baxter, Yuan and Jain 1992, Baxter *et al.* 1994, Yuan, Baxter and Jain 1991). We have used several physical and chemical agents to lower IFP in tumors (Kristjansen, Boucher and Jain 1993, Lee *et al.* 1994a, Lee, Boucher and Jain 1992, Lee *et al.* 1994b, Leunig *et al.* 1992a, Leunig *et al.* 1994a). Since microvascular and interstitial pressures in tumors are approximately equal, any change in one is followed rapidly by a similar change in the other, and thus the convective enhancement disappears rapidly (Boucher and Jain 1992, Netti *et al.* 1995, Zlotecki *et al.* 1995). By adapting a poroelastic model to solid tumors, we have calculated theoretically and confirmed experimentally that the time constant of pressure transmission across the tumor vasculature is on the order of 10 seconds (Netti *et al.* 1995). During such a short time, the convective enhancement is calculated to be very small (~ 1%). However, if vascular pressure is increased repeatedly and if the transvascular transport is unidirectional or if the molecule binds avidly in the extravascular region, then we can, in principle, increase drug delivery to solid tumors significantly.

In contrast, the physiologic barriers discussed here may be less of a problem for: (1) radioimmunodetection; (2) treating leukemias, lymphomas, and small tumors (*e.g.*, micrometastases) in which the physiological barriers are not yet fully established; (3) treatment of adequately perfused, low-pressure regions of large tumors; and, (4) treatment with antibodies or other agents directed against the host cells (*e.g.*, tumor endothelial cells, fibroblasts) or the sub-endothelial matrix. These physiologic barriers also may pose less problems for treatment with a molecule or cell that has nearly 100% specificity for cancer cells. Until such selective molecules or cells are developed, methods are urgently needed to overcome or exploit these physiologic barriers in tumors. It is hoped that an improved understanding of transport in tumors will help in developing these strategies (Jain 1996).

4.4 Acknowledgments

Research described here was primarily supported by grants from the National Cancer Institute, the National Science Foundation and the American Cancer Society.

An earlier version of this article was published as "1995 Whitaker Lecture: Delivery of Molecules, Particles and Cells to Solid Tumors", in the *Annals of Biomedical Engineering,* **24**:457-473 (1996). The author thanks the Biomedical Engineering Society for allowing him to reproduce this article.

4.5 References

Arbit, E., J. Lee, and G. DiResta. Interstitial hypertension in human brain tumors: possible role in peritumoral edema formulation. In: *Intracranial Pressure, Vol. 9,* (H. Nagai, K. Kamiya, and S. Ishi, eds.). Tokyo: Springer-Verlag, 1994, pp. 609-614.

Baish, J.W., Y. Gazit, D.A. Berk, M. Nozue, L.T. Baxter, and R.K. Jain. A novel approach to examine the role of vascular heterogeneity in nutrient and drug delivery for tumors: An invasion percolation model. *Microvasc. Res.* 51: 327-346, 1996.

Baxter, L.T., and R.K. Jain. Transport of fluid and macromolecules in tumors. I. Role of interstitial pressure and convection. *Microvasc. Res.* 37: 77-104, 1989.

Baxter, L.T., and R.K. Jain. Transport of fluid and macromolecules in tumors. II. Role of heterogeneous perfusion and lymphatics. *Microvasc. Res.* 40: 246-263, 1990.

Baxter, L.T., and R.K. Jain. Transport of fluid and macromolecules in tumors. III. Role of binding and metabolism. *Microvasc. Res.* 41: 5-23, 1991a.

Baxter, L.T., and R.K. Jain. Transport of fluid and macromolecules in tumors. IV. A microscopic model of the perivascular distribution. *Microvasc. Res.* 41: 252-272, 1991b.

Baxter, L.T., and R.K. Jain. Pharmacokinetic analysis of the microscopic distribution of enzyme-conjugated antibodies and prodrugs: comparison with experimental data. *Br. J. Cancer* 73: 447-456, 1996.

Baxter, L.T., F. Yuan, and R.K. Jain. Pharmacokinetic analysis of the perivascular distribution of bifunctional antibodies and haptens: comparison with experimental data. *Cancer Res.* 52: 5838-5844, 1992.

Baxter, L.T., H. Zhu, D.G. Mackensen, W.F. Butler, and R.K. Jain. Biodistribution of monoclonal antibodies: scale-up from mouse to man using a physiologically based pharmacokinetic model. *Cancer Res.* 55: 4611-4622, 1995.

Baxter, L.T., H. Zhu, D.G. Mackensen, and R.K. Jain. Physiologically based pharmacokinetic model for specific and nonspecific monoclonal antibodies and fragments in normal tissues and human tumor xenografts in nude mice. *Cancer Res.* 54: 1517-1528, 1994.

Beardsley, T. Trends in cancer epidemiology: a war not won. *Scien. Amer.* 270: 118-126, 1994.

Berk, D.A., F. Yuan, M. Leunig, and R.K. Jain. Fluorescence photobleaching with spatial Fourier analysis: measurement of diffusion in light-scattering media. *Biophys. J.* 65: 2428-2436, 1993.

Berk, D.A., F. Yuan, M. Leunig, and R.K. Jain. Direct *in vivo* measurement of targeted binding in a human tumor xenograft. *Proc. Natl. Acad. Sci. U.S.A.* 94: 1785-1790, 1997.

Boucher, Y., L.T. Baxter, and R.K. Jain. Interstitial pressure gradients in tissue-isolated and subcutaneous tumors: implications for therapy. *Cancer Res.* 50: 4478-4484, 1990.

Boucher, Y., and R.K. Jain. Microvascular pressure is the principal driving force for interstitial hypertension in solid tumors: implications for vascular collapse. *Cancer Res.* 52: 5110-5114, 1992.

Boucher, Y., M. Leunig, and R.K. Jain. Tumor angiogenesis and interstitial hypertension. *Cancer Res.* 56: 4264-4266, 1996.

Chary, S.R., and R.K. Jain. Direct measurement of interstitial convection and diffusion of albumin in normal and neoplastic tissues by fluorescence photobleaching. *Proc. Nat. Acad. Sci. U.S.A.* 86: 5385-5389, 1989.

Curti, B.D., W.J. Urba, W.G. Alvord, J.E. Janik, J.W. Smith, K. Madara, and D.L. Longo. Interstitial pressure of subcutaneous nodules in melanoma and lymphoma patients: changes during treatment. *Cancer Res.* 53: 2204-2207s, 1993.

Dedrick, R.L. Animal scale-up. *J. Pharmacokin. Biopharm.* 1: 435-461, 1973.

Dellian, M., G. Helmlinger, F. Yuan, and R.K. Jain. Fluorescence ratio imaging and optical sectioning: effect of glucose on spatial and temporal gradients. *Br. J. Cancer* 74: 1206-1215, 1996a.

Dellian, M., B.P. Witwer, H.A. Salehi, F. Yuan, and R.K. Jain. Quantitation and physiological characterization of bFGF and VEGF/VPF induced vessels in mice: effect of microenvironment on angiogenesis. *Am. J. Path.* 149: 59-72, 1996b.

Dellian, M., F. Yuan, V. Trubetskoy, V.P. Torchilin, and R.K. Jain. Dependence of microvascular permeability on molecular charge in a human tumor xenograft. *Int. J. Microcirc. Clin. Exp.* 16(Supp. 1): 152, 1996c.

Dudar, T.E., and R.K. Jain. Differential response of normal and tumor microcirculation to hyperthermia. *Cancer Res.* 44: 605-612, 1984.

Dvorak, H.F., L.F. Brown, M. Detmar, and A.M. Dvorak. Vascular permeability factor/vascular endothelial growth factor, microvascular hyperpermeability, and angiogenesis. *Am.J. Path.* 146: 1029-1039, 1995.

Endrich, B., H.S. Reinhold, J.F. Gross, and M. Intaglietta. Tissue perfusion inhomogeneity during early tumor growth in rats. *J. Natl. Cancer Inst.* 62: 387-395, 1979.

Eskey, C.J., A.P. Koretsky, M.M. Domach, and R.K. Jain. ^{2}H-nuclear magnetic resonance imaging of tumor blood flow: spatial and temporal heterogeneity in a tissue-isolated mammary adenocarcinoma. *Cancer Res.* 52: 6010-6019, 1992.

Eskey, C.J., A.P. Koretsky, M.M. Domach, and R.K. Jain. Role of oxygen *vs.* glucose in energy metabolism in a mammary carcinoma perfused *ex vivo*: Direct measurement by ^{31}P NMR. *Proc. Nat. Acad. Sci. USA* 90: 2646-2650, 1993.

Eskey, C.J., N. Wolmark, C.L. McDowell, M.M. Domach, and R.K. Jain. Residence time distributions of various tracers in tumors: implications for drug delivery and blood flow measurement. *J. Natl. Canc. Inst.* 86: 293-299, 1994.

Folkman, J. Tumor angiogenesis. In: *The Molecular Basis of Cancer* (J.M. Mendelsohn, M.A.P. Howley, and L.A. Liotta, eds.). Philadephia: W.B. Saunders, 1995, pp. 206-232.

Fukumura, D., H. Salehi, B. Witwer, R.F. Tuma, R.J. Melder, and R.K. Jain. TNFa-induced leukocyte-adhesion in normal and tumor vessels: effect of tumor type, transplantation site and host. *Cancer Res.* 55: 4824-4829, 1995.

Gazit, Y., D.A. Berk, M. Leunig, L.T. Baxter, and R.K. Jain. Scale-invariant behavior and vascular network formation in normal and tumor tissue. *Phys. Rev. Let.* 75: 2428-2431, 1995.

Gerlowski, L.E., and R.K. Jain. Physiologically based pharmacokinetic modeling: principles and applications. *J. Pharm. Sci.* 72: 1103-1127, 1983.

Gerlowski, L.E., and R.K. Jain. Microvascular permeability of normal and neoplastic tissues. *Microvasc. Res.* 31: 288-305, 1986.

Gullino, P.M. Techniques in tumor pathophysiology. In: *Methods in Cancer Research* (H. Busch, ed.). New York: Academic Press, 1970, pp. 45-92.

Hamberg, L.M., P.E. Kristjansen, G.J. Hunter, G.L. Wolf, and R.K. Jain. Spatial heterogeneity in tumor perfusion measured with functional computed tomography at 0.05 microliter resolution. *Cancer Res.* 54: 6032-6036, 1994.

Helmlinger G., F. Yuan, M. Dellian, and R.K. Jain. Interstitial pH and pO_2 gradients in solid tumors *in vivo*: high-resolution measurements reveal a lack of correlation. *Nature Med.* 3: 177-182, 1997.

Hobbs, S.K., F. Yuan, L.G. Cima, and R.K. Jain. Tumor microvascular pore cutoff size: implications for macromolecules and particle drug delivery. *Int. J. Microcirc. Clin. Exp.* 16(Supp. 1): 218, 1996.

Jain, R.K. Transport of molecules across tumor vasculature. *Cancer Metastasis Rev.* 6: 559-593, 1987a.

Jain, R.K. Transport of molecules in the tumor interstitium: a review. *Cancer Res.* 47: 3039-3051, 1987b.

Jain, R.K. Determinants of tumor blood flow: a review. *Cancer Res.* 48: 2641-2658, 1988.

Jain, R.K. Delivery of novel therapeutic agents in tumors: physiological barriers and strategies. *J. Natl. Canc. Inst.* 81: 570-576, 1989.

Jain, R.K. Barriers to drug delivery in solid tumors. *Scien. Amer.* 271: 58-65, 1994a.

Jain, R.K. Transport phenomena in tumors. *Adv. Chem. Eng.* 20: 129-200, 1994b.

Jain, R.K. Delivery of molecular medicine to solid tumors. *Science* 271: 1079-1080, 1996.

Jain, R.K., and L.T. Baxter. Mechanisms of heterogeneous distribution of monoclonal antibodies and other macromolecules in tumors: significance of elevated interstitial pressure. *Cancer Res.* 48: 7022-7032, 1988.

Jain, R.K., S.A. Shah, and P.L. Finney. Continuous noninvasive monitoring of pH and temperature in rat Walker 256 carcinoma during normoglycemia and hyperglycemia. *J. Natl. Canc. Inst.* 73: 429-436, 1984.

Jain, R.K., and K.A. Ward-Hartley. Tumor blood flow: characterization, modifications and role in hyperthermia. *IEEE Trans. in Sonics and Ultrasonics* 31: 504-526, 1984.

Jain, R.K., and J. Wei. Dynamics of drug transport in solid tumors: Distributed parameter model. *J. Bioengineering* 1: 313-329, 1977.

Johnson, E.M., D.A. Berk, R.K. Jain, and W.M. Deen. Diffusion and partitioning of proteins in charged agarose gels. *Biophys. J.* 68: 1561-1568, 1995.

Kaufman, E.N., and R.K. Jain. Quantification of transport and binding parameters using fluorescence recovery after photobleaching: potential for *in vivo* applications. *Biophys. J.* 58: 873-885, 1990.

Kaufman, E.N., and R.K. Jain. Measurement of mass transport and reaction parameters in bulk solution using photobleaching: reaction limited binding regime. *Biophys. J.* 60: 596-610, 1991.

Kristensen, C.A., M. Nozue, Y. Boucher, and R.K. Jain. Reduction of interstitial fluid pressure after TNF-α treatment of human melanoma xenografts. *Br. J. Cancer* 74: 533-536, 1996.

Kristjansen, P.E., Y. Boucher, and R.K. Jain. Dexamethasone reduces the interstitial fluid pressure in a human colon adenocarcinoma xenograft. *Cancer Res.* 53: 4764-4766, 1993.

Kristjansen, P.E., S. Roberge, I. Lee, and R.K. Jain. Tissue-isolated human tumor xenografts in athymic nude mice. *Microvasc. Res.* 48: 389-402, 1994.

Lee, I., Y. Boucher, T.J. Demhartner, and R.K. Jain. Changes in tumour blood flow, oxygenation and interstitial fluid pressure induced by pentoxifylline. *Br. J. Cancer* 69: 492-496, 1994a.

Lee, I., Y. Boucher, and R.K. Jain. Nicotinamide can lower tumor interstitial fluid pressure: mechanistic and therapeutic implications. *Cancer Res.* 52: 3237-3240, 1992.

Lee, I., T.J. Demhartner, Y. Boucher, R.K. Jain, and M. Intaglietta. Effect of hemodilution and resuscitation on tumor interstitial fluid pressure, blood flow, and oxygenation. *Microvasc. Res.* 48: 1-12, 1994b.

Less, J.R., M.C. Posner, Y. Boucher, D. Borochovitz, N. Wolmark, and R.K. Jain. Interstitial hypertension in human breast and colorectal tumors. *Cancer Res.* 52: 6371-6374, 1992.

Less, J.R., M.C. Posner, T. Skalak, N. Wolmark, and R.K. Jain. Geometric resistance to blood flow and vascular network architecture in human colorectal carcinoma. *Microcirculation*, in press, 1997.

Less, J.R., T.C. Skalak, E.M. Sevick, and R.K. Jain. Microvascular architecture in a mammary carcinoma: branching patterns and vessel dimensions. *Cancer Res.* 51: 265-273, 1991.

Leu, A.J., D.A. Berk, F. Yuan, and R.K. Jain. Flow velocity in the superficial lymphatic network of the mouse tail. *Am. J. Physiol.* 267: H1507-H1513, 1994.

Leunig, M., A.E. Goetz, M. Dellian, G. Zetterer, F. Gamarra, R.K. Jain, and K. Messmer. Interstitial fluid pressure in solid tumors following hyperthermia: possible correlation with therapeutic response. *Cancer Res.* 52: 487-490, 1992a.

Leunig, M., A.E. Goetz, F. Gamarra, G. Zetterer, K. Messmer, and R.K. Jain. Photodynamic therapy-induced alterations in interstitial fluid pressure, volume and water content of an amelanotic melanoma in the hamster. *Br. J. Cancer* 69: 101-103, 1994a.

Leunig, M., F. Yuan, D.A. Berk, L.E. Gerweck, and R.K. Jain. Angiogenesis and growth of isografted bone: quantitative *in vivo* assay in nuce mice. *Lab. Invest.* 71: 300-307, 1994b.

Leunig, M., F. Yuan, M.D. Menger, Y. Boucher, A.E. Goetz, K. Messmer, and R.K. Jain. Angiogenesis, microvascular architecture, microhemodynamics, and interstitial fluid pressure during early growth of human adenocarcinoma LS174T in SCID mice. *Cancer Res.* 52: 6553-6560, 1992b.

Lichtenbeld, H.C., F. Yuan, C.C. Michel, and R.K. Jain. Perfusion of single tumor microvessels: application to vascular permeability measurement. *Microcirculation* 3: 349-357, 1997.

Martin, G.R., and R.K. Jain. Noninvasive measurement of interstitial pH profiles in normal and neoplastic tissue using fluorescence ratio imaging microscopy. *Cancer Res.* 54: 5670-5674, 1994.

Melder, R.J., A.L. Brownell, T.M. Shoup, G.L. Brownell, and R.K. Jain. Imaging of activated natural killer cells in mice by positron emission tomography: preferential uptake in tumors. *Cancer Res.* 53: 5867-5871, 1993.

Melder, R.J., G. Koenig, B.P. Witwer, N. Safabakhsh, L.L. Munn and R.K. Jain. During angiogenesis, vascular endothelial growth factor and basic fibroblast growth factor regulate natural killer cell adhesion to tumor endothelium. *Nature Med.* 2: 992-997, 1996.

Milstone, D.S., D. Fukumura, R.C. Padget, P.E. O'Donnell, V.M. Davis, O.J. Benavidez, R.J. Melder, R.K. Jain, and M.A. Gimbrone. Mice lacking E-selectin show normal rolling but reduced arrest of leukocytes on cytokine-activated microvascular endothelium. Submitted, 1996.

Munn, L., G.C. Koenig, R.K. Jain, and R.J. Melder. Kinetics of adhesion molecule expression and spatial organization using targeted sampling fluorometry. *BioTechniques* 19: 622-631, 1995.

Munn, L.L., R.J. Melder, and R.K. Jain. Role of erythrocytes in leukocyte-endothelial interactions: Mathematical model and experimental validation. *Biophys. J.* 71: 466-478, 1996.

Netti, P.A., L.T. Baxter, Y. Boucher, R. Skalak, and R.K. Jain. Time dependent behavior of interstitial pressure in solid tumors: implications for drug delivery. *Cancer Res.* 55: 5451-5458, 1995.

Netti, P.A., S. Roberge, Y. Boucher, L.T. Baxter, and R.K. Jain. Effect of transvascular fluid exchange on arterio-venous pressure relationship: implication for temporal and spatial heterogeneities in tumor blood flow. *Microvasc. Res.* 52: 27-46, 1996.

Nozue, M., I. Lee, J.M. Manning, L.R. Manning, and R.K. Jain. Oxygenation in tumors bymodified hemoglobins. *J. Surgical Oncol.* 62: 109-114, 1996.

Nugent, L.J., and R.K. Jain. Extravascular diffusion in normal and neoplastic tissues. *Cancer Res.* 44: 238-244, 1984.

Patan, S., L. Munn, and R.K. Jain. Intussusceptive microvascular growth in solid tumors: a novel mechanism of tumor angiogenesis. *Microvasc. Res.* 51: 260-272, 1996.

Rippe, B., and B. Haraldsson. Fluid and protein fluxes across small and large pores in the microvasculature. Application of two-pore equations. *Acta Physiol. Scand.* 131: 411-428, 1987.

Roberts, W.G., and G. Palade. Neovasculature induced by vascular endothelial growth factor is fenestrated. *Cancer Res.* 57: 765-772, 1997.

Sevick, E.M., and R.K. Jain. Blood flow and venous pH of tissue-isolated Walker 256 carcinoma during hyperglycemia. *Cancer Res.* 48: 1201-1207, 1988.

Sevick, E.M., and R.K. Jain. Geometric resistance to blood flow in solid tumors perfused *ex vivo*: effects of tumor size and perfusion pressure. *Cancer Res.* 49: 3506-3512, 1989a.

Sevick, E.M., and R.K. Jain. Viscous resistance to blood flow in solid tumors: effect of hematocrit on intratumor blood viscosity. *Cancer Res.* 49: 3513-3519, 1989b.

Sevick, E.M., and R.K. Jain. Effect of red blood cell rigidity on tumor blood flow: increase in viscous resistance during hyperglycemia. *Cancer Res.* 51: 2727-2730, 1991a.

Sevick, E.M., and R.K. Jain. Measurement of capillary filtration coefficient in a solid tumor. *Cancer Res.* 51: 1352-1355, 1991b.

Swabb, E.A., J. Wei, and P.M. Gullino. Diffusion and convection in normal and neoplastic tissues. *Cancer Res.* 34: 2814, 1974.

Torres-Filho, I.P., M. Leunig, F. Yuan, M. Intaglietta, and R.K. Jain. Noninvasive measurement of microvascular and interstitial oxygen profiles in a human tumor in SCID mice. *Proc. Nat. Acad. Sci. USA* 91: 2081-2085, 1994.

Traykov, T.T., and R.K. Jain. Effect of glucose and galactose on red blood cell membrane deformability. *Int. J. Microcirc. Clin. Exp.* 6: 35-44, 1987.

Vaupel, P., and R.K. Jain (eds.). *Tumor Blood Supply And Metabolic Microenvironment: Characterization And Therapeutic Implications.* Gustav Fischer Publications, Stuttgart, 1991.

Ward, K.A., and R.K. Jain. Response of tumours to hyperglycaemia: characterization, significance and role in hyperthermia. *Int. J. Hyperthermia* 4: 223-250, 1988.

Yamada, S., T. Mayadas, F. Yuan, D. Wagner, R. Hynes, R.J. Melder, and R.K. Jain. Rolling in P-selectin deficient mice is reduced but not eliminated in dorsal skin. *Blood* 86: 3487-3492, 1995.

Yuan, F., L.T. Baxter, and R.K. Jain. Pharmacokinetic analysis of two-step approaches using bifunctional and enzyme-conjugated antibodies. *Cancer Res.* 51: 3119-3130, 1991.

Yuan, F., Y. Chen, M. Dellian, N. Safabakhsh, N. Ferrara, and R.K. Jain. Time-dependent changes in vascular permeability and morphology in established human tumor xenografts induced by an anti-VEGF/VPF antibody. *Proc. Nat. Acad. Sci. USA* 93: 14765-14770, 1996.

Yuan, F., M. Dellian, D. Fukumura, M. Leunig, D.A. Berk, V.P. Torchiliin, and R.K. Jain. Vascular permeability in a human tumor xenograft: molecular size-dependence and cut off size. *Cancer Res.* 55: 3752-3756, 1995.

Yuan, F., M. Leunig, D.A. Berk, and R.K. Jain. Microvascular permeability of albumin, vascular surface area, and vascular volume measured in human adenocarcinoma LS174T using dorsal chamber in SCID mice. *Microvasc. Res.* 45: 269-89, 1993.

Yuan, F., M. Leunig, S.K. Huang, D.A. Berk, D. Papahadjopoulos, and R.K. Jain. Microvascular permeability and interstitial penetration of sterically stabilized (stealth) liposomes in a human tumor xenograft. *Cancer Res.* 54: 3352-3356, 1994a.

Yuan, F., H.A. Salehi, Y. Boucher, U.S. Vasthare, R.F. Tuma, and R.K. Jain. Vascular permeability and microcirculation of gliomas and mammary carcinomas transplanted in rat and mouse cranial windows. *Cancer Res.* 54: 4564-4568, 1994b.

Zawicki, D.F., R.K. Jain, G.W. Schmid-Schoenbein, and S. Chien. Dynamics of neovascularization in normal tissue. *Microvasc. Res.* 21: 27-47, 1981.

Zlotecki, R.A., L.T. Baxter, Y. Boucher, and R.K. Jain. Pharmacologic modification of tumor blood flow and interstitial fluid pressure in a human tumor xenograft: Network analysis and mechanistic interpretation. *Microvasc. Res.* 50: 429-443, 1995.

4.6 Discussion

Intaglietta: Thank you, Rakesh, for this excellent and comprehensive explanation of what is going on in tumor therapy today. There are some questions. Maybe I could start by just bringing attention to a very important comment and line of research that you have undertaken, and that is that the special conditions of the tumor upregulate and express all kinds of molecules and even genes, and this could very well be for the future an important consideration. It is my understanding that the present thinking is that ischemia *per se*, which is of course what we are all chasing in developing artificial blood, has similar properties, and in fact they might be even more basic than the ones that appear in tumors. I was wondering if you or those in the audience would have some comments on this?

Jain: It is known that ischemia or hypoxia, which is one of the results of ischemia, upregulates a large number of genes. One of the genes it upregulates is VGEF which is one of the most potent angiogenic factors known today. It also upregulates heme oxygenase's one gene, H01, and several other genes. The tumor microenvironment definitely plays a key role from that point of view. The question is how does one alter this microenvironment, and I think to make several drugs effective, including radiation therapy, we need to do that. For example, we worked with Professor Jim Manning, as you know, at one time and using some of the hemoglobins he has made to examine if they will increase the pO_2 in tumors, and they do, but only marginally, by a couple mmHg. We also tried hemodilution, the work which we did in collaboration with you, and that showed some promise also. But what we need to do is go beyond what we have done so far, and that is the challenge facing the field.

Bonaventura: Two questions, and depending on an answer, perhaps a comment: 1) You indicated that you want to increase pO_2 in the tumor, and of course this applies primarily to radiation therapy. There are some therapies where you would want to lower the concentration. In collaboration with Mark Dewhurst, we have studied the effect of stroma- free hemoglobin solutions on microcirculation in tumors with the idea of doing what you have done with Jim Manning and others. We expected to see increased pO_2's in tumors, depending on what the oxygen affinity was. In fact, we used hemoglobins from Letterman to do this several years ago. Paradoxically, we found that the microcirculation responded by shutting down circulation and tremendously lowering the pO_2 in these tumors, so it was a disappointment with respect to radiation therapy, but an encouraging result with respect to certain chemotherapies. The question is about the potential role of extravasated drugs to increase the efficacy of treatment of solid tumors, those drugs being either ones which are the standard drugs or oxygen carriers. Do you have a comment about the potential utility of carrying oxygen by extravasation, which is a problem in blood substitutes, but may be a benefit to you.

Jain: I think that people have looked primarily at the intravascular pO_2 when they look at these blood substitutes, but I think using methods such as phosphorous quenching microscopy is important - electrodes are not going to answer that question. They are used, but they will have no meaning as far as I am concerned. I think the questions will have to be answered using phosphorous quenching microscopy where you see this material extravasating, use dual florescence, something which marks liposomes or carriers so you know where they are in the extravascular compartment. To my knowledge, these have not been answered to date. We are working on them currently to answer these kind of questions. What is the role of an extravasated carrier on pO_2? I don't think the way the University of Pennsylvania group does it with a very large tissue volume is satisfactory - you need microscopic imaging, and, to my knowledge, there are only about three laboratories in the country that have that. Marcos Intaglietta's lab started it, our laboratory can do it, and I think Dr. Pittman's laboratory has it as well.

Bonaventura: I think Dr. Dewhurst's laboratory at Duke also.

Jain: I have not seen anything published from there so I do not know.

Bonaventura: It might be very interesting to look at a low molecular weight oxygen carrier like pegylated myoglobin, or something like that, to greatly extravasate in the region where you want to deliver oxygen.

Jain: I think it would be a very useful thing to do, and we need strategies like this. What you need to remember is that when I showed you the extravasation, you saw that on one side of the blood vessels nothing is coming out. Those regions are going to have trouble no matter what you use. If it does not extravasate, and if it doesn't get there, you are in trouble.

Bonaventura: Yes, but you are looking at extravasation of a macromolecule. There are nonmacromolecule oxygen carriers with lower molecular weight than the compound you described.

Jain: The lowest molecular-weight oxygen carrier is oxygen itself, right? In our *Nature Medicine* article we show that a lot of blood vessels have plenty of blood flow but pO_2 of only 2 or 3 mmHg, so we have to keep that in mind. That's 32 molecular weight. Now if your stuff weighs more than that, be careful.

Johnson: In respect to this question of convective transport of oxygen by a carrier into the interstitium, wouldn't this be orders of magnitude different than diffusion over the short distances that we are talking about going from the vessel into the tissue?

Jain: Your point is well taken. I think what Dr. Bonaventura was asking was related to augmentation. That is, how much augmentation is there? Is it 2%, 5%, or 100%? And I think we can sit here and do a lot of mathematical modeling of it, but experiments have to be done. And that is what I imagine Dr. Bonaventura was asking.

Levin: You commented about white blood cells, but said nothing about blood platelets which may be a very important variable in blood flow, particularly since they tend to be elevated in people with tumors and can interact with white blood cells.

Jain: The question being asked is what do we know about platelets. Now, people have not used these window techniques so far to look at the behaviors of platelets in tumors. A post-doctoral fellow from Holland recently joined our lab who is looking at this very issue. What we do know is that platelets do roll on P-selectin, as reported in a paper last year by Denisa Wagner from Harvard in PNAS, and we are using some of her P-selectin deficient mice. If they are immunodeficient as well in rag 1 rag 2 background, then growing tumors on them would allow us to ask these kinds of questions. So I think we will learn about the role of platelets and a lot of these issues using some of these genetically-engineered mice where some of these molecules are missing and see how they affect the microcirculation or any other properties.

Levin: It would be easy to use fluorescently-labeled platelets to study interaction with blood vessels.

Jain: Exactly. We are using fluorescently-labeled platelets. We are looking at these models in these windows as to how platelets come in, what do they do, how do they direct in the tumor which has P-selectin and a host with P-selectin knocked out genetically. There was a lot of work done on that in Holland, by the way, about 15 or 20 years ago in the normal microcirculation. People have looked at the platelet, have visualized them. Rennemann and Tiglender are the people who have done a lot of work and published extensively in the 1970s and 1980s on that.

Intaglietta: Maybe I could end the discussion by posing a question to both Professor Jain and the audience. The issue is whether indeed an oxygen carrier can increase tissue oxygen independently of any other physiological alterations in the systems. In other words, is it possible by the introduction of additional oxygen carrying capacity in blood via liposomes, via fluorocarbons, via hemoglobins, actually increase the oxygen in the tissue? Is there any evidence that this can be done? Is there any experimental evidence that anybody has ever done this? The reason that I am asking is because we have not been able to do that.

Jain: You see, Marcos, that we have done only two studies, one with you with hemodilution and the other with Jim Manning, and in both cases the improvement is marginal. I know there are some studies in the literature, but you see the problem with those studies is that they give you an electrode pO_2 profile, and that really isn't enough. You remember, at least in cancer, you are dealing with a disease in which the 1% of cells which are protected are the ones that get us in trouble. So even if I were to give you a pO_2 profile histograph with electrode tracks, I need to find regions which are in critical need of oxygen and see if they are getting it. Our experience to date shows that almost any intervention we try when it comes to drug delivery, oxygen delivery, it works like Reaganomics; that means, the rich get richer and poor remain poor or get poorer. And what that means is that the regions that are pretty well oxygenated get even more oxygen. The trickle-down theory doesn't work, at least in the cases we have tried. Maybe somebody in the audience will show me some dramatic improvement.

Keipert: Certainly there is a lot of work that has been done in trying to look at tissue oxygenation, although we have not quite gotten down to the microscopic levels that you are describing here. We have studied several tissues, including gut, heart, muscle, liver and brain, as have people before us with Fluosol in other tissues using a variety of conventional polarographic electrodes, which are invasive and obviously poke holes into tissues. We have done a lot of work more recently with the multiwire surface and electrode system that was developed in Germany, and we have seen increases in tissue pO_2, at least at that global, macroscopic, or large-scale level. We have also seen functional biochemical consequences. We have looked at isolated heart studies. We have looked at the biochemistry, organic phosphate, high energy phosphate levels, and you can show some benefits in tissues that are clearly in need of oxygen, but whether what you are addressing in your last comment, whether those tiny areas that are in trouble, whether that particular area has gotten more, that remains to be seen using techniques like you have described.

Jain: Thank you. As I said, I am presenting only the point of view of cancer, and I think that is where the bottleneck has been in cancer. Maybe in other diseases that is not a problem.

Intaglietta: Peter, I don't mean to be critical, but you have seen your results when you increase the inhaled oxygen pO_2: you are on the hyperoxia, not on the conditions in which you just maintain the physiology constant. Is that true or maybe you could elaborate on that?

Keipert: Yes. Certainly fluorocarbons are designed to operate maximally under higher oxygen tension, but we always use an oxygen-breathing animal as the control condition and then look at what we see above and beyond that once we dose with fluorocarbon.

Hirsch: With respect to Dr. Intaglietta's comment, I just want to point out that last year we presented a paper where we showed we used an invertebrate hemoglobin in a guinea pig heart-perfusion model system where we can monitor directly using NMR spectroscopy, phosphocreatine and inorganic phosphate levels. We showed that the creatine phosphate levels were much greater than just using a normal buffer system, and this NMR technique, which we studied in collaboration with Linda Gelics and Bea Whittenberg at the Albert Einstein College of Medicine, seems to be quite promising in showing tissue oxygenation or energy maintenance in a direct way.

Intaglietta: But energy maintenance is not necessarily 100% local tissue pO_2, or am I completely mistaken?

Hirsch: I guess it is not a direct measure, but it would indicate the ATP levels, and it is involved in the whole metabolic pattern. I think it is a fairly direct way of showing the health and oxygenation of these tissues. It is obviously not direct, but you have to assume that that is the pathway.

Jain: May I add something to that ATP and energy level? It may be true that it may be an expression of oxygen in a lot of tissues, but in tumors, it is not. You take an isolated tumor, single artery and a single vein, and put an NMR coil so you can measure the ATP level, and then you begin to play with what is going into the tumor by the artery; you can control oxygen, glucose and everything. What you find is that you remove oxygen completely, make the perfusate totally anoxic, keep glucose decent, you find that ATP level doesn't change. Now you bring back oxygen, nothing happens. But if you remove glucose, the ATP level falls like you have done complete ischemia, and then when you put glucose back, it is back again. So, I think the answer is that it is very tissue-dependent whether ATP level is going to give you a level of oxygen or not.

I just wanted to address the earlier question which was raised about these oxygen carriers making a difference by extravasation. I just want to mention here that one of the reasons I am here is also because if any of you are interested in doing some of those studies in collaboration with us, please write to us, and if you have an agent and you are personally convinced this is going to work, and you can convince us, we will definitely try it and see if it really enhances or augments oxygenation in tumors. I mean, we are very open minded about this.

Cokelet: It seems to me that almost all of the experiments and the thinking is acute, and tumors are around for a while, and so you can do things over time sequentially. Is there no way you can use diffusion if it is all you've got? That is to impregnate a tumor with an oxygen carrier and then follow that with a hemoglobin carrying solution to just use diffusion. The tumor has got to be there for a few weeks or more.

Jain: Sure. You are raising a very good question. What you are saying is to implant something right into the tumor which will release whatever you want. There are a lot of companies that are trying to do that. But remember what I said to you earlier at the beginning my talk. Cancer is a systemic disease. It is not a local disease. If it were a local disease, between surgeons and radiation oncologists, we would have taken care of it by now. Ninety-five percent of the patients who die from cancer die because of wide-spread metastases. Now you cannot go ahead and implant these little devices in every little place in the body. As long as the disease is localized, even today, the surgeon and radiation oncologists do a pretty good job. And it is getting better with proton beam therapy, with local implantation of control release devices, you can take care of the local disease fairly well.

Chapter 5

The Pressor Effect of Hemoglobin—Good or Bad?

Robert J. Przybelski, M.D., Elaine K. Daily, R.N., B.S., FCCM, Marvin L. Birnbaum, M.D., Ph.D.

5.1 Introduction

When Bayliss infused hemolyzed blood into cats 75 years ago, he found that solution to "raise blood pressure, if it was low, and increase the secretion of urine" (Bayliss 1920). Amberson further explored this "vasoconstrictor action of dissolved hemoglobin," finding that infusions of hemoglobin "always raise the blood pressure" (Amberson 1937). He stated that in the case of large-volume infusions into animals "this pressor action may be ascribed in part to the high colloidal osmotic pressure of hemoglobin-saline solutions which draw fluid into the blood and so raise its volume." But even when small volumes were infused into humans, he "usually observed an elevation in blood pressure," concluding that "a chemical pressor effect is also present" (Amberson, Jennings and Rhodes 1949).

Over the past fifty years, this pressor effect has been reported with the administration of most hemoglobin solutions, including unmodified stroma-free hemoglobin (Hess, Macdonald and Brinkley 1993, Ning *et al.* 1992), cross-linked human hemoglobins (Keipert *et al.* 1993, Sharma and Gulati 1994a), polymerized cross-linked bovine hemoglobin (Matheson-Urbaitis *et al.* 1995, Lee *et al.* 1995, Lenz *et al.* 1991, Hughes *et al.* 1996) liposome-encapsulated hemoglobin (Rabinovici *et al.* 1990, Rabinovici, Rudolph and Feuerstein 1989), polyoxyethylene hemoglobin (Kida *et al.* 1995), and human recombinant hemoglobin (Loeb *et al.* 1995). While the potential benefit of the pressor effect of hemoglobin has been suggested in numerous animal models, the potential for toxicity has also been raised. This review examines the potential benefits and risks of the pressor effect in view of preclinical study data, presents recent human clinical data suggesting clinical utility, and discusses the possible mechanisms of this effect, including new concepts of vasoactivity, which might explain apparent contradictions posed by the hemoglobin pressor effect.

5.2 Pressor Potential Benefits

5.2.1 Increased perfusion

The major potential benefit of a hemoglobin solution pressor effect relates to the role of pressure as a major determinant of blood flow. Increasing the arterial pressure increases the arteriovenous perfusion gradient and, therefore, should enhance perfusion. Indirect evidence of improved tissue perfusion accompanying hemoglobin-induced increases in arterial blood pressure has been demonstrated in several hemorrhagic shock animal studies. In one study, anesthetized rats bled 30% of their total blood volume followed by resuscitation with 14% diaspirin cross-linked hemoglobin solution (half-volume or full-volume), autologous shed blood (full volume), or lactated Ringer's (two times the volume), demonstrated a prompt increase in the mean arterial pressure to above baseline levels in animals who received either volume of diaspirin cross-linked hemoglobin or blood (Przybelski *et al.* 1991). In addition, measurements of transcutaneous oxygen tension with a Clark-type, oxygen-consuming electrode were returned to normal levels only in the animals resuscitated with diaspirin cross-linked hemoglobin (half or full-volume) or blood.

In another study, awake rats bled to a venous base deficit of -15 (±2) mmol/L followed by resuscitation demonstrated a significantly higher central venous oxygen saturation one hour post-resuscitation with a 1:1 volume of diaspirin cross-linked hemoglobin compared to a 3:1 volume of lactated Ringer's (78.8% ± 1.6 *versus* 67.3% ± 2.1, respectively) (Powell, Schultz and Malcolm 1996). In a similar study, rats bled to a base deficit of -13 (±1) mmol/L demonstrated similar improvements in base deficit and restoration of base excess to baseline levels in animals resuscitated with whole blood or diaspirin cross-linked hemoglobin (half or full-volume) (Schultz, Hamilton and Malcolm 1993).

Direct assessment of changes in regional blood flow accompanying hemoglobin-induced increases in arterial blood pressure have been performed in several animal models. Swine hemorrhaged 30 ml/kg to a base deficit of -6.1 ±1.8 mEq/L, followed by resuscitation with 5 ml/kg of 7% diaspirin cross-linked hemoglobin (1/6th the blood-loss volume) demonstrated an immediate and significant increase in mean arterial pressure and cardiac output (McKenzie, Scandling and Ahle 1993). Measurement of regional blood flow by the radioactive microsphere technique demonstrated a significant increase to or above baseline levels to all tissues except the adrenal glands and the diaphragm (both of which remained unchanged) following diaspirin cross-linked hemoglobin infusion.

To determine the effect of hemoglobin solutions on brain and kidney perfusion following hemorrhage, anesthetized rats were bled to a mean arterial pressure of 35-40 mm Hg and a base deficit of -12 mmol/L, followed by resuscitation with 4 ml/kg diaspirin cross-linked hemoglobin or lactated Ringer's solution (Kumar, Sen and Gulati 1996). Using a laser Doppler flowmeter, perfusion, concentration of moving red blood cells, and red cell velocity in the brain and kidney were determined. Resuscitation with diaspirin cross-linked hemoglobin produced an increase in arterial pressure that was associated with improved arterial pH, pO_2, pCO_2 and improved perfusion to both the brain and kidney. The concentration of moving red blood cells in either organ was not altered by diaspirin cross-linked hemoglobin, but an increase in red cell velocity in the brain and kidney was observed following resuscitation with diaspirin cross-linked hemoglobin.

Several non-hemorrhage rat studies, in which hemoglobin solutions were administered as a top-load infusion, have demonstrated similar improvements in regional blood flow as determined by the radioactive microsphere technique (Gulati and Sharma 1994a, Sharma and Gulati 1994b, Barve, Sen and Gulati 1996, Loeb *et al.* 1995). Significant increases in blood flow to the heart, gastrointestinal tract, portal system and skin accompanied the diaspirin cross-linked hemoglobin-induced increase in arterial blood pressure. In addition, it appears that the observed increase in blood flow may be a dose-dependent effect of diaspirin cross-linked hemoglobin (Barve, Sen and Gulati 1996).

In some instances of hemoglobin solution infusion, the measured thermodilution cardiac output decreases, implicating increased resistance as the predominant mechanism for the increase in blood pressure. However, this is in discord with the findings of increased regional blood flow, indicating a paradox in the assessment of global *versus* regional blood flow. This may be related to the complex interaction of hemoglobin with nitric oxide (NO), whereby NO is taken up by the hemoglobin as it passes through the lung and released from the hemoglobin during arterial-venous transit (Jia *et al.* 1996). This could result in vasoconstriction of larger conduit vessels and vasodilation in smaller vessels or capillaries. This is discussed further below.

5.2.2 Blood pressure stability

In clinical conditions associated with frequent occurrences of hypotension which could lead to organ ischemia and dysfunction, or in conditions in which hypotension is recalcitrant despite maximum vasopressor therapy, hemoglobin solutions could provide blood pressure stability while preserving or enhancing organ perfusion. The discussion of the clinical utility of these applications is included in the Clinical Data section.

5.3 Pressor Potential Risks

5.3.1 Arterial hypertension

One of the possible risks associated with a rapid increase in blood pressure is the potential for development of an excessively high pressure that could result in a cerebrovascular accident. Fortunately, one unique feature of the hemoglobin pressor effect is that it appears to be self-limiting, with similar increases in pressure (30 to 40%) observed with both low and high doses (Malcolm *et al.* 1994, Nanavaty, Scanlan and McKenzie 1993). In addition, it has been shown that the effect of diaspirin cross-linked hemoglobin on blood pressure can be readily controlled by commonly used anti-hypertensive agents such as nitroglycerin, prazosin, nicardipine, or labetalol, as well as yohimbine (Bilello *et al.* 1994, Sharma and Gulati 1995, Gulati and Sharma 1994b).

In patients with active bleeding, there is concern that increased blood pressure could increase bleeding from injured vessels. In rats subjected to uncontrolled hemorrhage via a 50% tail transection, followed by resuscitation with 1:1 diaspirin cross-linked hemoglobin, 3:1 lactated Ringer's, 1:1 hypertonic saline, or 1:2 human serum albumin, restoration of mean arterial pressure to or above baseline levels was achieved only with the diaspirin cross-linked hemoglobin solution (Schultz *et al.* 1994). However, blood loss following resuscitation was less in the diaspirin cross-linked hemoglobin-treated animals than in any of the other treatment groups, but the difference was significant only when compared to the albumin group. A direct measurement of tissue perfusion via a subcutaneous tissue oxygen probe sensor demonstrated a fall in tissue oxygen tension following resuscitation with all solutions except the hemoglobin solution.

5.3.2 Pulmonary hypertension

Increases in pulmonary artery as well as systemic artery pressures have been reported with some hemoglobin solutions (Hess, Macdonald and Brinkley 1993). *In vitro* studies involving isolated porcine pulmonary artery rings indicate that the pressor effect of diaspirin cross-linked hemoglobin is also manifest in the pulmonary artery (Freas, Llave and Muldoon 1993). In a swine hemorrhagic shock study, diaspirin cross-linked hemoglobin resuscitation produced a significant increase in both systemic and pulmonary vascular resistance (McKenzie *et al.* 1993). While slight increases in pulmonary artery pressure could be beneficial in increasing the uniformity of pulmonary perfusion, the development of marked pulmonary hypertension resulting in increased capillary pressure could result in acute pulmonary edema.

5.3.3 Increased afterload

A potential effect of increases in pulmonary and systemic vascular resistance is the imposed increase in the work load of both the right and left ventricles. Excessive increases in afterload, unless accompanied by concomitant increases in contractility, are usually associated with decreases in cardiac output. The degree to which ventricular function becomes compromised, if at all, depends on the underlying physiologic status of the ventricles. In non-hemorrhaged swine, the administration of a top-load of diaspirin cross-linked hemoglobin resulted in a significant increase in mean arterial pressure and systemic vascular resistance and a slight decrease in thermodilution cardiac output. However, coronary vascular resistance remained unchanged, while coronary blood flow increased slightly (McKenzie, Scandling and West 1996). In a swine angioplasty study in which animals underwent 4 minutes of interrupted coronary blood flow during balloon inflation, infusion of diaspirin cross-linked hemoglobin increased mean arterial pressure to above control levels while significantly increasing left ventricular dP/dt and the rate pressure product (McKenzie *et al.* 1994). Coronary blood flow and coronary vascular resistance did not change from control values. These findings suggest that the increase in blood pressure with this particular modified hemoglobin solution does not negatively affect cardiac performance in these animal models.

5.3.4 Decreased tissue oxygenation

It has been suggested that vasoconstriction produced by hemoglobin solutions could cause changes in the distribution of oxygen within the microcirculation by lowering functional capillary density and tissue oxygenation (Tsai, Kerger and Intaglietta 1995). However, measurement of local tissue oxygen tension (tpO_2) in the striated skin muscle of hamsters following severe hemorrhage and resuscitation with autologous blood, diaspirin cross-linked hemoglobin, lactated Ringer's, or 6% Dextran demonstrated an increase in tpO_2 to 80%, 60%, 30%, and 40% of pre-shock values, respectively (Nolte *et al.* 1996). Moreover, tpO_2 showed a more even distribution across capillaries in the diaspirin cross-linked hemoglobin-resuscitated animals than in the blood-resuscitated animals.

In another hamster study, animals received diaspirin cross-linked hemoglobin as a top-load infusion, as an isovolemic exchange transfusion, or as a resuscitation infusion following acute hemorrhagic shock (Nolte *et al.* 1996). Following the top-load infusion, there was a brief (<10 minutes) period of arteriolar constriction in vessels 30-70 μm in diameter and a temporary decrease in spontaneous vasomotion. By 30 minutes after infusion, there was a significant increase in red blood cell velocity in postcapillary venules and no change in endothelial permeability or functional capillary density. Following diaspirin cross-linked hemoglobin resuscitation of acute hemorrhagic shock, there was a rapid restoration of red blood cell velocity to pre-hemorrhage levels. Functional capillary density, which was reduced following hemorrhagic shock, increased by approximately 44% following diaspirin cross-linked hemoglobin resuscitation. Again, variations in hemoglobin preparations and relative oxygen affinity could result in differences in microcirculatory effects and tissue oxygenation.

5.4 Clinical Data

A predictable pressor effect has been demonstrated consistently in humans receiving diaspirin cross-linked hemoglobin solution. In Phase I studies, volumes as low as ~20 ml of the 10% solution produced a 10-15 mm Hg rise in mean arterial pressure, with a greater effect on diastolic than systolic blood pressure (Przybelski *et al.* 1996). This solution was used to enhance cardiovascular stability during hemodialysis, where significantly fewer interventions for hypotension were required after prophylactic therapy with diaspirin cross-linked hemoglobin (Swan *et al.* 1995). Patients undergoing abdominal aortic repair who were treated with diaspirin cross-linked hemoglobin pre-operatively had fewer hypotensive episodes in the peri-operative period (Garrioch *et al.* 1996).

Human volunteers bled 15% of total blood volume followed by isovolemic hemodilution (3:1 lactated Ringer's) and infusion of either 16.5, 24.1, 30.2, 38, or 45 g of polymerized bovine hemoglobin or lactated Ringer's demonstrated an increase in arterial pressure and total peripheral resistance (Hughes *et al.* 1996). Calculated oxygen delivery varied directly with cardiac index which initially fell slightly following infusions of bovine hemoglobin solutions. However, metabolic cart measurements indicated a 10-24% increase in oxygen consumption in the hemoglobin-treated subjects and an up to 20% increase in oxygen diffusion capacity in subjects who received >30.2 g of bovine hemoglobin. Pulmonary function tests (including spirometry and flow volume loops) were unchanged during the study. The observed pressor effects of hemoglobin were not associated with compromised tissue oxygenation, but rather with enhanced diffusive or capillary oxygen transport.

Perhaps the most provocative application of the pressor effect of hemoglobin has been in the treatment of patients with sepsis syndrome and low systemic vascular resistance whose blood pressure could not be adequately maintained with conventional vasopressor agents (Rhea *et al.* 1996). Fourteen patients received up to 500 ml of diaspirin cross-linked hemoglobin over a 12-hour period, as needed, to maintain adequate mean arterial blood pressure. In all cases, a rapid and significant pressor response was observed, resulting in a 15 to 100% reduction in vasopressor drug requirements. Urine output, creatinine clearance and gastric mucosal pH_i either increased or remained unchanged. The cardiac output of these fluid-optimized patients showed little change compared to pre-infusion values. Mean APACHE II scores decreased from 30.1 (± 6.6) to 23.5 (±9.2) following diaspirin cross-linked hemoglobin infusion (p=0.002). None of these patients developed pulmonary hypertension or other serious adverse events due to the hemoglobin infusion.

5.5 Mechanisms of the Pressor Effect

The ability of hemoglobin to bind the endothelium-derived relaxation factor, nitric oxide, is well documented (Gibaldi 1993, Moncada, Palmer and Higgs 1991). *In vivo* animal studies have shown that the pressor effect of a modified human-derived product, diaspirin cross-linked hemoglobin, is similar to those produced by administration of a nitric oxide synthase inhibitor, L-NAME (Katsuyama *et al.* 1994) and blocked or reversed by the administration of L-arginine, an NO precursor (Sharma and Gulati 1994b, Schultz *et al.* 1993). However, with an unmodified, stroma-reduced hemoglobin, pre-treatment with L-arginine blocked the stroma-reduced, hemoglobin-induced decrease in blood flow to the kidneys, liver, and spleen of treated rats, but did not block the stroma-reduced, hemoglobin-induced increase in blood pressure (Sharma and Gulati 1994b).

Endothelin, a potent vasoconstrictor amino acid peptide, also has been shown to play a role in the pressor effect of hemoglobin. Rats pretreated with phosphoramidon, an inhibitor of proendothelin conversion to endothelin, had a significantly attenuated pressor response to diaspirin cross-linked hemoglobin administration (Schultz *et al.* 1993). The concentration of plasma endothelin-1 (ET-1) was significantly elevated in rats after receiving diaspirin cross-linked hemoglobin or unmodified stroma-reduced hemoglobin (Gulati *et al.* 1995). Although the pressor response of diaspirin cross-linked hemoglobin was significantly greater than that of stroma-reduced hemoglobin, the plasma ET-1 concentration was significantly greater in stroma-reduced hemoglobin (141%) than in diaspirin cross-linked hemoglobin (78%) treated rats (Gulati *et al.* 1995).

In another study, administration of diaspirin cross-linked hemoglobin or stroma-reduced hemoglobin in rats caused a prompt increase in arterial pressure and total peripheral resistance (Gulati, Sharma and Singh 1996). Stroma-reduced hemoglobin resulted in no change in cardiac output or stroke volume, while diaspirin cross-linked hemoglobin produced increases in cardiac output and stroke volume. Pretreatment with infusion of BQ-123, an endothelin-A receptor agonist, did not affect the stroma-reduced hemoglobin-induced increase in blood pressure but did attenuate the increase in total peripheral resistance in stroma-reduced hemoglobin-treated animals. In diaspirin cross-linked hemoglobin treated rats, increases in blood pressure and total peripheral resistance were significantly blocked by BQ-123. Thus, it appears that both hemoglobin products produce significant cardiovascular effects, but these effects are mediated through different mechanisms. While the exact role of ET-1 in the control of blood pressure is not clear, these data suggest that the pharmacologic effects of hemoglobin solutions may be influenced by the manufacturing process and purity of the product.

To determine the effects of diaspirin cross-linked hemoglobin on the peripheral vascular sensitivity of α-adrenoreceptors, various adrenergic antagonists were administered to rats pre-treated with diaspirin cross-linked hemoglobin (Gulati and Rebello 1994). Diaspirin cross-linked hemoglobin significantly potentiated (66.7%) the blood pressure response to norepinephrine and phenylephrine (40.6% increase). While administration of clonidine alone produced a fall in blood pressure, when pretreated with diaspirin cross-linked hemoglobin, the hypotensive effect of clonidine was blocked, and blood pressure increased. The specificity of diaspirin cross-linked hemoglobin-induced potentiation of the pressor effect of these agents was determined by the administration of phenoxybenzamine following norepinephrine infusion, prazosin following phenylephrine and clonidine infusions, and yohimbine prior to clonidine infusion. Phenoxybenzamine, prazosin and yohimbine all effectively blocked the pressor effect in diaspirin cross-linked hemoglobin, indicating that both α_1- and α_2-adrenoreceptors in the peripheral vascular system are sensitized by diaspirin cross-linked hemoglobin. This action may be direct or through endothelin mechanisms.

Increases in blood flow may also account for some of the observed increases in arterial pressure, particularly at higher doses of hemoglobin. In normovolemic rats, administration of 400 and 1200 mg/kg diaspirin cross-linked hemoglobin resulted in a 28.5 and 48.8% increase in cardiac output, respectively (Barve, Sen and Gulati 1996).

5.6 Vasoactivity: A Paradigm Shift

The pressor response to the administration of modified hemoglobin solution seems in part to contradict traditional views of physiology. On a global basis, the rise in systemic blood pressure associated with the administration of diaspirin cross-linked hemoglobin, for example, occurs in the face of a remarkably constant level of cardiac output, and hence, must be associated with an increase in total peripheral vascular resistance. Part of this response may be explained by arterial/arteriolar vasoconstriction in vessels leading to the musculoskeletal system, with redistribution of blood flow from the musculoskeletal system to the vital organs as has been observed in several animal studies (Gulati and Sharma 1994a, Sharma and Gulati 1994b).

Traditional concepts, however, cannot explain the effects of modified hemoglobin when administered during shock states where flow to the musculoskeletal system already is markedly attenuated. More recent evidence that explains the vascular responses in greater detail may be helpful in clarifying the physiologic mechanisms (Griffith 1995).

In order to understand these newer concepts of vascular reactivity, it is essential that the reactive tissue vascular beds be subdivided into three components: 1) conductance vessels, 2) resistance vessels, and 3) veins (Marcus *et al.* 1990). Conductance vessels often are called "feed" arteries or conduit vessels. The potential role of these conduit vessels in determining the distribution of the cardiac output and tissue perfusion is a relatively recent discovery (Marcus 1983, Chilian *et al.* 1989). In general, these conduit vessels are considered to be greater than 100-150 μm in diameter, while the resistance vessels are believed to be <100 μm in diameter (Marcus 1983, Chilian *et al.* 1989). Previously, it was thought that the resistance vessels provided the primary resistance to flow in any organ. However, it now is believed that the conduit vessels may contribute as much as 50% of the total resistance to flow in some organs (Griffith *et al.* 1989, Marcus *et al.* 1990, Segal and Duling 1986, Meininger, Fehr and Yates 1987).

Often these vessels operate in a heterogeneous fashion: with some stimuli, the conduit vessels may constrict while the resistance vessels may dilate and *vice versa* (Griffith *et al.* 1989). Some humoral substances only cause constriction of the resistance vessels (*e.g.*, vasopressin), while others cause constriction only of the conduit vessels (*e.g.*, serotonin) (Marcus *et al.* 1990; Griffith *et al.* 1989). Sympathetic stimulation, activation of alpha receptors, and infusions of norepinephrine result in constriction of coronary vessels >150 μm and dilatation of the vessels <100 μm in diameter (Chilian *et al.* 1989). Nitroglycerin administration causes dilatation of the conduit coronary arteries >200 μm in diameter and has little effect on the smaller arteries (Kanatsuka *et al.* 1988). Cholinergic stimulation is mediated by the release of NO, and this results in relatively homogeneous dilatation of arterial and venous vessels (Marcus 1983).

Constriction of the conduit vessels for a fixed flow (cardiac output on the global basis) produces an increase in velocity through the conduit vessel. With the increased resistance and the same flow rate, it is possible that the intravascular pressure as the blood exits the conduit vessel and enters the resistance vessels downstream may be the same as it is with lower vascular tone in the conduit vessel. Central arterial pressure, as measured in the large arteries, therefore, may increase without a decrease in overall organ blood flow. In fact, some studies have demonstrated as much as a two-fold increase in tissue flow to some organs when the principal constriction occurred in the conduit vessels (Segal and Duling 1986, Griffith *et al.* 1989). This may account for the increase in regional blood flow to the metabolically-active organs seen following diaspirin cross-linked hemoglobin infusions (McKenzie, Scandling and Ahle 1993, Gulati and Sharma 1994a, Sharma and Gulati 1994a).

Thus, it is necessary to consider the dynamics of the vascular system when attempting to understand the pressor responses induced by the infusion of a modified hemoglobin solution. Rather than just a simple increase in total peripheral resistance and shifts in distribution of blood flow, there now are explanations for the increases in tissue flow and improved oxygenation observed in the face of "vasoconstriction" with such products.

5.7 Conclusion

The pressor effect of hemoglobin solution cannot be viewed as either good or bad—it is different: different from what was expected of a "blood substitute", and different in action from other pressor agents. In clinical indications, such as hemodialysis, surgical anesthesia, or shock, where an increase in blood pressure and perfusion are beneficial and desirable, the pressor effect will be considered an attribute. In normotensive or hypertensive patients merely requiring enhanced oxygen carrying capacity, this effect could be considered adverse. In considering the "good or bad" question of the pressor effect of hemoglobin, it is hoped that the current information at least challenges one to reconsider previous assumptions about the vasoactivity of these unique, pharmacologically-active, hemoglobin-based, oxygen-carrying solutions.

5.8 References

Amberson, W.R. *Blood Substitutes*, 48-85, 1937.

Amberson, W.R., J.J. Jennings, and C.M. Rhode. Clinical experience with hemoglobin saline solutions. *J. Appl. Physiol.* 1: 469-489, 1949.

Barve, A., A. Sen, and A. Gulati. Dose-dependent effect of diaspirin cross-linked hemoglobin on the systemic and regional blood circulation in rats. *FASEB J.* 10: A600, 1996.

Bayliss, W.M. Is haemolysed blood toxic? *Brit. J. Exp. Pathol.* 7-8, 1920.

Bilello, K., S. Schultz, C. Powell, J. Jaffin, F. Cole, and D. Malcolm. Diaspirin cross-linked hemoglobin (DCLHb™): Control of pressor effect with anti-hypertensive agents. *Artif. Cells, Blood Substit., Immobil. Biotech.* 22: 819-825, 1994.

Chilian, W.M., S.M. Layne, C.L. Eastham, and M.L. Marcus. Heterogeneous microvascular coronary α-adrenergic vasoconstriction. *Circ. Res.* 64: 376-388, 1989.

Freas, W., R. Llave, and S.M. Muldoon. Effect of diaspirin cross-linked hemoglobin solution on isolated porcine pulmonary artery and vein rings. *FASEB J.* 7: A314, 1993.

Garrioch, M., R. Larbuisson, J.F. Brichant, M. Lamy, E. Daily, and R. Przybelski. The hemodynamic effects of diaspirin cross-linked hemoglobin (DCLHb) in the operative setting. *Crit. Care Med.* 24: A39, 1996.

Gibaldi, M. What is nitric oxide and why are so many people studying it? *J. Clin. Pharmacol.* 33: 488-496, 1993.

Griffith, T.M. Endothelium-derived relaxing factor and the control of flow in conduit and resistance arteries. In: *Flow-Dependent Regulation of Vascular Resistance*, New York: Oxford University Press, 1995, pp. 178-213.

Griffith, T.M., D.H. Edwards, R.L. Davies, and A.H. Henderson. The role of EDRF in flow distribution: a microangiographic study of the rabbit isolated ear. *Microvasc. Res.* 37: 162-177, 1989.

Gulati, A., and S. Rebello. Role of adrenergic mechanisms in the pressor effect of diaspirin cross-linked hemoglobin. *J. Lab. Clin. Med.* 124: 125-133, 1994.

Gulati, A., and A.C. Sharma. Effect of stroma-free hemoglobin and diaspirin cross-linked hemoglobin on the regional circulation and systemic hemodynamics. *Life Sci.* 55: 827-837, 1994a.

Gulati, A., and A.C. Sharma. Prazosin blocks the pressor but not the regional circulatory effects of diaspirin crosslinked hemoglobin. *Life Sci.* 55: 121-130, 1994b.

Gulati, A., A. Sharma, and G. Singh. Role of endothelin in the cardiovascular effects of diaspirin crosslinked and stroma-reduced hemoglobin. *Crit. Care Med.* 24: 137-147, 1996.

Gulati, A., G. Singh, S. Rebello, and A. Sharma. Effect of diaspirin crosslinked and stroma-reduced hemoglobin on mean arterial pressure and endothelin-1 concentration in rats. *Life Sci.* 56: 1433-1442, 1995.

Hughes, G.S., E.J. Antal, P.K. Locker, S.F. Francom, W.J. Adams, and E.E. Jacobs. Physiology and pharmacokinetics of a novel hemoglobin-based oxygen carrier in humans. *Crit. Care Med.* 24: 756-764, 1996.

Hess, J.R., V.W. Macdonald, and W.W. Brinkley. Systemic and pulmonary hypertension after resuscitation with cell-free hemoglobin. *J. Appl. Physiol.* 74: 1769-1778, 1993.

Jia, L., C. Bonaventura, J. Bonaventura, and J.S. Stamler. S-nitrosohaemoglobin: A dynamic activity of blood involved in vascular control. *Nature* 380: 221-226, 1996.

Kanatsuka, H., K.G. Lamping, C.L. Eastham, and M.L. Marcus. Non-uniform effect of nitroglycerin on different size coronary arterial vessels. *FASEB J.* 2: A496, 1988.

Katsuyama, S.S., D.J. Cole, J.C. Drummond, and K. Bradley. Nitric oxide mediates the hypertensive response to a modified hemoglobin solution (DCLHb™) in rats. *Artif. Cells, Blood Substit., Immobil. Biotech.* 22: 1-7, 1994.

Keipert, P.E., A. Gonzales, C.L. Gomez, V.W. Macdonald, J.R. Hess, and R.M. Winslow. Acute changes in systemic blood pressure and urine output of conscious rats following exchange transfusion with diaspirin-crosslinked hemoglobin solution. *Transfusion* 33: 701-708, 1993.

Kida, Y., M. Maeda, S. Iwata, Y. Iwashita, K. Goto, and K. Nishi. Effects of pyridoxylated hemoglobin polyoxyethylene conjugate and other hemoglobin-related substances on arterial blood pressure in anesthetized and conscious rats. *Artif. Organs* 19: 117-128, 1995.

Kumar, A., A.P. Sen, and A. Gulati. Effect of diaspirin crosslinked hemoglobin on the brain and kidney perfusion of hemorrhaged rats using a laser-Doppler flowmeter. *Artif. Cells, Blood Substit., Immobil. Biotech.* 24: 370, 1996.

Lee, R., K. Neya, T.A. Svizzero, and G.J. Vlahakes. Limitations of the efficacy of hemoglobin-based oxygen-carrying solutions. *J. Appl. Physiol.* 79: 236-242, 1995.

Lenz, G., H. Junger, R. van den Ende, B. Brotman, and A.M. Prince. Hemodynamic effects after partial exchange transfusion with pyridoxylated polyhemoglobin in chimpanzees. *Biomat., Artif. Cells, Immobil. Biotech.* 19: 708-718, 1991.

Loeb, A.L., L.J. McIntosh, B.S. Raj, and D.E. Longnecker. Effects of recombinant human hemoglobin (rHb1.1) on systemic and regional hemodynamics in the anesthetized rat. *Anesthesiology* 84: A642, 1995.

Malcolm, D.S., I. Hamilton, S. Schultz, F. Cole, and K. Burhop. Characterization of the hemodynamic response to intravenous diaspirin cross-linked hemoglobin solution in rats. *Artif. Cells, Blood Substit., Immobil. Biotech.* 22: 91-107, 1994.

Marcus, M.L. Neural control of the coronary circulation. In *The Coronary Circulation in Health and Disease.* New York: McGraw-Hill Book Co., 1983, 128-146.

Marcus, M.L., W.M. Chilian, H. Kanatsuka, K.C. Dellsperger, C.L. Eastham, and K.G. Lamping. Understanding the coronary circulation through studies at the microvascular level. *Circ.* 82: 1-7, 1990.

Matheson-Urbaitis, B., Y.S. Lu, C. Fronticelli, and E. Bucci. Renal and systemic-hemodynamic response to isovolemic exchange transfusion with hemoglobin cross-linked with bis(3,5-dibromosalicyl) fumarate or albumin. *J. Lab. Clin. Med.* 126: 250-260, 1995.

McKenzie, J.E., E.A. Cost, D.M. Scandling, N.W. Ahle, and R.W. Savage. Effects of diaspirin crosslinked hemoglobin during coronary angioplasty in the swine. *Cardiovasc. Res.* 28: 1188-1192, 1994.

McKenzie, J.E., D.M. Scandling, and N.W. Ahle. Diaspirin cross-linked hemoglobin (DCLHb™): Improvement in regional blood flow following administration in hypovolemic shock in the swine. Vth International Symposium on Blood Substitutes (ISBS), San Diego, 1993 (Abstract).

McKenzie, J.E., D.M. Scandling, M.J. Rohrer, and J.L. Jacot. Diaspirin cross-linked hemoglobin (DCLHb™) during hypovolemic shock in the swine. Vth International Symposium on Blood Substitutes (ISBS), San Diego, 1993 (Abstract).

McKenzie, J.E., D.M. Scandling, and S.D. West. Diaspirin crosslinked hemoglobin (DCLHb™): Effects on myocardial blood flow and cardiac function during increased cardiac performance. *Artif. Cells, Blood Substit., Immobil. Biotech.* 24: 387, 1996.

Meininger, G.A., K.L. Fehr, and M.B. Yates. Anatomic and hemodynamic characteristics of the blood vessels feeding the cremaster skeletal muscle in the rat. *Microvasc. Res.* 33: 81-97, 1987.

Moncada, S., R.M.J. Palmer, and E.A. Higgs. Nitric oxide: Physiology, pathophysiology, and pharmacology. *Pharmacol. Rev.* 43: 109-142, 1991.

Nanavaty, M., D.M. Scanlan, and J. McKenzie. Diaspirin cross-linked hemoglobin (DCLHb™): Characterization of blood pressure response in the swine. Vth International Symposium on Blood Substitutes (ISBS), San Diego, CA, 1993.

Ning, J., L.M. Peterson, P.J. Anderson, and G.P. Biro. Systemic hemodynamic and renal effects of unmodified cell-free hemoglobin solution in dogs. *Biomat., Art. Cells, Immob. Biotech.* 20: 723-727, 1992.

Nolte, D., R. Botzlar, R. Hecht, C. Csapo, M.D. Menger, and K. Messmer. Diaspirin cross-linked hemoglobin: Evaluation of effects on the microcirculation of striated muscle. *Artif. Cells, Blood Substit., Immobil. Biotech.* 22: 587-592, 1994.

Nolte, D., S. Pickelmann, A. Botzlar, and K. Messmer. Effects of diaspirin cross-linked hemoglobin (DCLHb™) on local tissue oxygen tension in striated skin muscle after resuscitation from severe hemorrhagic shock. *Shock* 5: 16, 1996.

Powell, C., S. Schultz, and D. Malcolm. Diaspirin cross-linked hemoglobin (DCLHb™): More effective than lactated Ringer's solution in restoring central venous oxygen saturation after hemorrhagic shock in rats. *Biomat., Artif. Cells, Immobil. Biotech.* 24: 25-29, 1996.

Przybelski, R.J., E.K. Daily, J.C. Kisicki, C. Mattia-Goldberg, M.J. Bounds, and W.A. Colburn. Phase I study of the safety and pharmacologic effects of diaspirin cross-linked hemoglobin solution (DCLHb™). *Crit. Care Med.* 24: 1993-2000, 1996.

Przybelski, R.J., D.S. Malcolm, D.G. Burris, and R.M. Winslow. Cross-linked hemoglobin solution as a resuscitative fluid after hemorrhage in the rat. *J. Lab. Clin. Med.* 117: 143-151, 1991.

Rabinovici, R., A.S. Rudolph, and G. Feuerstein. Characterization of hemodynamic, hematologic, and biochemical responses to administration of liposome-encapsulated hemoglobin in the conscious, freely moving rat. *Circ. Shock* 29: 115-132, 1989.

Rabinovici, R., A.S. Rudolph, T.L. Yue, and G. Feuerstein. Biological responses to liposome-encapsulated hemoglobin (LEH) are improved by a PAF antagonist. *Circ. Shock* 31: 431-445, 1990.

Rhea, G., A. Bodenham, A. Mallick, R. Przybelski, and E. Daily. Vasopressor effects of diaspirin cross-linked hemoglobin (DCLHb™) in critically ill patients. [abstract] *Crit. Care. Med.* 24: A39, 1996.

Schultz, S.C., B. Grady, F. Cole, I. Hamilton, K. Burhop, and D. Malcolm. A role for endothelin and nitric oxide in the pressor response to diaspirin cross-linked hemoglobin. *J. Lab. Clin. Med.* 122: 301-308, 1993.

Schultz, S.C., I.N. Hamilton, and D.S. Malcolm. Use of base deficit to compare resuscitation with lactated Ringer's solution, Haemaccel, whole blood, and diaspirin cross-linked hemoglobin following hemorrhage in rats. *J. Trauma* 35: 619-626, 1993.

Schultz, S.C., C.C. Powell, D.G. Burris, H. Nguyen, J. Jaffin, and D.S. Malcolm. The efficacy of diaspirin crosslinked hemoglobin solution resuscitation in a model of uncontrolled hemorrhage. *J. Trauma* 37: 408-412, 1994.

Segal, S.S., and B.R. Duling. Communication between arteries and microvessels in hamster striated muscle: Segmental vascular responses are functionally coordinated. *Circ. Res.* 59: 283-290, 1986.

Sharma, A.C., and A. Gulati. Effect of diaspirin cross-linked hemoglobin and norepinephrine on systemic hemodynamics and regional circulation in rats. *J. Lab. Clin. Med.* 123: 299-308, 1994a.

Sharma, A.C., and A. Gulati. Role of nitric oxide in cardiovascular effects of diaspirin cross-linked hemoglobin (DCLHb™) and stroma-reduced hemoglobin (SRHb). *FASEB J.* 8: A625, 1994b.

Sharma, A.C., and A. Gulati. Yohimbine modulates diaspirin crosslinked hemoglobin-induced systemic hemodynamics and regional circulatory effects. *Crit. Care Med.* 23: 874-884, 1995.

Swan, S.K., C.E. Halstenson, A.J. Collins, W.A. Colburn, J. Blue, and R.J. Przybelski. Pharmacologic profile of diaspirin cross-linked hemoglobin in hemodialysis patients. *Am. J. Kid. Dis.* 26: 918-923, 1995.

Tsai, A.G., H. Kerger, and M. Intaglietta. Microcirculatory consequences of blood substitution with hemoglobin. In *Blood Substitutes: Physiological Basis of Efficacy* (R.M. Winslow, K.D. Vandegriff, and M. Intaglietta, Eds.) New York: Birkhäuser, 1995.

5.9 Discussion

Baldwin: Am I right in thinking that when you inject 25 mg/kg of hemoglobin, you get an increase in blood pressure?

Przybelski: Yes.

Baldwin: I have found in rats that I get a dose-dependent response with 25 mg/kg. I actually get a reduction in blood pressure, and then when I increase the dose, I get an increase in blood pressure. Have you found this is other species?

Przybelski: We have never seen that, although it has been reported historically. There have been decreases and increases, although they have not been identified as articulately as you have. I assume you are working with product that does not have any endotoxin in it - that would be the first thing I would think of. The lowest that I have ever looked at was 25 mg/kg. In animals, the lowest we've looked at was 62 mg/kg, so you may be seeing something that we've never seen.

Baldwin: You talked about an increase in vascular resistance. We are looking at the microcirculation of the intestine, and with that dose we see a marked increase in blood flow and also vasodilation.

Przybelski: In microvasculature work we have done, primarily with Professor Messmer's lab in Germany, we have used higher doses than that, and although we don't see vasoconstriction, I don't think we can say we've seen vasodilation. That's really interesting.

Winslow: Dr. Baldwin, could you clarify which hemoglobin you are working with because I think this may be an important issue.

Baldwin: I found the same thing happens with PEG hemoglobin and with two different cross-linked hemoglobins.

Winslow: As I understand it then, Bob, at the doses you are reporting, you are really looking at a pharmacologic effect and probably not so much of an oxygen- transport effect. Is that correct?

Przybelski: I think that's true for the majority of the data. Certainly with volumes in the range of 250 ml up to a liter or so, which we are using in our studies in the United States now, I've got to believe we have a significant oxygen load. If you have a patient, let's say, that hemorrhaged and still has three liters of their own blood, and you are putting in a product that is vasoactive and has hemodynamic effects, it is hard to separate those out. It's really hard to say whether the effect is due to perfusion, the additional oxygen that it might be imparting, a little bit of right shift, or is it the kind of things you've talked about before in your book about its proximity to the tissue *versus* where the red cells are. It is so complicated and exciting at the same time, it's hard to answer your question. All of what you've said is true, but we certainly are looking at the oxygen-carrying aspects of it, *per se*.

Winslow: I wonder if you would care to comment on the volumes that you are planning on using because it may be that we are really not talking about a blood substitute, *per se*, in terms of an oxygen transporter, but purely a pharmacologic effect, and I wonder if you would expect to see different things at higher doses where you actually might increase the DO_2.

Przybelski: I think the first thing you'd see is that a lot of the hemodynamic effects would go away. In some of Diana Malcolm's animal work, and even the work that we've done with the higher doses, like 1-1/2 volume resuscitation, you don't see some of these effects. It's as if the need for the hemodynamic response is not there. So the compensatory mechanisms that are invoked initially are either down-regulated or something later on.

Winslow: From a practical or a clinical point of view, one thinks about a blood substitute as being used as blood is used: the patient is bleeding, so you give the product. It seems to me that you are really talking about something different, dissociating volume and the oxygen-carrying effect from the pharmacologic hemodynamic effect, and maybe we should be making that distinction more than we do.

Przybelski: From the standpoint of understanding it, I think you are right. And I think it is exciting because in my mind that is where the controversy is that you are identifying. Are they linked, are they separate, are both required or are both beneficial in the same setting? Can you differentiate them? Can you create a hemoglobin that has no pharmacodynamic effect but that just carries oxygen, or one at doses we just heard about that may have certain properties that are desirable at certain doses? That's where the issues are I think.

Winslow: If you were thinking not so much about designing clinical protocol, but specifically in treating a patient, let's say, in hypovolemic shock, would you imagine using this product to restore volume as well as blood pressure, or would you imagine using some other colloid or even a crystalloid in conjunction with hemoglobin, and if so, in what sequence or what combination? How do you actually see it being used?

Przybelski: My own experience with large-volume resuscitation has been kind of negative. When you have the five liters per minute of Ringer's lactate going in, you see in humans what we saw in rats: the response drops very quickly, whether it is because we are massively hemodiluting what red cells are left, or whatever. I don't see a favorable response. In a study that we will be starting in Europe soon, patients in Class III and IV shock will first receive between 500 ml and 1 liter of the hemoglobin solution at the site of the accident and then additional volume beyond that as needed, including red cells if they are available. If there is going to be any benefit demonstrated (it is hard to show a benefit unless you are looking at mortality or significant morbidity), it is going to come with early intervention, hopefully in lieu of crystalloids and colloids, but certainly never in lieu of red cells.

Gould: I think I'm probably the only surgeon in the room, so I'm sure I've lost more blood than anybody else in this room, and I want to pick up on the theme that Bob Winslow started which is the pharmacoactivity *versus* the volume-expansion oxygen-carrying capacity, because as a surgeon, we are traditionally taught several basic principles. The treatment of hypovolemic hemorrhagic shock, as Bob said, traditionally, and I'll be glad to comment on the Mattox study, but still currently is rapid volume expansion. Actually, what is not often said, because it is just assumed, is what saves the patient's life is stopping the hemorrhage, so we shouldn't ignore that. I think you gave a wonderful review of the data that has been generated with this product, and it has really intriguing and fascinating pharmacologic activity. Our approach has been different, more along the line of what Bob was trying to get out, that in large-volume hemorrhage, it makes sense to expand volume. We have tried to develop a solution that is not pharmacologically active because there are times in the operating room when the surgeon and the anesthesiologist don't want to have to worry about additional properties of what they are giving, and I am going to show some of those data this afternoon. It's not to say that one is better or worse. I think that the value of this afternoon's program is that we may see a couple of different approaches, but what I want to get at is what I always teach my residents and students. Ultimately, when bleeding patients die, while it may be from inadequate volume, at some point you reach a critically low hemoglobin level, and I would be interested if you might comment on more than just volumes, Bob, on the hemoglobin increments that you can achieve. Somewhere along the way, even though you are maintaining a blood pressure with a pharmacologically active agent, there has to be a sufficient circulating hemoglobin mass, and that comes back to our approach to replace the lost hemoglobin. These are fascinating data, they have been all along, and if I can put it in the form of a question, maybe you can extend what Bob was asking. How do you decide whether you are more concerned with maintaining hemodynamics for a period of time, and where do you look at the circulating hemoglobin level, which is an important part of that whole oxygen delivery equation?

Przybelski: I can reflect on our cardiac surgery experience, in which we've tried to get the surgeons to use a transfusion trigger. We have selected 7.0 g/dl based on the literature and their feelings, so at that time of randomization or just before randomization, a decision is made whether these patients will be treated with either red cells as a control or the hemoglobin solution, for whatever volume they are allowed to use in that protocol. In answer to your question, we typically see an increase of 0.5 to 1.0 g hemoglobin in the process, which is not as much on a unit-per-unit basis as you would expect to see with red cells. I think the reason for this is because of the oncotic properties of these solutions. Now to get more to answer your question, I don't think this product is made for large-volume hemorrhages. It is made to support the majority of patients through what would typically be a two or three unit transfusion as an alternative. Certainly, at best, it would be a bridge to transfusion, so to speak. I'm glad you point out the difference in approaches because they are complementary. We are looking for an initial hemodynamic response; I think you are looking more for the absolute larger volume.

Gould: Yes. Just in case anyone in the audience is not familiar, as Bob asked Dr. Baldwin, there are different products and so what we've heard is the approach of a low volume to a bioactive approach with pretty intriguing results, but there are other ways, and I think that is part of the problem that often comes up - that people are confused by the different data and not paying sufficient attention to the different natures of the preparations.

Przybelski: Right. And the different approaches. We definitely have different clinical/regulatory or clinical strategies in developing our products.

Winslow: We found, using the Army's αα-hemoglobin, some differences in hemodynamics in anesthetized animals depending upon the anesthetic agent - barbiturates are quite different from gas anesthetics - and I wonder if you have seen any of that, or if you had really designed the protocols around specific anesthetic agents and surgical patients?

Przybelski: We did a study (Cole, you cited one of his papers earlier in your review) in which we studied isoflurane MAC to see whether or not there was effect on that gas, and there wasn't. It is also true of our clinical studies. With phenobarbital, we've seen drops in blood pressure, in particular, with animals.

Winslow: And survival?

Przybelski: I don't know about survival. We saw a difference in survival with chloral hydrate, and I don't know if anybody else has any experience with it, but there may be an interaction between the products and chloral hydrate which is not used in human situations much any more, certainly not as an anesthetic agent, but in some of the rat models we looked at. We had a study in which two out of the six animals died in the anesthesia, probably as a result of some kind of interaction.

Winslow: The other question was about catecholamines. You mentioned in your septic shock patients that you were able to decrease norepinephrine. I think that there is a paper from Gulati about catecholamine release, and I wonder if you would remind us, is catecholamine release associated with administration of DCLHB, and is that why you can decrease norepinephrine?

Przybelski: I really thought that was the case a long time ago when we did that first rat study, because of the responses we were seeing. We measured catecholamine metabolites in probably half a dozen models and in humans in the stroke study. We see receptor changes and that might be what you are referring to. There is a potentiation of the norepinephrine response which corresponds with the human data I showed you. But we don't see release of catecholamines. It would have been a nice explanation for that.

Gonzales: I was just wondering if there are any evaluations or observations on psychological or neurological effects in some of your subjects.

Przbelski: In a hemodialysis study we looked at profile of mood scales because I was interested to know whether a blood pressure response like that is associated with anxiety, agitation, that kind of thing. We didn't see it, although it wasn't with the larger volumes that we are using now. Of course with the trauma and the surgical patients, since our treatments are perioperative, it probably would be somewhat difficult, at least acutely. We are not running any specific neurological tests other than to look for routine adverse events, so I guess all I can say is no, we haven't really looked that carefully at either neurological or psychological effects. That's actually what got Bob Winslow and me interested in the rat studies that we set up at Walter Reed. There were prior reports of neurological toxicity using early solutions. We looked for it pretty carefully in the rat studies, but in the human studies other than looking for adverse events we have not done that.

Winslow: Bob, thank you very much for that excellent review.

Chapter 6

Perflubron-based Emulsion: Efficacy as Temporary Oxygen Carrier

Stephen F. Flaim, Ph.D.

6.1 Introduction

Perfluorochemicals (PFCs) are inert, primarily fluorine-substituted hydrocarbons. These materials have been studied extensively over the past 15-20 years primarily as the basic chemical platform for synthetic blood substitutes (Spence 1996).

PFCs are clear fluids which dissolve O_2 and other gases in accordance with Henry's law (Riess and LeBlanc 1982). The relationship between PFC-dissolved O_2 and the partial pressure of O_2 at ambient conditions is linear and unlike the chemically based O_2-hemoglobin association which demonstrates saturation kinetics. O_2 dissolved in PFCs is not affected by pH, pCO_2, 2,3-diphosphoglycerate (2,3-DPG; responsible for the regulation of the release of O_2 from hemoglobin), temperature, or other physiological conditions. The specific solubility of O_2 in PFCs depends on the chemical structure of the PFC and ranges between 30 and 50 vol % for the clinically useful agents (Lowe, 1991). When prepared for parenteral use, PFCs distribute in the acellular phase of the blood thereby enhancing the O_2-carrying capacity of the blood compartment normally occupied solely by plasma. These unique characteristics are considered to be the basis of the mechanism whereby PFCs effectively facilitate the transfer of O_2 to the tissues.

PFCs are water insoluble and, therefore, must be emulsified for intravenous use. The first PFC emulsion approved in the United States for medical use was *Fluosol®*. This product, developed by *Green Cross Corp.* of Japan, was a 20% w/v PFC emulsion (14 g/dL perfluorodecalin and 6 g/dL perfluorotripropylamine) containing emulsifying agents (egg yolk phospholipid [EYP] and poloxamer-188) (Ohyanagi *et al.* 1979). *Fluosol* has been used commercially in the United States and in the United Kingdom as an intracoronary agent to enhance O_2 delivery to the myocardium during percutaneous transluminal coronary angioplasty. Unfortunately, due to poor sales, *Fluosol* has recently been removed from the market. Despite the limited success, the preclinical and clinical experience with the first generation PFC emulsions, culminating in the development of *Fluosol*, has served to validate PFC emulsions as a safe and effective means to enhance O_2 delivery to tissue (Spence 1996).

Riess and Le Blanc (1988) initiated the effort that has resulted in the development of the second generation PFC emulsion products. The goal of this development effort has been to define products with increased O_2 solubility, reduced tissue retention and fast excretion, minimal clinically significant side-effects, high definition and purity, and large-scale commercial availability. The most promising among the resulting products is perflubron-based emulsion (developed by *Alliance Pharmaceutical Corp.* initially under the tradename, *Oxygent*™) (Spence 1996). Perflubron (perfluorooctyl bromide; $C_8H_{17}Br$) is an 8-carbon linear chain molecule which is fluorine saturated with the exception of a single bromine atom on the terminal carbon. The current formulation (AF0144) of perflubron-based emulsion is a 60% w/v PFC emulsion (58% w/v perflubron with 2% w/v perfluorodecyl bromide) containing 3.6% w/v EYP as the emulsifier. AF0144, which is being developed as a temporary O_2 carrier for use during surgical procedures, is currently in Phase IIb clinical trials and is being developed jointly by *Alliance Pharmaceutical Corp.*, San Diego, CA and *Johnson & Johnson* subsidiaries the *Robert Wood Johnson Pharmaceutical Research Institute* and *Ortho Biotech Inc.*, Raritan, NJ. The pharmacokinetics and side-effects of perflubron-based emulsion have been summarized previously (Flaim 1994). Perflubron-based emulsion does not cause activation of the complement or plasma contact systems, it does not induce immunogenic or allergic reactions, it does not induce leukocyte adhesion, vasoconstriction, or disturbances of the microcirculation. Numerous preclinical safety and pharmacokinetic (distribution, metabolism, and elimination) studies have been completed on perflubron-based emulsion and the results from these studies have successfully supported the ongoing clinical development program.

The material reviewed in this chapter, components of which have been presented previously (Flaim *et al.* 1994), is intended to summarize the preclinical efficacy experience with perflubron-based emulsion as a temporary O_2 carrier for enhancement of O_2 delivery to tissues. Unless otherwise indicated throughout the remainder of this chapter, the term "PFC" will indicate specifically perflubron and "PFC emulsion" will refer specifically to perflubron-based emulsion.

6.2 Enhanced O_2 Delivery Mechanisms

The mechanisms by which PFC emulsions deliver O_2 to tissues are associated with both the physical characteristics of the emulsion system (O_2 solubility in the PFC, emulsion particle size) and the convective delivery of the O_2-loaded PFC emulsion to the capillary bed. These concepts have been clearly described by Faithfull (1993). Because of their small particle size (diameter approximately 0.2 μm), these O_2-carrying emulsion particles travel in the plasma phase of the blood (thereby increasing plasma O_2 solubility) without causing microvascular disturbances (Lang *et al.* 1994) (Figure 6.1). This effect is expected to be enhanced in vessels

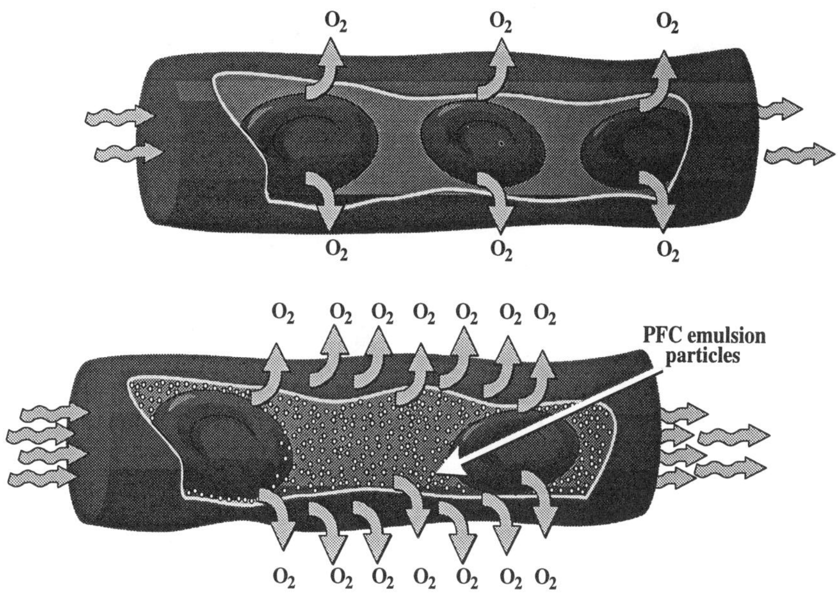

Figure 6.1. Diagrammatic illustration of a potential mechanism of enhancement of O_2 delivery to tissue at the level of a microvessel or capillary by PFC emulsion. In the upper figure without PFC emulsion, O_2 transport across the vessel wall and into the tissue largely occurs at sites on the vessel wall near erythrocytes. When the PFC emulsion is present in the plasma space (lower figure), O_2 transport across the vessel wall may occur not only at sites near erythrocytes but also over areas of the vessel wall in contact with plasma-containing the PFC emulsion.

with rapid flow where erythrocyte streaming leaves a near-wall plasma excess (Figure 6.2). Additionally, because of its small particle size, PFC emulsion is capable of reaching capillary regions that may exclude erythrocytes but possess a sustained plasma flow (e.g. capillary beds which are "shut down" due to physiological or pathological conditions). In these regions, PFC emulsions increase microvascular PO_2 thereby increasing the effective surface area for diffusion of O_2 from blood to tissue. Additionally, PFC emulsions may improve blood flow by increasing erythrocyte flexibility which is known to be reduced in low-O_2, acidotic conditions.

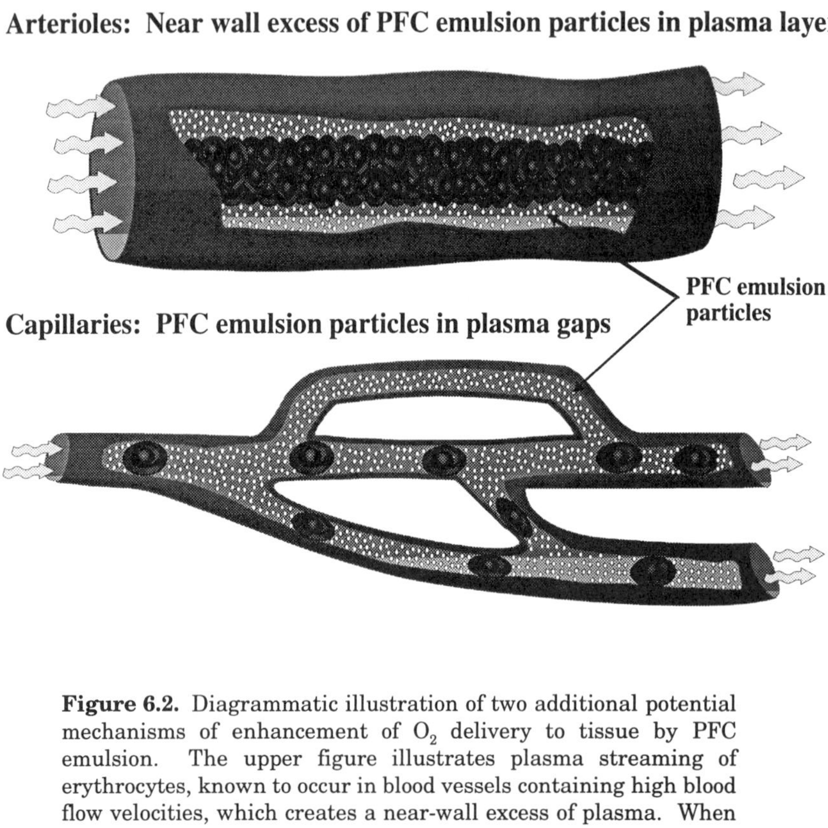

Figure 6.2. Diagrammatic illustration of two additional potential mechanisms of enhancement of O_2 delivery to tissue by PFC emulsion. The upper figure illustrates plasma streaming of erythrocytes, known to occur in blood vessels containing high blood flow velocities, which creates a near-wall excess of plasma. When PFC emulsion is present, this near-wall excess of plasma may enhance O_2 transport across the vessel wall and into the surrounding tissue. The lower figure illustrates the possibility that PFC emulsion-containing plasma, which continues to flow through microvessels or capillary regions that effectively exclude erythrocytes for physiologic or pathophysiologic reasons (commonly thought to be vascular regions which are "shut down"), may continue to support O_2 transport to tissue.

In summary, the mechanism of enhanced O_2 delivery to tissues by PFC emulsion is thought to be associated with at least two distinct functions: (a) a modulation of O_2 diffusion barriers between the erythrocyte and the tissue cells, and (b) an increase in convective O_2 transport. The theoretical basis for each of these mechanisms is described below.

6.2.1 O_2 diffusion barriers

The capillary bed is the principal site of diffusive gas exchange between blood and tissue. The geometric features of a given capillary bed determine the amount and distribution of blood available for gas exchange, as well as the diffusive pathway for O_2 from blood to mitochondria. The PO_2 fall per unit length of the O_2 diffusion pathway from blood to mitochondria defines the overall PO_2 gradient. This gradient can be subdivided into four sites of resistance (a) the gradient from the interior to the surface of the red cell, (b) the gradient across the extracellular carrier-free region (CFR; the O_2 diffusion path through plasma, endothelium, and interstitium where there is no specific O_2 carrier available under normal circumstances), (c) the gradient over the average diffusion path from sarcolemma to mitochondria, and (d) the gradient around the individual mitochondrion. A major barrier to effective O_2 diffusion is that which occurs as a result of the CFR (b above). By distributing in the plasma compartment of the blood, PFC emulsions are thought to diminish this barrier by providing a specific O_2 carrier to the CFR.

6.2.2 O_2 transport

The interrelationship between various parameters of O_2 transport are illustrated in Figure 6.3 in which O_2 content is plotted against PO_2 to create an oxyhemoglobin dissociation curve (ODC) for a normal, 70-kg man at rest with a hemoglobin concentration of approximately 15 g/dL (hematocrit of 45%). The data for the ODC in this figure were generated by a model developed by R.M. Winslow (Winslow 1985) that calculates the total O_2 content dissolved in the plasma and bound to hemoglobin (Faithfull *et al.* 1994). For a given arterial and venous PO_2 of 100 and 40 mm Hg, respectively, the arterial to venous O_2 content difference (CaO_2 - CvO_2) is 5 mL/dL. At a normal cardiac output of 5 L/minute, the O_2 consumption ($\dot{V}O_2$, represented by the shaded area) is approximately 250 mL/minute or 3.5 mL/kg/min. The relevance of this computer model to predict outcome in a dog model and in the clinical setting has been demonstrated (Keipert *et al.* 1996).

When $\dot{V}O_2$ is not supply-limited (i.e., when an increase in $\dot{D}O_2$ does not result in an increase in $\dot{V}O_2$), changes in O_2 content of the arterial blood can be compensated for by physiological mechanisms. For example, in anemia, cardiac output increases, as does the level of red cell 2,3-DPG. An increase in red cell 2,3-DPG shifts the ODC to the right, indicating a reduced affinity of O_2 for hemoglobin and an increased P_{50} (PO_2 at which hemoglobin is half saturated with O_2). A similar compensatory mechanism (with respect to cardiac output) occurs during acute normovolemic hemodilution (ANH). As hematocrit decreases during hemodilution, blood viscosity also decreases, which allows cardiac output to increase without a significant change in the work load on the heart. In this way, total $\dot{D}O_2$ and, therefore, $\dot{V}O_2$ can be maintained. This is illustrated in Figure 6.3, Panels A and B, where $\dot{V}O_2$ from hemoglobin under air-breathing conditions (" $\dot{V}O_2$ on air" area of shading) is the same in both

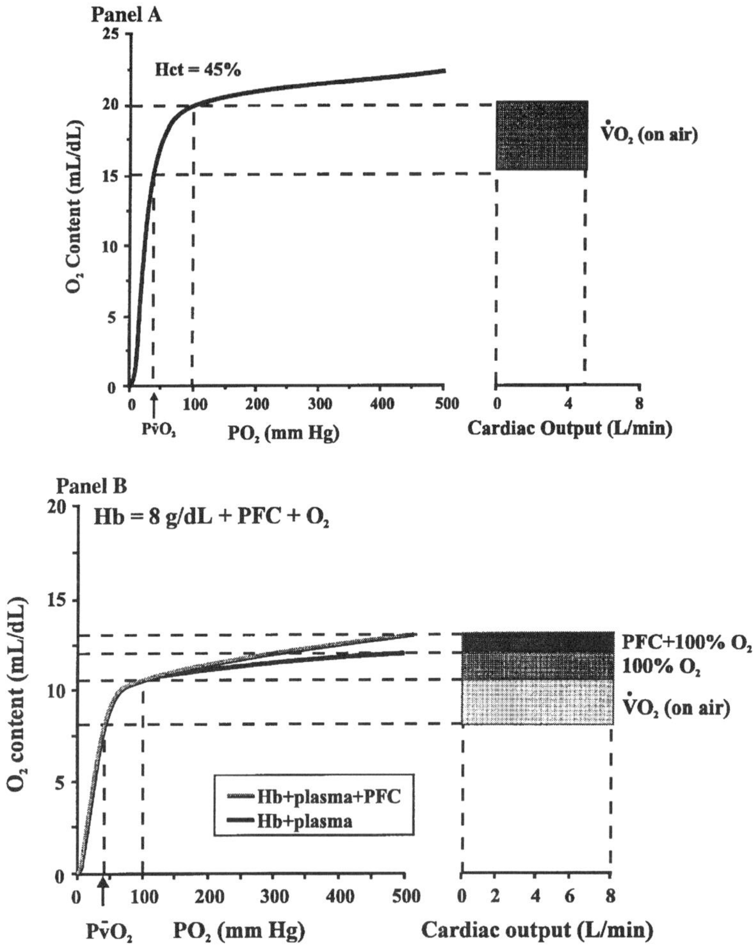

Figure 6.3. Panel A: Relationship between the O_2 delivery from hemoglobin in blood and cardiac output under normal conditions (hematocrit = 45%). Total O_2 utilization (or consumption; $\dot{V}O_2$) is equal to cardiac output times the arterial-venous O_2 content difference, and is indicated by the shaded area. Panel B: Oxygen delivery and total O_2 consumption following acute normovolemic hemodilution (to a hematocrit of 25%) and injection of 2.7 g PFC/kg while breathing 100% O_2. The potential contributions to total $\dot{V}O_2$ by the individual compartments (i.e., the red cells, plasma, and the PFC emulsion) are shown by the different shaded areas. At a cardiac output of 8 L/min., (and an arterial PO_2 of 500 mm Hg), the total amount contributed to $\dot{V}O_2$ by the plasma and PFC phase approximately equals normal $\dot{V}O_2$ (Winslow 1985, 1995, Faithfull *et al.* 1994).

Panels (Panel A representing conditions prior to hemodilution and Panel B indicating conditions after hemodilution) (Winslow 1995).

Figure 6.3, Panel B illustrates the increase in potential $\dot{D}O_2$ that can be achieved by elevating the O_2 content of blood by breathing 100% O_2 (shaded area defined as 100% O_2). This additional contribution to $\dot{D}O_2$ is primarily due to the increased amount of O_2 dissolved in the plasma compartment of the blood. $\dot{D}O_2$ can be further increased by the addition of a PFC emulsion under these conditions, which provides an even greater margin of safety (shown by the extra shaded area in the figure). The presence of an additional O_2 carrier, such as a PFC in the plasma, increases the total O_2 content of the plasma compartment and facilitates the diffusion of O_2 from the red cell into the tissues. According to the model (Figure 6.3, Panel B), the addition of a single dose (2.7 g PFC/kg body weight [BW]) of a PFC emulsion will result in an increase in the total O_2 content in the plasma. $\dot{V}O_2$ may come preferentially from the PFC in the plasma compartment since this O_2 is physically dissolved and therefore may be more easily utilized compared to the O_2 that is bound as a ligand to hemoglobin. Oxygen will not be released from hemoglobin until the PO_2 in tissues has fallen below the value at which hemoglobin is fully saturated with O_2 (± 120 mm Hg). Under these conditions, the remaining O_2 carried by the red cells represents an available reserve of extra O_2 that can supply additional O_2 during high-demand and low-supply conditions to prevent tissue hypoxia.

6.3 Efficacy to Enhance O_2 Delivery

In order to demonstrate that a temporary O_2 carrier such as PFC emulsion improves tissue oxygenation, it is important to show, in critical tissues such as the brain and heart, that the product increases tissue oxygenation as well as protects or improves tissue metabolic status, resulting in the protection of, or improvement in, organ function. Studies in both normal and surgical animal models have shown PFC emulsion to be efficacious for the enhancement of O_2 delivery to critical tissues, enhancement of tissue PO_2 levels, enhancement or protection of tissue metabolic status, and ultimately the preservation or recovery of critical organ function. These benefits are reviewed here in four categories of studies demonstrating (a) the efficacy of PFC emulsion for improved O_2 delivery, tissue metabolic status, and organ function, (b) the efficacy of PFC emulsion as an adjunct during cardiac surgical procedures, (c) the efficacy of PFC emulsion as a temporary O_2 carrier, and (d) the use of $P\bar{v}O_2$ as a component of the "transfusion trigger".

6.3.1 Tissue and organ function

The ability of first generation intravenous (IV) perfluorodecalin emulsions to increase tissue PO_2 was demonstrated by multiple investigators

(Kessler, Hoper and Pohl, 1982, Clark *et al.* 1989). Similar studies conducted with PFC emulsion have demonstrated improvements in tissue oxygenation in an isolated skeletal muscle preparation and in *in vivo* and *in vitro* models of two critical tissues, the brain and the heart. The results of these studies, summarized below, further indicate that the increased delivery of O_2 by PFC emulsion is associated with an improvement in tissue metabolic status and ultimately in sustained or enhanced organ function under conditions of hypoxia or ischemia.

6.3.1.1 Skeletal muscle

Hogan *et al.*(1992) assessed the ability of PFC emulsion to increase the O_2 diffusing capacity (D_mO_2) of a working skeletal muscle by increasing O_2 plasma solubility. This study was based on the assumption that an increase in D_mO_2 would be reflected in an increase in skeletal muscle $\dot{V}O_2$ above that expected by simply increasing $\dot{D}O_2$. $\dot{V}O_2$ was measured in a maximally working *in situ* canine gastrocnemius muscle perfused (IA, 120 mL/min/100g) with diluted blood (8-9 g/dL hemoglobin) containing 5.4 g PFC/kg PFC emulsion or an equivalent volume of vehicle under hyperoxic conditions ($PaO_2 \cong 500$ mm Hg). Muscle O_2 delivery and $\dot{V}O_2$ were significantly improved, while muscle O_2 extraction and estimated D_mO_2 were unaffected by PFC emulsion. These results indicate that PFC emulsion increased plasma O_2 solubility and $\dot{V}O_2$ through enhanced convective O_2 transport. Most importantly, this study demonstrates an increase in maximal O_2 consumption when O_2 delivery to the muscle was increased by PFC emulsion.

6.3.1.2 Brain

The retina is a neurosensory tissue and is considered to be part of the central nervous system (CNS). To a limited extent, therefore, oxygenation of retinal tissue can be considered to reflect oxygenation of CNS tissue. Retinal tissue oxygenation can be assessed by measuring the partial pressure of O_2 diffusing from the retinal microcirculation through the retinal tissue into the vitreous humor of the eye. The vitreous humor is a nonvascular, noncellular fluid which is continuous with the interstitial fluid "third" space of the body. O_2 reaching this space, therefore, represents a reasonable approximation of CNS tissue oxygenation. Braun, Linsenmeier, and Goldstick (1992) used a double-barreled, recessed cathode O_2 microelectrode to assess retinal tissue oxygenation in anesthetized cats under conditions of air and 100% O_2 breathing. The O_2 microelectrode (tip diameter 5-10 μm) was inserted into the eye and positioned within the vitreous humor 150-mm anterior to the retinal surface (far from major blood vessels) for measurement of pre-retinal PO_2. As discussed, PO_2 measured at this location represents interstitial fluid O_2 tension, which is governed by O_2 delivered to the retinal capillary bed.

PO_2 measurements were made prior to, during, and following peripheral vein infusion of small doses of PFC emulsion (three consecutive 1 g PFC/kg IV doses) during ventilation with room air and while breathing 100% O_2. Some animals were also assessed following infusion of equivalent volumes of emulsion vehicle and all measurements were made under dark-adapted conditions to minimize tissue functional and metabolic changes. In addition to pre-retinal PO_2, electroretinograms (ERG) were evaluated as an indication of retinal function.

Intravenous PFC emulsion greatly enhanced pre-retinal PO_2 during 100% O_2 breathing: mean pre-retinal PO_2 on 100% O_2 breathing was approximately 40 mm Hg at baseline (pre-infusion), and increased to 53 and 60 mm Hg following the first and second consecutive doses of PFC emulsion, respectively. Overall, the cumulative effect of three 1 g PFC/kg doses of PFC emulsion was to double pre-retinal PO_2 under these 100% O_2-breathing conditions.

Intravenous infusion of vehicle had little effect on the PO_2 response to 100% O_2, indicating that the increased PO_2 associated with PFC emulsion infusion was not simply due to an increase in blood flow as a result of fluid load or hemodilution. The small volumes of PFC emulsion infused in this study also argue against increased blood flow as an explanation for the observed PO_2 enhancement. There were no significant changes in either the b- or c-wave components of the ERG following PFC emulsion infusion, indicating that the increased pre-retinal PO_2 observed following PFC emulsion was not the result of changes in tissue metabolism or function. Taken together, these results provide clear evidence that peripheral IV infusion of PFC emulsion can effectively increase O_2 delivery to a peripheral circulatory bed and that this additional O_2 has diffused from the vasculature into the tissue, resulting in an increase in tissue oxygenation in the CNS.

van Rossem *et al.* (1997) demonstrated the effect of PFC emulsion on local tissue PO_2 in the cerebral cortex of conscious rabbits during room air and 100% O_2 breathing. Cortical tissue PO_2 was continuously monitored with chronically implanted polarographic O_2 sensors at three locations in the somatosensory cortex (interelectrode distance of 2 mm) during the following protocol: 15 minutes on room air, 5 minutes on 100% O_2, 5 minutes on room air, infusion of 5.4 g PFC/kg perflubron-based emulsion or vehicle, switch to 100% O_2 at 30 minutes post-infusion. Results were recorded as O_2 electrode current (iO_2), which is directly and linearly related to tissue PO_2.

Oxygen breathing alone (without infusion of PFC emulsion) was associated with an increase in iO_2 in all cases with high variability between animals and between different locations within a single animal. PFC emulsion infusion during room air breathing was not associated with a significant change in iO_2, but with 100% O_2 breathing, iO_2 values rose approximately 2.6 times higher than those observed with 100% O_2

breathing alone. Vehicle infusion had no effect on iO_2 regardless of inspired O_2 concentration. These results further support the conclusion that PFC emulsion can significantly enhance cerebral tissue oxygenation under conditions of 100% O_2 breathing.

In order to determine if the increased cerebral tissue oxygenation induced by IV PFC emulsion results in an improvement of cerebral tissue metabolic status, the effect of IV PFC emulsion on local cerebral blood flow (LCBF; iodo[^{14}C]antipyrine) and local cerebral glucose utilization (LCGU; 2[^{14}C]deoxy-D-glucose) was assessed in a conscious rat model of severe hemorrhage and fluid resuscitation (Waschke *et al.* 1994). Hemorrhage (total blood loss of 40 mL/kg or approximately 2/3 of circulating blood volume) was induced in Sprague-Dawley rats by controlled arterial bleeding and was followed by 30 minutes of hemorrhagic hypovolemia. Animals were then placed on 100% O_2 breathing and assigned to either the control hydroxyethyl starch (HES: intravascular volume replaced by infusion of 6% HES) or the HES-PFC (intravascular volume replaced by infusion of 6% HES plus 2.7 g PFC/kg PFC emulsion) groups. Physiologic variables were assessed prior to and at the end of hemorrhage and at 15 minutes and 2 hours following fluid resuscitation. At the two-hour time point, LCBF and LCGU were determined in 34 discrete brain structures using autoradiography.

Hemorrhage resulted in a decrease in mean arterial pressure and arterial O_2 content, the development of metabolic acidosis, and an increase in plasma glucose in all animals. There were no differences between groups during the course of the study in any physiologic parameter with the exception of arterial O_2 tension which was higher in HES-PFC compared to HES. It is important to note that there were no measurable differences between HES-PFC and HES with respect to arterial O_2 content or hemoglobin concentration throughout the course of the study. LCBF was significantly greater in HES-PFC compared to HES in 32 of the 34 brain structures assessed (average LCBF was 30% higher in HES-PFC vs. HES). Lower values of LCGU were found in HES-PFC *versus* HES, with significant differences occurring in 19 of the 34 brain structures assessed. Therefore, the addition of PFC emulsion to the resuscitation fluid was associated with a leftward (decreased LCGU) and upward (increased LCBF) shift of the regression line as compared to HES alone. Thus, PFC-emulsion-treated tissues were supported in a higher aerobic state (less glucose utilization) than tissues of the control HES-treated group. It should be noted that a single molecule of glucose, metabolized under aerobic conditions, yields 38 molecules of adenosine triphosphate (ATP), whereas only 2 ATPs are yielded from 1 molecule of glucose metabolized under anaerobic conditions. The higher aerobic state in the HES-PFC group was associated with a decreased glucose metabolic requirement. The results of this study were compared to those of a historical group in which LCBF and LCGU were assessed in untreated (i.e., no hemorrhage and no fluid resuscitation) animals. In general, LCBF was lower in untreated controls *versus* HES, whereas LCGU was unchanged. Perhaps the best way to compare the effects of hemodilution with HES alone and with HES-PFC is to evaluate the overall ratio of LCBF/LCGU. The LCBF/LCGU ratio was increased from 1.5 mL/mol in untreated animals (historical controls) to 2.2 mL/mol in the HES group due to the increased blood flow effects of hemodilution alone. The LCBF/LCGU ratio was further increased to 3.4 mL/mol in the HES-PFC group due to the additive effects of the hemodilution-induced increase in blood flow, the PFC-induced improvement in aerobic metabolic state, and the consequent decrease in LCGU. Thus, IV PFC emulsion increases cerebral tissue oxygenation and this change is associated with an actual improvement in cerebral tissue aerobic metabolic status.

In order to conclude that treatment with IV PFC emulsion has a functional tissue-oxygenation benefit, it is necessary to demonstrate not only that the tissue receives more O_2 with a resulting improvement in metabolic status, but it must also be possible to demonstrate an improvement in organ function as a result of PFC emulsion treatment. To this end, a study was conducted in a canine model of temporary brainstem ischemia and reperfusion (Guo, White and Batjer 1995). In this model, the bifurcation of the basilar artery and the superior cerebellar artery was occluded with cyanoacrylate glue, and temporary brainstem ischemia was induced by clipping the bilateral vertebral arteries and the ventral spinal artery. This study was based on the assumptions that (a) brain infarction occurs only in those areas in which residual blood flow drops below some critical level for a relatively prolonged interval, and (b) that if the residual blood flow is able to provide enough metabolic substrate to maintain integrity and clear metabolic by-products, permanent infarction will not occur. Brainstem auditory evoked potentials (BAEP) were monitored in this study as an indicator of brainstem ischemic insult and recovery of brainstem function. Animals received 1.35 g PFC/kg PFC emulsion or an equivalent volume of 0.9% saline (controls) prior to 20 minutes of isolated brainstem ischemia under 100% O_2 breathing conditions (ventilation was adjusted as needed to maintain a PaO_2 of approximately 630 mm Hg and a $PaCO_2$ of approximately 40 mm Hg). BAEP and regional cerebral blood flow (rCBF: measured by a laser doppler flowmeter placed on the ventrolateral surface of the medulla near the emergence of the hypoglossal nerve) were assessed prior to ischemia, at 5, 10, and 20 minutes during ischemia, and for five hours following reperfusion. rCBF decreased significantly to less than 10 mL/min/100g during ischemia in both groups. Following reperfusion, rCBF in both groups showed a similar short period of reactive hyperemia and returned to baseline by 30 minutes post-reperfusion with no further change during the remaining 4.5 hours of the study (Figure 6.4, Panel A). During the ischemic period, both control and PFC emulsion-treated animals experienced dramatic declines in BAEP to under 10% of baseline values. Upon reperfusion, BAEP increased in both groups to between 50% and

70% of baseline. In the PFC emulsion group, BAEP continued to recover to 80% of baseline by 1 hour and to 88% of baseline by 5 hours. In con-

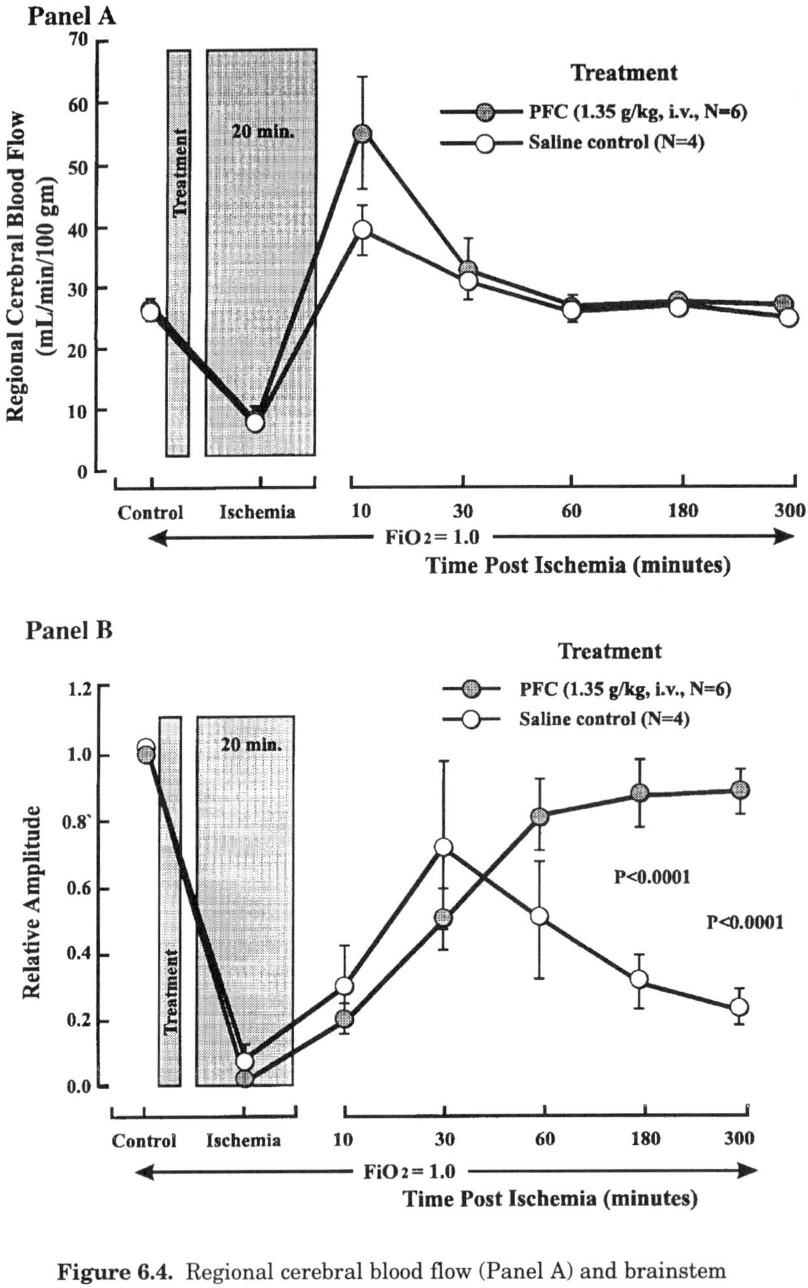

Figure 6.4. Regional cerebral blood flow (Panel A) and brainstem auditory evoked potentials (Panel B) during and following partial brainstem ischemia in dogs (Guo, White and Batjer 1995). Data are means ± SEM.

trast, the control animals suffered a drop in BAEP to 23% of baseline after the brief postischemic peak (Figure 6.4, Panel B). The improvement in cerebral function assessed by BAEP in this study is attributed to an improved O_2 delivery to tissues by the PFC emulsion during ischemia and reperfusion. The finding that rCBF was not different between groups indicates that the improvement in brain function was not related to changes in blood flow, which supports the hypothesis that improved O_2 delivery in the perflubron-based emulsion-treated group was responsible for the observed recovery of organ function. It is also possible that a component of the improvement in cerebral function in the PFC emulsion group was related to other effects such as a PFC-mediated reduction of reperfusion injury.

Collectively, these four studies indicate that PFC emulsion increases O_2 delivery to cerebral tissue, that this increased tissue oxygenation results in an improvement in cerebral tissue metabolic status, and that this overall benefit results in an improvement in cerebral function.

6.3.1.3 Cardiac muscle

Another critical tissue where the benefit of IV PFC emulsion should be demonstrable is cardiac muscle. A series of *in vitro* and *in vivo* studies have been conducted to assess the potential benefits of PFC emulsion on cardiac muscle tissue oxygenation, metabolic status, and organ function. The results of these studies demonstrate that PFC emulsion increases O_2 delivery to cardiac muscle tissue, that this results in an improvement in tissue metabolic status which is translated into a concomitant improvement in cardiac function. These benefits have been observed under both warm- and cold-perfusion conditions and in both normally perfused hearts and in hearts under various ischemic conditions.

A study was conducted to measure the effects of PFC emulsion on myocardial tissue O_2 levels during no-flow ischemia using electron paramagnetic resonance (EPR) spectroscopy to determine continuous myocardial tissue PO_2. Isolated rat hearts were perfused with crystalloid solution (Krebs-Henseleit [KH] buffer) and equilibrated at 37°C with 95% O_2/5% CO_2 in the presence or absence (historical control) of a 50% v/v dilution of a 100% w/v PFC emulsion. Coronary perfusion was then arrested and the time course of the decay in PO_2 in the myocardium was assessed with EPR oximetry. Baseline tissue PO_2 in this no-flow preparation has been shown to be approximately 0.45 mm Hg (Zweier *et al.* 1994). In control, KH-perfused hearts during no-flow ischemia, PO_2 fell rapidly to approximately 0.21 mm Hg over the first 7 minutes of ischemia and then fell at a slower rate to approximately 0.15 mmHg over the final 35 minutes of the study (Zweier *et al.* 1994). In a heart pretreated with PFC emulsion, the initial transient fall in PO_2 during no-flow ischemia was entirely absent. PO_2 gradually fell to approximately 0.36 mm Hg over the first 30 minutes of no-flow ischemia and declined further to approximately 0.20 mm Hg over the final 20 minutes of ischemia (J. Zweier, Johns Hopkins University School of Medicine, unpublished data). The results of this study demonstrated that the presence of PFC emulsion in the coronary vascular bed resulted in a sustained level of cardiac tissue oxygenation for 20-30 minutes following arrest of coronary perfusion under 37°C conditions. These findings indicate that PFC emulsion sustains tissue oxygenation during no-flow ischemia in cardiac muscle.

A study was conducted to assess the effects of intracoronary (IC) PFC emulsion in an isolated, perfused non-recirculating rabbit heart Langendorff preparation (del Balzo *et al.* 1996c). Hearts were perfused, with PFC emulsion (1:10 v/v dilution of a 100% w/v PFC emulsion), vehicle alone (1:10 v/v dilution) in KH buffer, or control KH buffer at a constant pressure (60 mm Hg). Coronary flow, cardiac function and myocardial O_2 delivery and consumption were assessed at various times throughout the study for each group of hearts. Significant increases in perfusate PO_2, O_2 delivery, and O_2 consumption in PFC-emulsion-treated hearts were accompanied by improvements in cardiac function (left ventricular [LV] systolic and diastolic pressures [LVSP and LVDP], LV +dP/dt and -dP/dt, and rate-pressure product [RPP]) relative to the control groups. The increase in perfusate PO_2 reflected a greater amount of dissolved O_2 per unit volume of solution due to the higher solubility of O_2 in the PFC emulsion compared to vehicle or KH buffer. Coronary flow in the PFC emulsion group was reduced compared to the control groups presumably due to a diminished autoregulatory demand secondary to the improvement in O_2 supply. A similar effect in isolated, perfused hearts has been previously reported by Biro, Masika and Korecky (1989). The increased O_2 delivery from the PFC emulsion resulted in improved myocardial tissue oxygenation and left ventricular performance and caused an increased O_2 consumption. It is well known that hearts perfused with crystalloid solutions are O_2 supply limited. By adding PFC emulsion to the perfusate, O_2 supply was significantly increased, and this was reflected in improved cardiac function in this *in vitro* preparation.

Taken together, these findings clearly indicate that PFC emulsion increases O_2 supply to cardiac muscle tissue.

A study was conducted to determine if PFC emulsion improved O_2 delivery and supported normal metabolic function in hearts during cold cardioplegic arrest (del Balzo *et al.* 1995a; 1995b). Isolated rabbit hearts were perfused (retrograde Langendorff apparatus) with KH buffer (gassed with 95% O_2-5% CO_2) under normothermic (37°C), aerobic conditions at constant pressure (70 mm Hg) for 20-30 minutes to establish baseline conditions. Subsequently, hearts were subjected to 150 minutes of hypothermic (20°C) cardioplegic arrest. During arrest, hearts were intermittently perfused (20 minutes; 15 mL, 20°C) with oxygenated control-cardioplegia solution (crystalloid cardioplegia; 25 mEq/L KCl,

290-310 mosmol/L, pH=7.4) or PFC-cardioplegia (crystalloid cardioplegia containing 10% v/v PFC emulsion). Hearts were then subjected to 45 minutes of aerobic reperfusion at 37°C. During cardioplegic arrest, the intraventricular balloon was emptied to simulate an arrested, vented heart. Assessment was made of cardiac function and myocardial oxygenation at various times throughout the study for both groups of hearts. At the end of cardioplegic arrest or following reperfusion, the hearts were frozen for analysis of high-energy metabolites by an enzymatic assay method. During 20°C cardioplegic arrest, PFC-cardioplegia delivered significantly higher myocardial O_2 and supported increased O_2 consumption compared to controls. In addition, both coronary arterial PO_2 and coronary sinus venous O_2 content were increased compared to crystalloid cardioplegia solution alone, even in the face of increased myocardial O_2 consumption. PFC-cardioplegia provided for an improved preservation of high-energy phosphates both during the ischemic arrest and at reperfusion. Following reperfusion, recovery of LV function (as assessed by RPP and LV +dP/dt) was significantly enhanced in hearts treated with PFC-cardioplegia compared to hearts receiving crystalloid cardioplegia alone. The left ventricular pressure-volume relationship, assessed in each heart at the end of the reperfusion period, confirmed the improved functional benefit in the PFC-cardioplegia treated hearts. These results demonstrate that the improved myocardial O_2 delivery resulting from the addition of PFC emulsion to the perfusate better sustained aerobic metabolism in myocardial tissue during cold cardioplegia and that this benefit resulted in a more efficient use of myocardial energy stores, preserving high-energy phosphates and ultimately resulting in the improvement in functional recovery of the heart after reperfusion. Similar beneficial results have been reported in an isolated, blood-perfused swine heart preparation (Martin *et al.* 1991).

To confirm the results obtained in the isolated hearts, a study was performed in dogs to assess the benefits of PFC emulsion administered as an adjunct to cardioplegia on myocardial oxygenation and functional recovery in hearts previously exposed to a period of warm ischemia (Mosca *et al.* 1996). Anesthetized mongrel dogs were instrumented for hemodynamic and cardiac function assessment in conjunction with total cardiopulmonary bypass (CPB). Normothermic (37°C) CPB was instituted and baseline conditions were established. Normothermic global myocardial ischemia was then initiated and maintained for 15 minutes followed by 75 minutes of cold (10°C) cardioplegic arrest using 15 mL/kg of control blood cardioplegia solution (hematocrit approximately 5%) or cardioplegia solution supplemented with PFC emulsion (6-11 g PFC/kg of a 60% w/v PFC emulsion). Cardioplegia solution was administered at 15 minute intervals. Hearts then underwent a 30-minute period of normothermic reperfusion. Myocardial tissue PO_2 was measured directly by a polarographic needle electrode in the myocardium, and cardiac functional recovery (stroke work) was assessed. As was observed in the isolated-heart studies, PFC emulsion treated canine hearts demonstrated a significantly higher tissue PO_2 compared to control hearts during cold cardioplegia. This improved tissue oxygenation secondary to PFC emulsion treatment was associated with improved stroke work recovery following reperfusion.

The results of these studies demonstrated the ability of PFC emulsion to deliver O_2 and support myocardial function under reduced temperature conditions. These observations are supported by the work of Bass (1991) who demonstrated that perflubron dissolves O_2 (and is, therefore, capable of delivering O_2 to tissue) as well as, if not slightly better, at lower temperatures compared to normal body temperature. The following series of studies were conducted, therefore, to determine if PFC emulsion is capable of supporting cardiac oxygenation and function under normal body temperature conditions.

Myocardial oxygenation and function were evaluated following 37°C low-flow global ischemia in isolated, Langendorff perfused rabbit hearts (del Balzo *et al.* 1994). Hearts were perfused at constant pressure (60 mm Hg) with KH buffer for approximately 20 minutes, subjected to low-flow global ischemia (1.5 mL/min) for 60 minutes and then reperfused at constant pressure for another 60 minutes. PFC emulsion (1:10 v/v dilution of a 100% w/v PFC emulsion) or vehicle was administered as an IC perfusion during the terminal 30 minutes of ischemia and through the initial 30 minutes of reperfusion. Cardiac function and myocardial oxygenation were assessed during both low-flow ischemia and reperfusion and following 60 minutes of reperfusion. Frank-Starling function curves were determined at the end of the reperfusion period. PFC emulsion significantly increased O_2 delivery both during ischemia and reperfusion. As noted previously, the increase in O_2 delivery resulted in an attenuation of reactive hyperemia during early reperfusion and improved left ventricular developed pressure (Figure 6.5, Panel A) and RPP (Figure 6.5, Panel B). The ratio of O_2 consumption to RPP was reduced at most time points indicating improved myocardial metabolic-functional efficiency in the PFC emulsion hearts. Finally, the left ventricular developed pressure at any given left ventricular end diastolic pressure (LVEDP) at the end of the reperfusion period was significantly improved in the PFC emulsion group indicating an overall improvement in myocardial function. In a separate study, hearts were subjected to the same experimental conditions but assayed for high-energy phosphates at the termination of the reperfusion period (del Balzo *et al.* 1996e, Symons *et al.* 1995). PFC emulsion treated hearts were found to have significantly increased adenine ribonucleotides, energy charge, creatine, and creatine phosphate as well as reduced lactate levels compared to control untreated hearts. In a further study, PFC emulsion was found to attenuate the rate of development and the magnitude of ischemic contracture which occurred during 120 minutes of low-flow ischemia (del Balzo *et al.* 1995b). Together, these studies in low-flow, warm ischemic hearts demonstrate that increased O_2 delivery with PFC emulsion under normothermic conditions results in enhanced myocardial metabolic efficiency and a

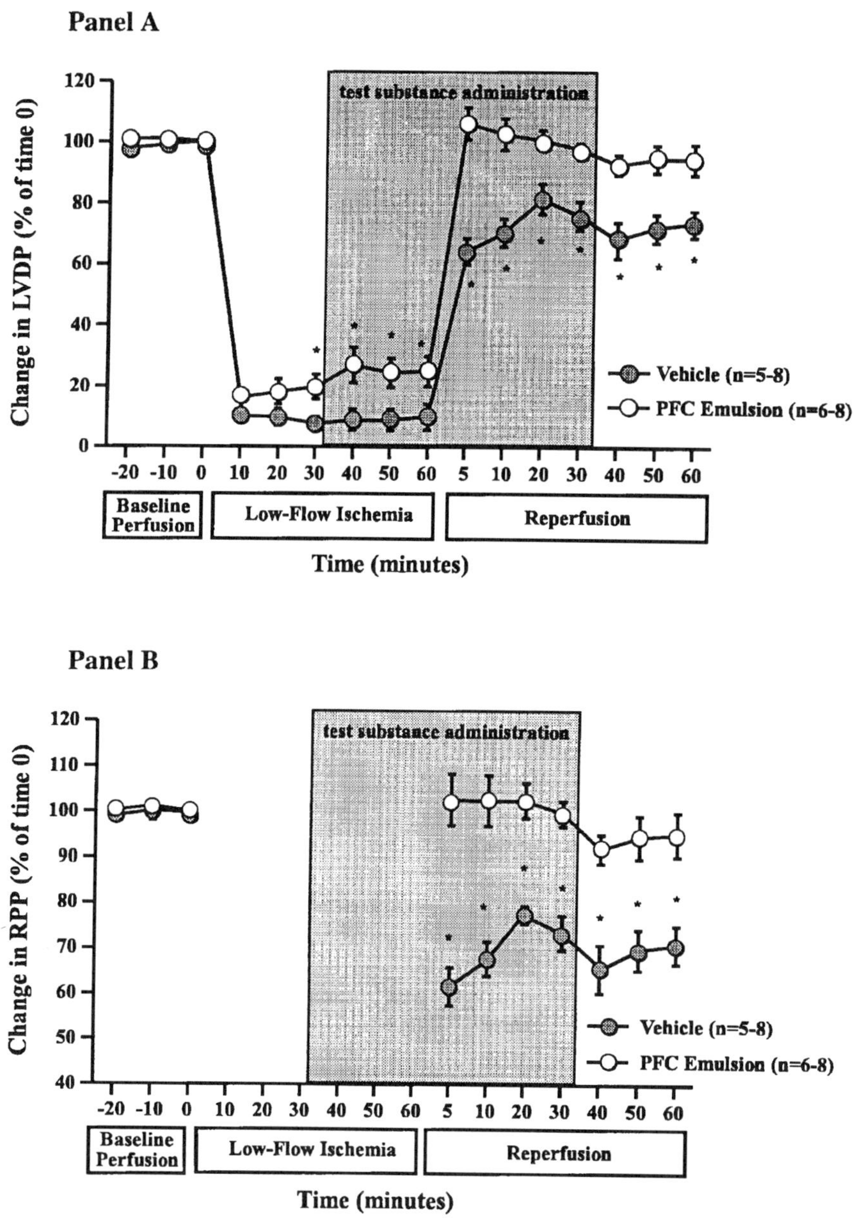

Figure 6.5. Effects of PFC emulsion compared to vehicle control administered during low-flow ischemia and reperfusion on left ventricular developed pressure (Panel A) and on rate-pressure product (Panel B) in isolated Langendorff perfused rabbit heart. Data are means ± SEM.

preservation of energy charge. These benefits provide protection against the detrimental biochemical and functional effects of myocardial ischemia and improve myocardial post-ischemic functional recovery.

The previous studies demonstrated the benefit of PFC emulsion administered during ischemia on cardiac oxygenation and functional recovery. A follow-up study was designed to test the benefit of PFC emulsion administered at the onset of reperfusion after a period of no-flow global ischemia (del Balzo *et al.* 1996c). Following 20 minutes of perfusion with KH buffer, hearts were subjected to 20 minutes of no-flow global ischemia followed by 60 minutes of constant pressure reperfusion with KH buffer alone or KH buffer supplemented with PFC emulsion (1:10 v/v of a 100% w/v PFC emulsion). Perfusate PO_2, O_2 delivery, and myocardial O_2 consumption were significantly improved in the PFC emulsion group suggesting that tissue PO_2 was better maintained in these hearts. This improved O_2 delivery and consumption was accompanied by a significant improvement in cardiac function during reperfusion as measured by RPP (Figure 6.6). Thus, PFC emulsion can significantly benefit myocardial recovery during reperfusion after no-flow global ischemia.

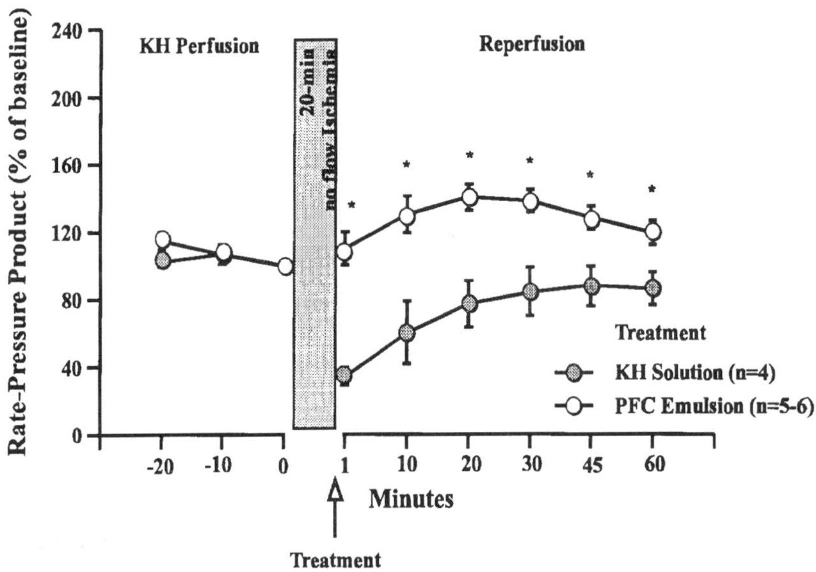

Figure 6.6. Effects of PFC emulsion compared to Krebs-Henseleit solution control administered after 20 minutes of no-flow global ischemia at the onset of reperfusion on rate-pressure product in isolated Langendorff perfused rabbit hearts (del Balzo et al. 1996d). Data are means ± SEM.

Intracoronary PFC emulsion has also been associated with an improvement in cardiac wall motion *in vivo* during acute coronary artery ligation in the canine (Ogilby *et al.* 1993). Canine hearts were instrumented for assessment of hemodynamic and cardiac functional parameters. The left anterior descending or circumflex coronary arteries were isolated, a carotid artery bypass established, and animals were instrumented for intracoronary low-flow perfusion. After baseline conditions were established, and a 20-second successful test occlusion was achieved, the carotid-coronary bypass was partially occluded for 2 minutes during which the coronary bed distal to the occlusion was perfused at a low-flow rate (24 mL/min) with control oxygenated autologous blood or oxygenated PFC emulsion (21.6 g PFC/min) to create a low-flow regional ischemic zone. Wall motion was assessed using ultrasonic crystallography to determine regional systolic shortening at baseline, during low-flow ischemia, and during reperfusion in both non-ischemic zones and in the ischemic zones distal to the partial occlusion. Systolic shortening remained unchanged in the non-ischemic zones throughout the experiment. In the ischemic zones during low-flow perfusion distal to the occlusion, systolic shortening was significantly greater during PFC emulsion treatment compared to autologous blood perfusion. These results demonstrate the efficacy of PFC emulsion to support cardiac muscle function during decreased O_2 delivery due to low-flow ischemia in the *in vivo* setting.

Manning and coworkers (1996) have used PFC emulsion to selectively perfuse the coronary circulation (via retrograde aortic arch perfusion) during ventricular fibrillation-induced cardiac arrest and cardiopulmonary resuscitation (CPR) in canines. They measured coronary perfusion pressure as an index of spontaneous recovery of cardiac function and determined survival in animals treated with PFC emulsion versus controls. The results of these studies demonstrated that IC PFC emulsion during CPR caused a more rapid recovery of cardiac function and significantly increased survival rate compared to animals receiving CPR without PFC emulsion infusion.

Buddemeier *et al.*(1994) evaluated the potential benefits of PFC emulsion to protect the coronary microvasculature from reperfusion injury in closed-chest dogs. The left anterior descending coronary artery was occluded (PTCA balloon inflation) for 90 minutes followed by a 72-hour reperfusion period. Treated dogs received IV PFC emulsion 15 minutes prior to reperfusion, and control dogs received placebo. All animals were maintained on 100% O_2 breathing during the first 4 hours of reperfusion. Coronary flow velocity was measured and vasodilator reserve calculated pre-occlusion, 2, and 72 hours post-reperfusion in the presence of an endothelial-dependent (acetylcholine) and an endothelial-independent (papaverine) coronary vasodilator. PFC emulsion preserved both endothelial-dependent and independent coronary vasodilator reserve compared to the control group. This finding suggests that oxygenated PFC emulsion protects the microvasculature from reperfusion injury, and this effect may contribute to the benefits observed with this product in models of ischemia and reperfusion.

Collectively, these studies demonstrate that PFC emulsion enhances O_2 delivery to critical tissues and improves the metabolic and functional status of the tissue. These benefits are translated into an overall improvement in critical organ function especially under conditions of limited O_2 supply.

In order to demonstrate more clearly the clinical benefits of PFC emulsion and to understand how to measure these benefits in the clinical setting, a series of studies have been conducted in large animal models of high blood loss that mimic the clinical surgical setting. The systemic and hemodynamic effects of PFC emulsion have been studied in animal models of cardiopulmonary bypass. Additionally, PFC emulsion has been administered as a temporary O_2 carrier in the setting of intraoperative surgical blood loss.

6.3.2 Cardiac surgical procedures

One proposed clinical application of PFC emulsion is to augment O_2 availability to systemic and cardiac tissues during CPB procedures. During CPB, the patient becomes hemodiluted due to the volume of pump-priming solution required to fill the extracorporeal bypass circuit. In addition to this hemodilution, it is not uncommon during CPB for 1 to 3 units of whole blood to be collected during the peri-operative period (i.e., immediately prior to or at the initiation of bypass) to provide autologous blood for transfusion during or following the procedure, if needed. In this application, PFC emulsion may be used to maintain and enhance systemic oxygenation in the setting of decreased hematocrit (i.e., loss of red blood cells) and thereby to reduce or eliminate the need for allogeneic (donor) blood transfusions. A series of animal studies have been conducted to demonstrate the utility and efficacy of PFC emulsion as an adjunct to current priming fluid administration during CPB surgery.

Studies were conducted to assess the efficacy of PFC emulsion to enhance and maintain O_2 delivery to the systemic circulation during and following CPB (del Balzo *et al.* 1996b). In these studies, PFC emulsion was added directly to the pump priming-solution at the initiation of bypass. Anesthetized open-chest swine were intubated and mechanically ventilated with room air. Venous return to the CPB circuit was provided by a cannula positioned in the right atrium. Oxygenated blood from the CPB circuit was returned to the animal through a cannula placed in the ascending aorta. The extracorporeal circuit was primed with standard crystalloid solution containing either PFC emulsion (2.7 or 3.6 g PFC/kg) or *Plasma-Lyte* (control) at equal volume (3 mL/kg). Hematocrits in the control and treated groups were equivalent throughout the study. CPB was instituted for 2 hours (body temperature of 30-32°C) and following CPB, animals were rewarmed to 36-38°C. Hemodynamic parameters, cardiac function, and arterial blood gases and pH were assessed at baseline, during CPB, and for 2 hours following CPB. PFC emulsion increased PaO_2 compared to control during and following CPB despite equivalent hematocrits. PFC emulsion also improved myocardial regional contractile function and maintained global left ventricular function (LV systolic pressure and +dP/dt) at higher levels following 1 hour of CPB.

The efficacy of PFC emulsion to improve overall systemic oxygenation status has also been assessed in a canine model of CPB following severe hemodilution by Holman *et al* (1995). In this model, systemic O_2 delivery during bypass was regulated by bypass pump flow rate and was limited by anemia (due to hemodilution) and the hypothermia-induced increase in hemoglobin O_2 affinity. Animals were hemodiluted to a hematocrit of approximately 15% prior to initiation of CPB. A standard priming solution was used, and animals received PFC emulsion (1.35 g PFC/kg) or an equal volume of crystalloid solution as an additive to the venous line of the bypass circuit immediately following initiation of CPB. During bypass, animals were maintained at a body temperature of 32°C. The effects of PFC emulsion during bypass on mixed venous O_2 tension ($P\bar{v}O_2$) were determined at different (randomized) bypass pump flow rates (0.25, 0.5, 1.0, 1.5, 2.0, and 3.0 L/min/m^2). $P\bar{v}O_2$ in the PFC emulsion group was elevated compared to control during CPB at all bypass flow rates. This difference was statistically significant at flow rates of 1.5, 2.0 and 3.0 L/min/m^2 (Figure 6.7, Panel A). Similar increases were observed in coronary sinus PO_2. Following CPB, $P\bar{v}O_2$ of the PFC emulsion group remained consistently higher than that of the control group. There were no significant differences between groups with respect to hematocrit or O_2 consumption, but O_2 extraction from hemoglobin was consistently higher in the control group indicating that PFC emulsion had a sparing effect on hemoglobin-bound O_2 (Figure 6.7, Panel B). While there was no significant difference in cardiac index between the groups following CPB, PFC emulsion improved positive LV dP/dt during recovery from CPB. These improvements were also associated with a significant (22%) increase in survival in the PFC emulsion group compared to control. Similar post-CPB cardiac functional recovery benefit with perflubron emulsion has been reported elsewhere (del Balzo *et al.* 1996a; 1996d). A $P\bar{v}O_2$ of approximately 30 mm Hg is considered to be the critical lower limit for adequate tissue oxygenation during bypass under control conditions. In the control group in Holman's study (Holman *et al.* 1995), the critical lower PO_2 limit was reached at and below bypass pump flow rates of 1.5 L/min/m^2 (Figure 6.7, Panel A). In the presence of PFC emulsion, the critical lower limit of $P\bar{v}O_2$ was reached at a bypass pump flow rate of 0.5 L/min/m^2. There is a clear clinical benefit to maintaining the bypass pump at the lowest acceptable flow rate since it is well known that higher bypass pump flow rates are associated with increased blood cellular damage due to increased fluid shear forces. Thus, these results suggest that PFC emulsion, used as an adjunct to CPB priming solution, not only enhances tissue oxygenation, as assessed by $P\bar{v}O_2$, at various flow rates but also may provide greater flexibility in the management of the bypass pump flow rate.

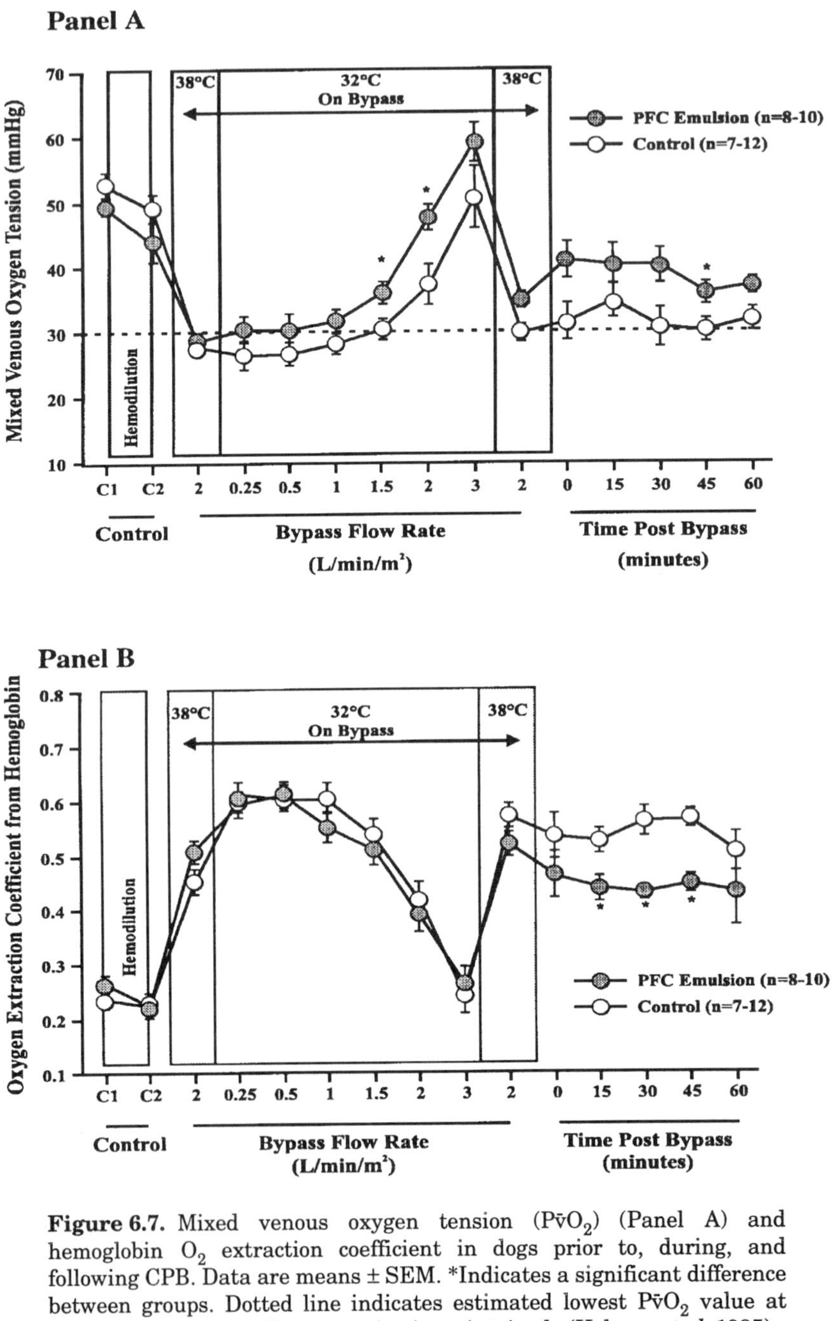

Figure 6.7. Mixed venous oxygen tension ($P\bar{v}O_2$) (Panel A) and hemoglobin O_2 extraction coefficient in dogs prior to, during, and following CPB. Data are means ± SEM. *Indicates a significant difference between groups. Dotted line indicates estimated lowest $P\bar{v}O_2$ value at which adequate overall oxygenation is maintained (Holman *et al.* 1995).

Collectively these studies in animal models of CPB indicate that PFC emulsion is associated with the maintenance or improvement of overall systemic and cardiac oxygenation status during bypass and improved cardiac functional recovery and animal survival following bypass. These results support those discussed earlier and further illustrate the efficacy of PFC emulsion for improved O_2 delivery, tissue metabolic status, and organ function. Additionally, these results support the conclusion that PFC emulsion will reduce the need for blood transfusion during high blood-loss surgeries such as CPB. Finally, these results suggest that PFC emulsion may provide an additional benefit during CPB by supporting adequate O_2 delivery at lower bypass flow rates, thereby reducing the need for higher flow rates and decreasing consequent potential for blood cellular damage due to increases in fluid shear forces.

6.3.3 Intraoperative surgical bleeding and hemodilution

Another potential application of PFC emulsion, which is currently under clinical investigation, is to augment O_2 availability to tissues during the active bleeding phase of surgical procedures as an adjunct to autologous transfusion techniques (i.e., predonation and intraoperative ANH). Predonation involves withdrawal and storage of several units of a patient's blood during a 6-week period prior to surgery. ANH involves withdrawal of several units of blood from the patient just prior to surgery and simultaneous replacement of the blood with either a crystalloid or a colloid plasma-volume expander. The autologous blood collected by either technique is then available for transfusion during or following surgery. As is the case with CPB, PFC emulsion is expected to maintain and enhance tissue oxygenation in the setting of decreased hematocrit (i.e., loss of red blood cells) due to intraoperative surgical bleeding and thereby to reduce or eliminate the need for allogeneic (donor) blood transfusions. A series of animal studies have been conducted to demonstrate the utility and efficacy of PFC emulsion as a temporary O_2 carrier in the setting of intraoperative surgical bleeding and hemodilution.

A study was conducted to evaluate the O_2 delivery capability of PFC emulsion during profound normovolemic hemodilution (Keipert *et al.* 1994a). Dogs were subjected to ANH (to a hematocrit of approximately 10 to 12%), ventilated with 100% O_2, and then treated intravenously with PFC emulsion (3 g PFC/kg). In this study, the efficacy of PFC emulsion as an O_2 carrier was assessed, and $P\bar{v}O_2$ was monitored as an indicator of overall systemic oxygenation status. PFC emulsion significantly increased $P\bar{v}O_2$ (Figure 6.8) compared to control (infusion of Ringer's lactate). Similar effects have been reported at higher doses of PFC emulsion in swine (Stern *et al.* 1995) and in dogs subjected to less profound hemodilution (Johnson *et al.* 1995). Calculations of $\dot{D}O_2$ and $\dot{V}O_2$ indicated that while the percent of total $\dot{D}O_2$ contributed by PFC-dissolved O_2 was only 8-10%, approximately 25-30% of total $\dot{V}O_2$ was provided by the PFC-dissolved O_2 (Keipert *et al.* 1994a). The percentage of total $\dot{V}O_2$ contributed by the hemoglobin-carried O_2 was significantly less in dogs treated with PFC emulsion than in controls indicating a sparing of O_2 bound to hemoglobin in PFC-emulsion-treated dogs. The results of this study demonstrate that PFC emulsion significantly increases O_2 transport and supports O_2 consumption in a surgical model of blood loss and hemodilution.

A study in hemodiluted dogs was conducted to investigate the efficacy of PFC emulsion, administered prior to volume-compensated blood loss, for the maintenance of overall systemic tissue oxygenation in the setting of prolonged surgical blood loss (Keipert *et al.* 1994b). Purpose-bred beagles were anesthetized, ventilated with room air, and instrumented for assessment of hemodynamic parameters, administration of fluids, and collection of blood (arterial and mixed venous) samples. All parameters were monitored prior to (under air-breathing conditions) and following (under air-breathing conditions and on 100% O_2) isovolemic hemodilution with *Hespan* to a hemoglobin of approximately 8.0 g/dL.

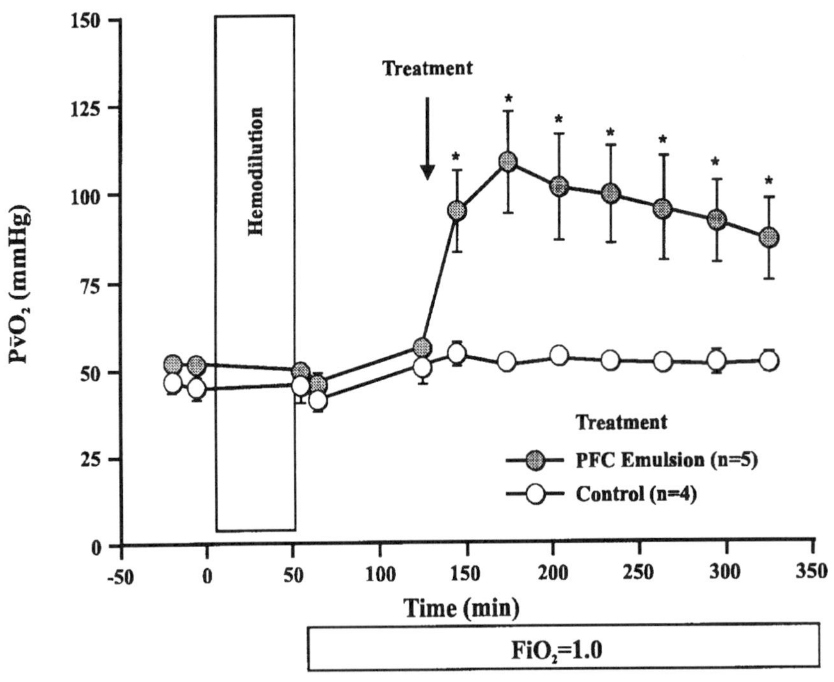

Figure 6.8. Mixed venous oxygen tension ($P\bar{v}O_2$) in anesthetized dogs during and following acute normovolemic hemodilution. *Indicates a significant difference between groups (Keipert *et al.* 1994a). Data are means ± SEM.

Animals were then treated with PFC emulsion (1.35 g PFC/kg) or an equivalent volume of *Plasma-Lyte* (controls), and parameters were assessed during progressive volume-compensated blood loss

(0.75 mL/kg/min on 100% O_2) to a final hemoglobin of approximately 2.0 g/dL. $P\bar{v}O_2$ values measured during 100% O_2 ventilation just prior to injection of either PFC emulsion or *Plasma-Lyte* were used to establish the "O_2-breathing baseline" against which changes in $P\bar{v}O_2$ following treatment were assessed. Total hemoglobin levels were similar for both groups over the course of the study. This was expected as the rate of hemorrhage was held constant at 0.75 mL/min/kg by design, and the initial target of approximately 8.0 g/dL hemoglobin was achieved in all cases prior to volume-compensated bleeding (Figure 6.9, Panel A). $P\bar{v}O_2$ of both groups remained above the established O_2-breathing baseline during volume-compensated blood loss to a total hemoglobin of approximately 7.0 g/dL. At this point, mean $P\bar{v}O_2$ of the control group dropped below the O_2-breathing baseline while that of the PFC-emulsion group remained above the O_2-breathing baseline to a final hemoglobin of approximately 2 g/dL (Figure 6.9, Panel B). In the presence of 1.35 g PFC/kg it was possible to further hemodilute (as volume-compensated blood loss) for an average of 90 minutes (equivalent to a blood loss of about 65 mL/kg BW or approximately 70% of the total blood volume) before $P\bar{v}O_2$ approached the O_2-breathing baseline levels. Expressed as hemoglobin equivalents, this represented an average drop of approximately 4.1 g/dL hemoglobin. By comparison, control animals reached the O_2-breathing baseline after only approximately 20 minutes (equivalent to a blood loss of about 15 mL/kg BW and a hemoglobin drop of approximately 1.5 g/dL). Therefore, in this study, PFC emulsion provided a margin of safety in that $P\bar{v}O_2$ was maintained during greater blood loss in the presence of the PFC than was possible in the control animals. If the O_2-breathing baseline is representative of a potential "transfusion trigger" (i.e., the hemoglobin level at which transfusion of red cells may be required in order to maintain good tissue oxygenation), the presence of PFC emulsion safely lowered the "transfusion trigger" for these animals. In summary, PFC emulsion was shown, in these canine models of hemodilution and blood-loss, to have a sparing effect on the reserve of O_2 available in the red cells, and to provide a margin of safety in that a normal $P\bar{v}O_2$ was maintained during greater blood loss in the presence of the PFC.

A key unanswered question was whether PFC emulsion can maintain effective diffusive gradients for O_2 in the face of blood loss, thereby extending the limits of tolerable surgical anemia and delaying the initiation of blood transfusion. A study in hemodiluted dogs was conducted to mimic the clinical situation of surgical blood loss in which PFC emulsion would be used in conjunction with autologous blood transfusion strategies (Batra *et al.* 1996a). The hypothesis tested in this study was that PFC-emulsion-treated animals would tolerate greater surgical blood loss compared to control animals without compromising hemodynamics or systemic oxygenation. Canines were anesthetized, ventilated (100% O_2) and isovolemically hemodiluted to approximately 8.0 g/dL hemoglobin.

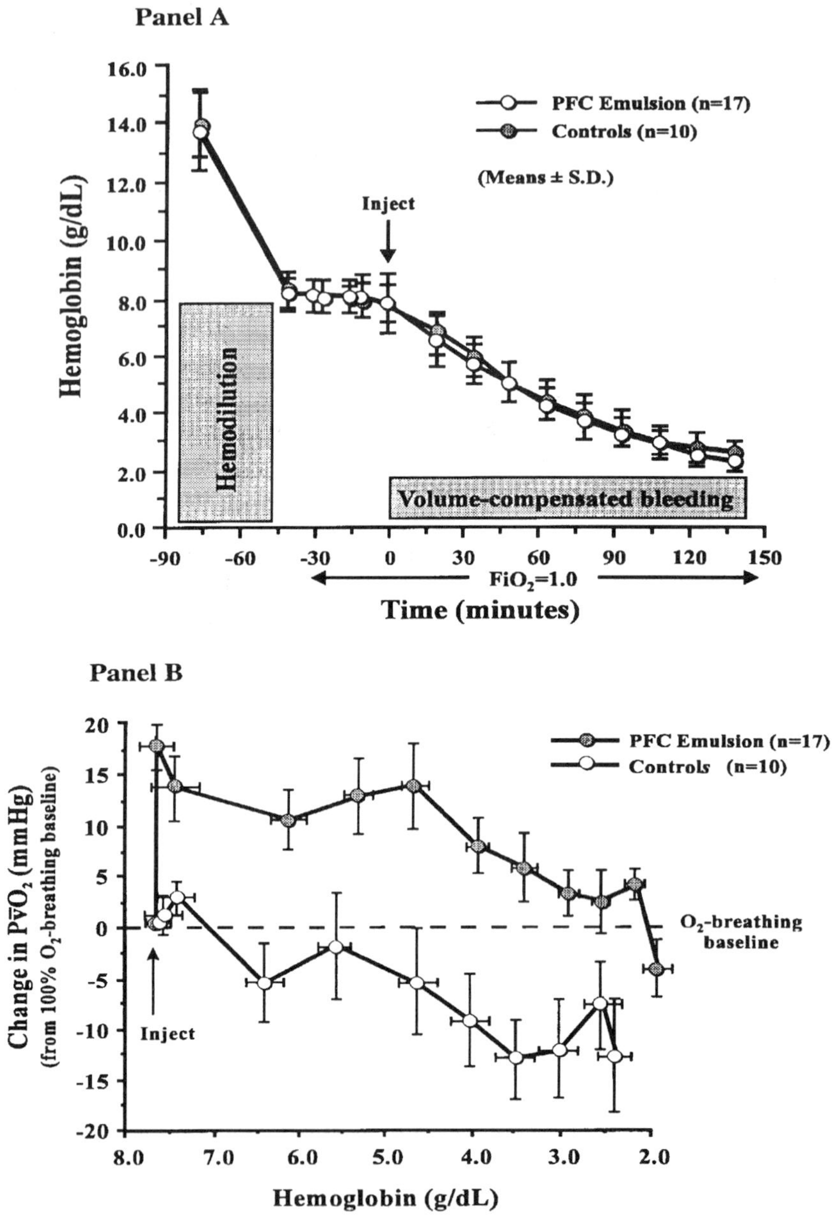

Figure 6.9. Total hemoglobin levels (Panel A) and change in $P\bar{v}O_2$ (relative to the O_2-breathing baseline) (Panel B) in dogs during volume-compensated blood loss to a total hemoglobin of 2.0 g/dL. Animals received either PFC emulsion or *Plasma-Lyte* following hemodilution to a hemoglobin of 8 g/dL and were then subjected to progressive volume-compensated blood-loss. Data are means ± SEM.

The autologous blood collected during this hemodilution was centrifuged into packed red cells and divided into "units" (1 unit = 10% of the estimated blood volume) for later transfusion. Animals received either 1 unit of packed red cells (controls) or PFC emulsion (1.35 or 2.7 g PFC/kg) and were then subjected to volume-compensated blood loss (normovolemia maintained with 1:1 replacement with *Hespan*). The PFC emulsion animals were bled to approximately 5 g/dL hemoglobin while control animals received an additional unit of pack red cells each time their hemoglobin reached approximately 8 g/dL (which resulted in an increase in hemoglobin of approximately 1.2 g/dL/unit). The transfusion triggers of 5 g/dL and 8 g/dL were established by study design for the PFC emulsion and control groups, respectively. At the end of the blood-loss phase of the study, all remaining autologous units were returned to the animals. For control animals, these units were those not transfused during the blood-loss phase; for PFC-emulsion-treated animals, all units collected during initial hemodilution were available for transfusion at the end of the study. A net savings of blood (i.e., red cells) was defined as the difference in total hemoglobin between control and PFC-emulsion-treated animals following transfusion of all remaining units. $P\bar{v}O_2$ increased significantly after treatment in both PFC emulsion groups and remained consistently higher in these animals compared to controls throughout volume-compensated blood loss (Figure 6.10) despite the significantly greater drop in hemoglobin concentration. These findings indicated a maintenance of global oxygenation status in the presence of intravascular PFC despite a greater loss of red blood cells. Following transfusion of all available units at the end of the study, there resulted a significantly higher total hemoglobin calculated in the PFC-emulsion

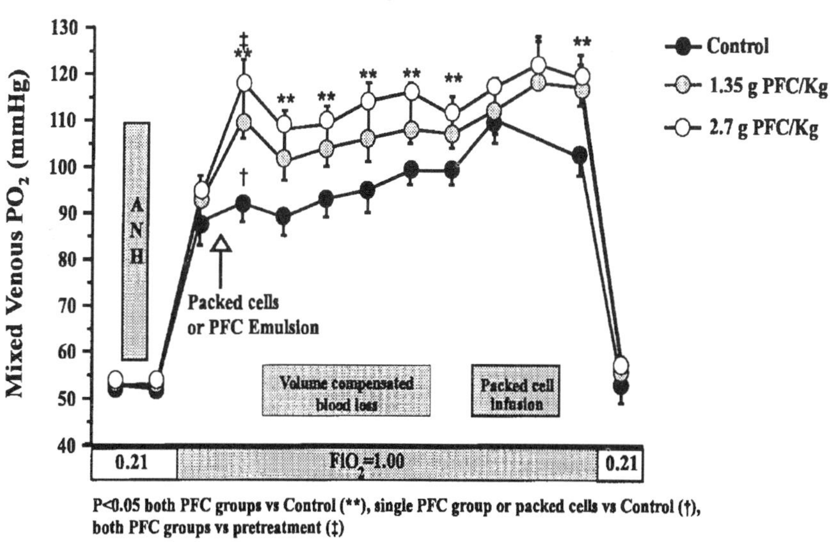

Figure 6.10. Mixed venous PO_2 ($P\bar{v}O_2$) over the course of the experiment described in the text. Data are means ± SEM.

group compared to control animals indicating that the control group experienced a significantly greater net loss of hemoglobin over the course of the study than did those animals treated with PFC emulsion. The PFC emulsion treatment resulted in an overall savings of 1.5-2 units of blood in this model.

The results of these studies in models of hemodilution and surgical blood loss indicated that IV PFC emulsion increases the margin of safety for ANH and can, therefore, potentially decrease the need for transfused blood by lowering the transfusion trigger during surgical procedures. In these studies, PFC emulsion was associated with an increase in $P\bar{v}O_2$ and was shown to contribute significantly to O_2 consumption.

6.3.4 Transfusion trigger

$P\bar{v}O_2$ is considered to be the most reliable estimate of systemic tissue oxygenation status. However, there has been little direct evidence demonstrating the relevance of $P\bar{v}O_2$ as a component of the transfusion trigger in the setting of PFC emulsion transfusion during surgical hemodilution and blood loss. To address this issue, two dog studies have been conducted to assess the correlation of tissue PO_2 with changes in $P\bar{v}O_2$ during PFC emulsion treatment in the setting of hemodilution.

A dog study was conducted to determine if the PFC-emulsion-induced changes in, or maintenance of, $P\bar{v}O_2$ during 100%-O_2 breathing and progressive hemodilution positively correlated with changes in specific indices of tissue oxygenation (S. Cain, University of Alabama at Birmingham, unpublished data). Tissue oxygenation status of gut and muscle was measured directly using multiwire MDO surface O_2 electrodes placed on the surface of the gut and on a hindlimb skeletal muscle as described previously (Lund, Odman and Lewis 1980). Anesthetized, paralyzed, mechanically ventilated dogs were isovolemically hemodiluted with 5% albumin to a hemoglobin of approximately 8 g/dL and maintained on 100% O_2 breathing for the remainder of the study. Multiwire MDO O_2 electrodes were used to monitor gut serosal and hindlimb skeletal muscle tissue PO_2. Vascular catheters were used to monitor $P\bar{v}O_2$ and O_2 tension of the venous blood draining the skeletal muscle and gut tissue regions assessed by the MDO O_2 electrodes. Baseline measurements were made, and PFC emulsion (1.35 g PFC/kg, IV) was administered followed by a 90-minute phase of progressive isovolemic hemodilution to a hemoglobin of approximately 3 g/dL. During 100% O_2 breathing, PFC emulsion increased both $P\bar{v}O_2$ and the PO_2 of the venous blood draining the hindlimb skeletal muscle and the gut. The enhancement of $P\bar{v}O_2$, gut venous PO_2, and skeletal muscle PO_2 were of a similar degree and were maintained throughout the entire bleeding phase of the protocol. The percent increase in both skeletal muscle (Figure 6.11, Panel A) and gut (Figure 6.11, Panel B) tissue PO_2 values, as measured by the MDO electrodes, were similar in magnitude and duration to the increase observed in $P\bar{v}O_2$ and organ venous drainage PO_2. These results indicate that PFC emulsion increases tissue oxygenation during hemodilution

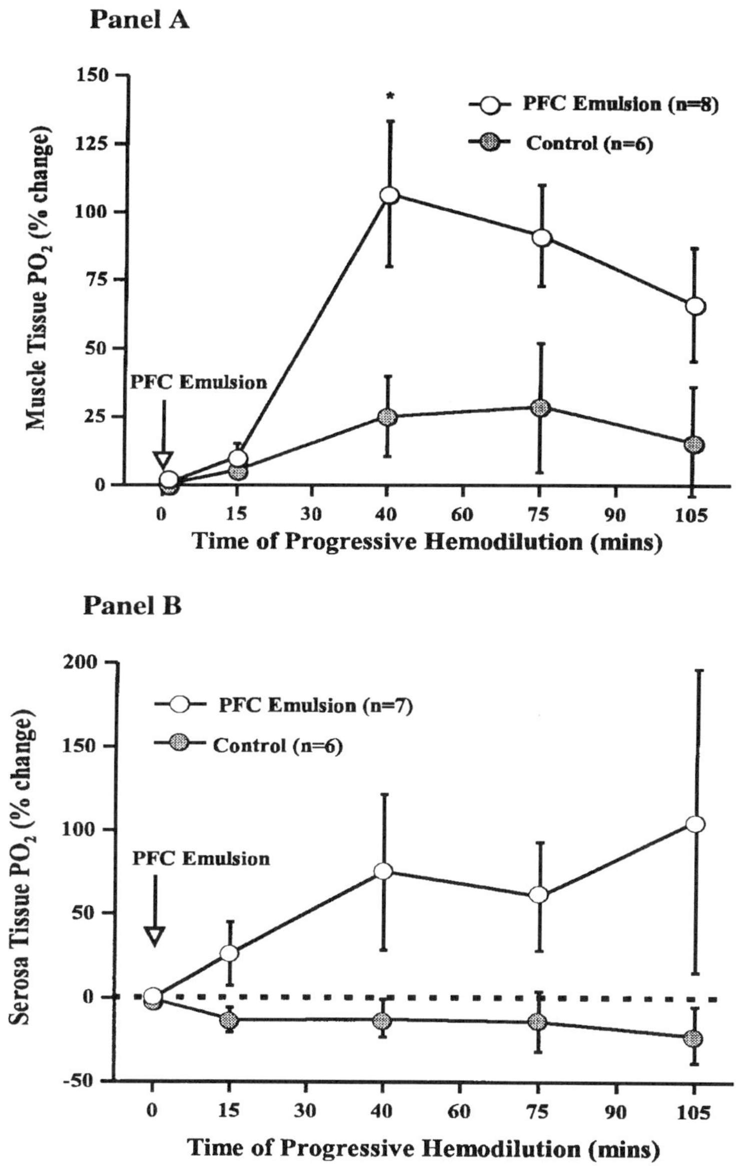

Figure 6.11. Changes in hindlimb skeletal muscle (Panel A) and gut serosa (Panel B) PO_2 as directly assessed by multiwire MDO O_2 electrodes in a canine model of surgical blood loss. Improved muscle and gut serosa PO_2, as assessed by O_2 electrodes, correlated with improved venous drainage PO_2 and with $P\bar{v}O_2$ in the PFC emulsion group. Data are means ± SEM. (Courtesy of S. Cain, University of Alabama at Birmingham, Birmingham, AL)

and these changes are reflected both in increases in local tissue venous drainage PO_2 and in $P\bar{v}O_2$ levels. Thus, increases in $P\bar{v}O_2$ correlate with improved tissue oxygenation during hemodilution. These data support the conclusion that $P\bar{v}O_2$, therefore, is a meaningful component of the "transfusion trigger" in the clinical setting.

A second study was conducted in canines to confirm that tissue oxygenation during treatment with PFC emulsion in hemodilution correlates positively with changes in $P\bar{v}O_2$ (Batra *et al.* 1996b). Anesthetized, mechanically ventilated canines were surgically instrumented to monitor systemic and pulmonary pressures and to obtain arterial and mixed venous blood samples. Tissue PO_2 was polarographically measured on the surface of the gracilis muscle and gut serosa by multiwire surface MDO O_2 electrodes and in the parietal cortex by a motor driven Eppendorf needle electrode. On room-air breathing, animals were isovolemically hemodiluted to a hemoglobin concentration of 8 g/dL using *Hespan*. Animals were then placed on 100% O_2 breathing and were subsequently administered a single dose of PFC emulsion (1.8 g PFC/kg) or an equal volume of *Plasma-Lyte*. $P\bar{v}O_2$, tissue PO_2, and the PO_2 of venous blood draining those tissue regions, assessed by the O_2 electrodes, were measured throughout the protocol. $P\bar{v}O_2$ and tissue PO_2 values were not significantly different between the PFC emulsion and control groups prior to or following hemodilution. There were significant increases in $P\bar{v}O_2$ and tissue PO_2 in gracilis, gut serosa and parietal cortex when animals were placed on 100% O_2 breathing, but there were no statistically significant differences between the PFC emulsion and control groups. Following administration of PFC emulsion, changes in tissue PO_2 levels were significantly greater compared to the control group in the parietal cortex (Figure 6.12, Panel A), the surface of the gut serosa (Figure 6.12, Panel B), and the gracilis muscle (Figure 6.12, Panel C). Again, these increases correlated with a PFC emulsion induced increase in $P\bar{v}O_2$ (Figure 6.12, Panel D). The results of this study confirm that administration of PFC emulsion is associated with an increase in tissue oxygenation.

The increase in oxygenation at the tissue level contributes to the increase in $P\bar{v}O_2$ observed subsequent to treatment with PFC emulsion. Additionally, these results suggest that the increase in $P\bar{v}O_2$ following infusion of PFC emulsion may be used as a reliable indicator of a PFC emulsion induced improvement in tissue oxygenation and may, therefore, be considered as a useful component of the "transfusion trigger".

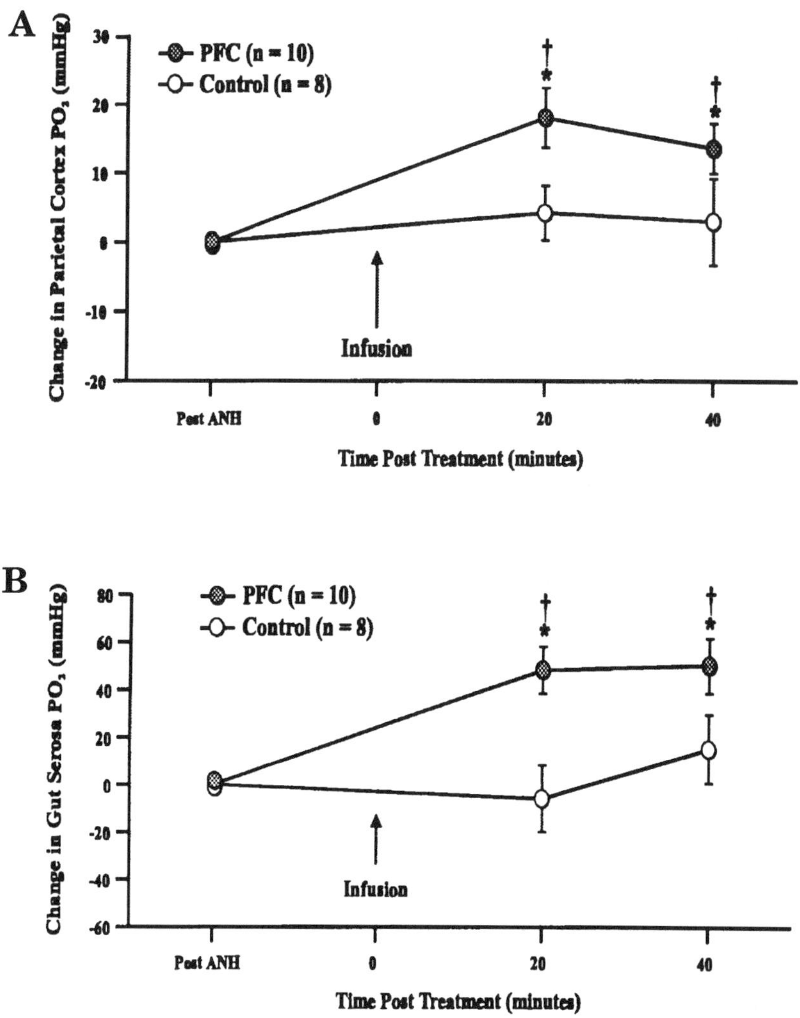

Figure 6.12. Panel A and B

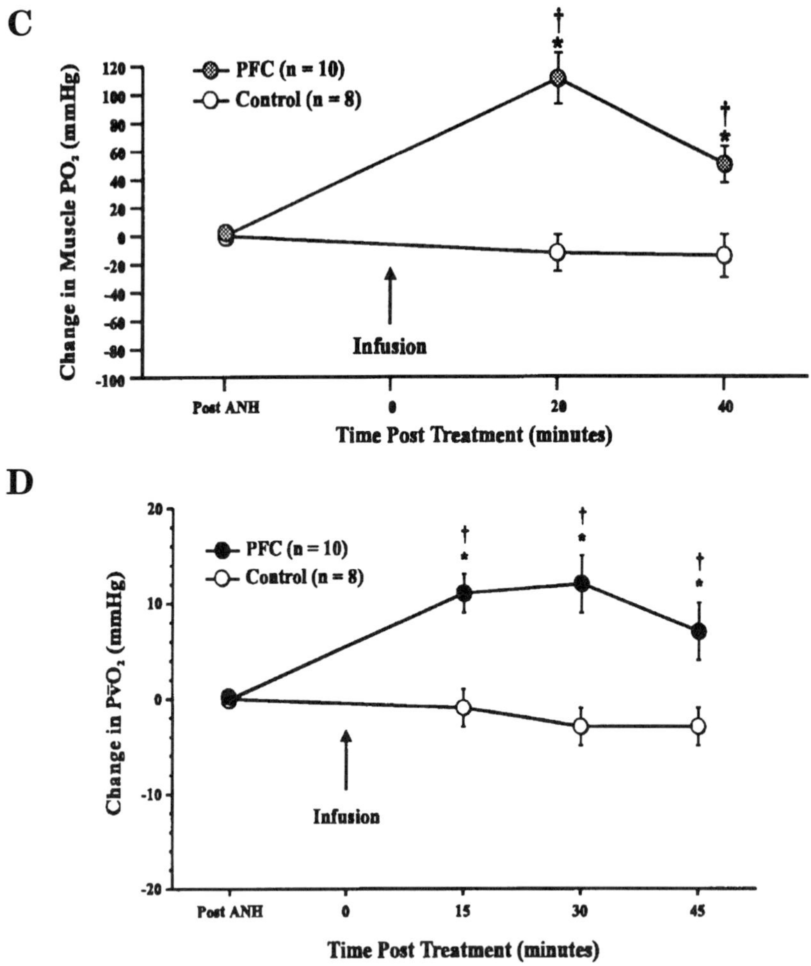

Figure 6.12. Panel C and D

Changes in parietal cortex PO_2 as directly assessed by a polarographic needle electrode (Panel A), gut serosa PO_2 as directly assessed by multiwire MDO O_2 electrodes (Panel B), gracilis muscle surface PO_2 as directly assessed by multiwire MDO O_2 electrodes (Panel C) and mixed venous PO_2 (Panel D) in a canine model of surgical blood loss. Improved tissue PO_2 levels as assessed by O_2 electrodes correlated with improved $P\bar{v}O_2$ in the PFC emulsion group. Similar changes were also measured in the venous blood draining the tissues of interest (Batra *et al.* 1996b). Data are means ± SEM;* $P<0.05$ *versus* post-ANH; † $P<0.05$ *versus* respective control.

6.4 Summary and Conclusion

The data summarized in this chapter constitutes the preclinical efficacy experience with perflubron-based emulsion. These data support the conclusion that IV perflubron-based emulsion improves tissue oxygenation in critical tissues such as heart and brain, that the increased O_2 is available to support the metabolic processes which occur at the mitochondrial level in these tissues, and that this improved metabolic status does, indeed, translate into an improvement in organ function. These studies also demonstrate the efficacy of IV perflubron-based emulsion to support systemic oxygenation during hemodilution and intraoperative surgical bleeding as well as in the setting of cardiopulmonary bypass surgery. Finally, these results indicate that improvements in tissue oxygenation status as a result of treatment with perflubron-based emulsion are reflected by increases in systemic $P\bar{v}O_2$, suggesting that $P\bar{v}O_2$ can be considered as a potentially useful component of a transfusion trigger during perflubron-based emulsion treatment in the clinical setting of hemodilution and transfusion.

6.5 Acknowledgments

The author wishes to recognize the support and encouragement of Drs. Ughetta del Balzo, Sanjay Batra, JoAnn Bradley, and Peter Keipert, the technical and editorial assistance of Mrs. Dorothy C. Saewert and the administrative assistance of Mrs. Shaun Alvarez and Ms. Shannon Pipes.

6.6 References

Bass, C.W. Solubilities of gases in perfluorocarbons as a function of temperature. Ph.D. dissertation, University of California, San Diego and San Diego State University, 1991.

Batra, S., P.E. Keipert, J.D. Bradley, N.S. Faithfull, and S.F. Flaim. Use of perflubron emulsion to extend the limits of surgical hemodilution and delay autologous transfusion. *Crit. Care Med.* 24: A36, 1996a.

Batra, S., B.P. Peters, J.D. Symons, D.Y. Hazard, U. del Balzo, J.D. Bradley, and S.F. Flaim. Perflubron emulsion increases tissue oxygenation in a canine model of hemodilution. *Biomat. Artif. Cells. Immob. Biotech.* 24: 307, 1996b.

Biro, G.P., M. Masika, and B. Korecky. Oxygen delivery and performance in the isolated, perfused rat heart: Comparison of perfusion with aqueous and perfluorocarbon-containing media. *Adv. Exp. Med. Biol.* 248: 509-516, 1989.

Braun, R., R.A. Linsenmeier, and T.K. Goldstick. New perfluorocarbon emulsion improves tissue oxygenation in cat retina. *J. Appl. Physiol.* 72: 1960-1968, 1992.

Buddemeier, K.J., T.L. Hursey, R.F. Kelly, J.C. Okner, J.E. Parrillo, and G.L. Schaer. *Oxygent* (oxygen-carrying perfluorochemical emulsion) preserves endothelial dependent and independent vasodilator responses after experimental myocardial infarction and reperfusion. *J. Invest. Med.* 42: 164A, 1994.

Clark, Jr., L.C., R.B. Spokane, R.E. Hoffmann, and R. Sudan. The nature of fluorocarbon enhanced cerebral oxygen transport. *Adv. Exp. Med. Biol.* 248: 341-355, 1989.

del Balzo, U., R.A. Harrell, S.K. Hedley, J.J. Clymer and S.F. Flaim. Perflubron emulsion improves post-ischemic functional recovery in the isolated perfused rabbit heart. *FASEB J.* 8: A559, 1994.

del Balzo, U., R.A. Harrell, M.T. Duggan, and S.F. Flaim. Perflubron cardioplegia and myocardial protection. *Ann. Thorac. Surg.* 60: 866, 1995a.

del Balzo, U., E.S. Kornbrust, C.A. Strnat, M.T. Duggan, R.A. Harrell, and S.F. Flaim. Hemostasis and hemodynamic study of cardiopulmonary bypass with perflubron emulsion: A 7-day recovery model. *J. Invest. Med.* 44: 415A, 1996a.

del Balzo, U., E.S. Kornbrust, C.A. Strnat, R.A. Harrell, and S.F. Flaim. Hemostasis, hemodynamic and cardiac effects of cardiopulmonary bypass with perflubron emulsion. *J. Invest. Med.* 44: 415A, 1996b.

del Balzo, U., C.A. Strnat, R.A. Harrell, and S.F. Flaim. Myocardial protection with perflubron emulsion cardioplegia. *FASEB J.* 9: A622, 1995b.

del Balzo, U., C.A. Strnat, R.A. Harrell, S.K. Hedley and S.F Flaim. Perflubron emulsion: Effect on post-ischemic ventricular function in the isolated rabbit heart. *J. Invest. Med.* 44: 415A, 1996c.

del Balzo, U., J.D. Symons, C. Strnat, R. Harrell, and S.F. Flaim. Efficacy of perflubron emulsion in a canine model of cardiopulmonary bypass. *Biomat. Artif. Cells. Immob. Biotech.* 24: 305, 1996d.

del Balzo, U., J.D. Symons, X. Sun, R.A. Harrell, and S.F. Flaim. Perfusion with perflubron emulsion attenuates high-energy phosphates depletion during low-flow ischemia in isolated rabbit hearts. *FASEB J.* 10: A319, 1996e.

Faithfull, N.S. Oxygen delivery from fluorocarbon emulsions - aspects of convective and diffusive transport. In *Blood Substitutes and Oxygen Carriers,* (T.M.S. Chang, ed.). New York: Marcel Dekker, Inc., 1993, pp. 569-576.

Faithfull, N.S., G.E. Rhoades, P.E. Keipert, A.S. Ringle, and A. Trouwborst. A program to calculate mixed venous oxygen tension - a guide to transfusion? *Adv. Exp. Med. Biol.* 361: 41-49, 1994.

Flaim, S.F. Pharmacokinetics and side effects of perfluorocarbon-based blood substitutes. *Art. Cells Blood Subs. and Immob. Biotech.* 22: 1043-1054, 1994.

Flaim, S.F., S. Batra, J. Bradley, P. Keipert, S. Faithfull, and K.E. Flaim. Fluorocarbons. *Int. J. Microcirc. Clin. Exptl.* 14: 184, 1994.

Guo, J., J.A. White, and H.H. Batjer. Intravenous perflubron emulsion administration improves the recovery of auditory evoked potentials after temporary brain stem ischemia in dogs. *Neurosurg.* 36: 350-357, 1995.

Hogan, M.C., D.C. Willford, P.E. Keipert, N.S. Faithfull, and P.D. Wagner. Increased plasma O_2 solubility improves O_2 uptake of *in situ* dog muscle working maximally. *J. Appl. Physiol.* 73: 2470-2475, 1992.

Holman, W., R. Spruell, E. Ferguson, J. Clymer, W. Vicente, C.P. Murrah, and A. Pacifico. Tissue oxygenation with graded dissolved oxygen delivery during cardiopulmonary bypass. *J. Thorac. Cardiovasc. Surg.* 119: 774-785, 1995.

Johnson, E.C., B.K. Erickson, A. Podolsky, E.K. Birks, P.E. Keipert, N.S. Faithfull, and P.D. Wagner. Effects of a perfluorocarbon emulsion for enhanced O_2 solubility on hemodynamics and O_2 transport in dogs. *J. Appl. Physiol.* 79: 1777-1786, 1995.

Keipert, P.E., N.S. Faithfull, J.D. Bradley, D.Y. Hazard, J. Hogan, M.S. Levisetti, and R.M. Peters. Oxygen delivery augmentation by low-dose perfluorochemical emulsion during profound normovolemic hemodilution. *Adv. Exp. Med. Biol.* 345: 197-204, 1994a.

Keipert, P.E., J.D. Bradley, N.S. Faithfull, D.Y. Hazard, M. Spooner, K.M. Mackley, P.D. Rusheen, S. Batra, and S.F. Flaim. Effects of *Oxygent™* (perflubron emulsion) on O_2 transport in a dog model of hemodilution and surgical bleeding. *FASEB J.* 8: A901, 1994b.

Keipert, P.E., N.S. Faithfull, D.J. Roth, J.D. Bradley, S. Batra, P. Jochelson, K.E. Flaim. Supporting tissue oxygenation during acute surgical bleeding using a perfluorochemical-based oxygen carrier. *Adv. Exp. Med. Biol.* 388: 603-609, 1996.

Kessler, M., J. Hoper, and U. Pohl. Tissue oxygen supply of liver, pancreas, kidney and skeletal muscle. In *Oxygen Carrying Colloidal Blood Substitutes,* (R. Frey, H. Beisbarth and K. Stosseck, eds.). Munich: Zuckschwerdt, 1982, pp. 99-107.

Lang, M., D. Nolte, A. Botzlar, R. Hecht, and K. Messmer. Effects of a perfluorocarbon-based oxygen carrier (perflubron emulsion) on the microcirculation in striated skin muscle of the hamster. *Int. J. Microcirc. Clin. Exptl.* 14: 25, 1994.

Lowe, K.C. Synthetic oxygen transport fluids based on perfluorochemicals: applications in medicine and biology. *Vox. Sang.* 60: 129-140, 1991.

Lund, N., S. Odman, and D.H. Lewis. Skeletal muscle oxygen pressure fields in rats. *Acta Anaesth. Scand.* 24: 155-160, 1980.

Manning, J.E., D.N. Batson, F.B. Payne, N. Adam, C. Murphy, S.G. Perretta, and E.A. Norfleet. Selective aortic arch perfusion during cardiac arrest: Enhanced resuscitation using oxygenated perflubron emulsion with and without aortic arch epinephrine. *Ann. Emerg. Med.* (in press), 1996.

Martin, S.M., D.G. Stein, H. Laks, D.C. Drinkwater, E.R. Capouya, S.W. Barthel, and P. Chang. Amino acid-enriched perfluorochemical cardioplegia reperfusion improves myocardial recovery after prolonged hypothermic global ischemia. *Surg. Forum* 42: 250-252, 1991.

Mosca, R.S., T.J. Rohs, R.R. Waterford, K.F. Childs, L.A. Brunsting, and S.F. Bolling. Perfluorocarbon supplementation and postischemic cardiac function. *Surgery* 120: 197-204, 1996.

Ogilby, J.D., S. Noma, G. DiLoretto, and G. Stets. Preservation of myocardial function during ischemia with intracoronary perfluorooctylbromide (*Oxygent*™). In *Blood Substitutes and Oxygen Carriers,* (T.M.S. Chang, ed.). New York: Marcel Dekker, Inc., 1993, pp. 728-732.

Ohyanagi, H., K. Toshima, M. Sekita, T. Itoh, and T. Mitsuno. Clinical studies of perflurorochemical whole blood substitutes: safety of *Fluosol-DA* (20%) in normal human volunteers. *Clin. Ther.* 2: 306-312, 1979.

Riess, J.G. and M. LeBlanc. Solubility and transport phenomena in perfluorochemicals relevant to blood substitution and other medical applications. *Pure. Appl. Chem.* 54: 2383-2406, 1982.

Riess, J.G. and M. Le Blanc. Preparation of perfluorochemical emulsions for biomedical use: principles, materials and methods. In *Blood Substitutes: Preparation, Physiology and Medical Applications,* (K.C. Lowe, ed.). Chichester: Ellis Horwood Ltd., 1988, pp. 94-100.

Spence, R.K. Perfluorocarbons. In *Principles of Transfusion Medicine,* (E.C. Rossi, T.L. Simon, G.S. Moss, and S.A. Gould, eds.). Baltimore: Williams & Wilkins, 1996, pp. 189-196.

Stern, S.A., S.C. Dronen, A.J. McGoron, X. Wang, K. Chaffins, R. Millard, P.E. Keipert, and N.S. Faithfull. Effect of supplemental perfluorocarbon administration on hypotensive resuscitation of severe uncontrolled hemorrhage. *Am. J. Emerg. Med.* 13: 269-275, 1995.

Symons, J.D., R.A. Harrell, S.F. Flaim, and U. del Balzo. Perflubron emulsion increases tolerance to myocardial ischemia in the isolated rabbit heart. *FASEB J.* 9: A622, 1995.

van Rossem, K., H. Vermarien, N.S. Faithfull, L. Wouters, and K. Decuyper. Effects of perflubron emulsion and 100% oxygen breathing on local tissue PO_2 in brain cortex of unanesthetized rabbits. *Adv. Exp. Med. Biol.* (in press), 1997.

Waschke, K.F., M. Riedel, D.M. Albrecht, K. van Ackern, and W. Kuschinsky. Effects of a perfluorocarbon emulsion on regional cerebral blood flow and metabolism after fluid resuscitation from hemorrhage in conscious rats. *Anesth. Analg.* 79: 874-882, 1994.

Winslow, R.M. A model for red cell O_2 uptake. *Int. J. Clin. Monitor. Comp.* 2: 81-93, 1985.

Winslow, R.M. A physiologic basis for the transfusion trigger. In *Blood Substitutes: Physiological Basis of Efficacy,* (R.M. Winslow, K.D. Vandegriff, and M. Intaglietta, eds.). Boston: Birkhäuser, 1995, pp. 25-41.

Zweier, J.L., M. Chzhan, U. Ewert, G. Schneider, and P. Kuppusamy. Development of a highly sensitive probe for measuring oxygen in biological tissues. *J. Mag. Reson.* 105: 52-57, 1994.

6.7 Discussion

Woodson: How long does it take the ICAM expression to drop after perflubron comes on the scene, and what do you know about the mechanism?

Flaim: You are asking questions about things that we don't know yet. This is an area that we're actively investigating, and I'm afraid I don't have answers to those questions at this point.

Meiselman: I'm sorry, I came in a couple of minutes late, so perhaps what I'm asking is part of your earlier presentation. Let me start off, however, by disagreeing with you with the artistic drawing that you had for the arterioles. There is absolutely no evidence to suggest under normal conditions that you will have an axial core with a cell-free region at the wall. At best, it would be statistically cell- poor. You might see an axial accumulation with a cell-poor region on the venous side under low-flow, low-shear conditions, but not on the arterioles.

Flaim: I agree with you very much.

Meiselman: My real question has to deal with the emulsifying agent which you are now using. I didn't hear it. The reason I'm very interested is that there are data in the literature for the emulsifying agent pleuronic F68 or for poloxamer 188 showing that agent is as effective as Fluosol® in changing rheological properties, etc. There are current data that suggest that it is effective in reducing red-cell adhesion to endothelial cells, and white-cell adhesion to endothelial cells. Last year we published some material indicating that the commercially viable form, which is RheothRx, is able to essentially totally eliminate red-cell mediated platelet aggregation which, of course, you might see in the pump system. So, I guess my bottom-line question is how much of the effect you are seeing is specific to the oxygen-carrying capacity of material, and how much of it is related to the rather substantial rheological effects and beneficial effects that we now know exist because of the poloxamer, whatever ones you are using?

Flaim: Actually, you did miss part of this talk. We do not use poloxamers in our surfactant preparation. It's entirely egg-yolk phospholipid, and we've done control studies with the surfactant by itself, and we see none of the benefits that we see with the final product. So we're convinced that the benefits that we see, especially in the area of oxygen delivery, are due to the perfluorocarbon material.

Meiselman: You don't believe any of the rheological effects, cell-adhesion, or PMN-endothelial cell interactions are an effect of the myocyte but rather of the oxygen-carrying capacity?

Flaim: Right. In those last slides, there was a vehicle control that showed no benefit at all.

Cokelet: I think it's probably too early to know the answer to my question. It's known quite well that when we have a completely ischemic preparation, you have a no-reperfusion phenomena which is, in some quarters anyway, attributed to various functions of the white cells, and perhaps free radicals. I was wondering in your reperfusion experiments, have you looked at, or are you looking at the possibility that the benefit gained is not from the oxygen-carrying but rather from the effect of the perfluorocarbon on white-cell function in free radicals?

Flaim: I believe personally that that's probably going to be a player in this story, and we are, in fact, looking at those issues, but unfortunately, I don't have any data I can share with you at the moment. I think that's a very important comment.

Bonaventura: I'm curious. You're in phase II clinical trials, but you showed only one slide with human data.

Flaim: I apologize for that. Our partner, Johnson & Johnson, prefers that we don't discuss clinical data, and that slide is what I can show you at this point. The only other thing I can tell you is that, as I indicated, as a result of an interim analysis of that trial, Johnson & Johnson paid Alliance a $15 million dollar milestone payment.

Bonaventura: Should I do like Winston Churchill, then, and say the more I learn from man, the more I like dogs? I mean, are dogs better in your product or humans? I mean, who responds better, animals or humans, or is that really beyond the limit of what you can...

Flaim: I think I tried to make the point that certainly the human results are following our preclinical assessments.

Bonaventura: And then when your product is approved, what would you predict that I'll read in a PDR for indications, contra-indications and adverse effects?

Flaim: This is a tough question to answer at this point. Certainly in terms of indications, we and Johnson & Johnson are pursuing the use of the product during cardiopulmonary bypass as an adjunct to the reservoir crystalloid-priming solution, and the other major indication we are pursuing is use of the product as a temporary oxygen carrier during high blood loss surgeries. Those are the primary indications. Beyond that, I think that I really can't comment further at this point.

Bonaventura: If we assume, and I think it's a reasonable assumption, that HBOCs, if that's what we are to call them, and your type of materials, fluorocarbons or non-proteinaceous oxygen carriers, assuming they're complementary, and I think that they are, how do you define what is a unit and what is the cross-over unit? What is the equivalence, and is there a standard if we want to divide it - your industry versus the HBOC industry?

Flaim: I think there are probably two ways of answering that. One is a pricing approach, and we believe that a unit of this material will be competitive with a unit of blood, essentially.

Bonaventura: Price-wise, you mean?

Flaim: Pricing, right.

Bonaventura: What if we're not worried about price, which ought not to be...

Flaim: Then you're worried about efficacy, and the unit would be one that gives us a benefit along the lines of what you're seeing here in the preclinical studies.

Bonaventura: May I do one final, quick, technical question? I'm interested in your data on nitric oxide, as you might imagine, and I'm surprised that your figure for solubility at 22 degrees is only eight times that of water. Water is about 1.8 millimolar under standard conditions. I don't know about neat fluorocarbons, but if you look at hexane, for example, it's an order of magnitude higher than Adax. So, are the data that you show for solubility of your product or of something else?

Flaim: The data you saw was the solubility measured in neat perflubron for nitric oxide.

Bonaventura: Not the emulsion?

Flaim: Not the emulsion.

Bonaventura: And how is the NO measured? What's the chemical analytical method?

Flaim: I don't have an answer to that. I can find out, and we can talk later.

Woodson: I have a question from a physiological point of view. As I know you know very well, venous PO_2 can be increased for a number of reasons, and these reasons would include diffusion across from arteries to veins which would indicate that the oxygen molecules to some degree bypassed the metabolizing tissues. Do you have any direct evidence that oxygenation is improved in proportion to raising the arterial oxygen content with perflubron?

Flaim: We have spent a lot of time looking at that issue, and I tried very hard to summarize our view in this talk. We've shown that, by any method that we can measure, MDO surface electrodes, Eppendorf electrodes, and so forth, that we've measured a rise in tissue PO_2, especially in critical organs. At the same time, we saw a rise in venous blood oxygen partial pressure draining those regions where we're measuring tissue levels using different methods, and those changes are not only in the same direction but they're in proportion. On top of that, we see the same direction and the same proportional increase in mixed venous PO_2 returning to the heart. Beyond that, what I showed you were data showing that in tissues with critical function - the brain and the heart - there is direct evidence that the product increases metabolic function that correlates to an improvement in organ function, especially in ischemic and hypoxic conditions.

So, the way I would answer your question is that if there was a substantial amount of short circuiting of oxygen from arteriole to venule, bypassing the capillary beds, I would certainly not expect to see metabolic function in the end organ being improved. That's essentially a "steal" phenomenon from the standpoint of oxygen. We actually see a benefit in metabolic function that correlates with the increase in tissue oxygenation and organ function.

Woodson: I guess I'm asking, is the increment in metabolic activity, such as oxygen consumption, absolutely linear with a 45-degree slope with the increase in arterial oxygen content, or is it something less than 45 degrees? I'm sure it's up, and I'm sure that metabolic data you cite is evidence for that, but I'm asking for the proportionality of the two effects.

Flaim: We really haven't made that correlation. I don't know the answer to that. I know it's positive, but I don't know whether it's a 1:1 relationship.

Woodson: Do you have any observations, not with electrodes, but with fluorometric indicators of oxygen in tissue?

Flaim: We have not attempted those experiments yet with fluorometric assessment.

Woodson: Then the last little question is what's the definition of a unit that you used in answering Joe's question a moment ago?

Flaim: That's a tough question to answer. As I tried to answer it before, a unit would be based upon a pricing issue as well as on an efficacy benefit. If you are looking for a volume, or if you're looking for a concentration, I don't really have an answer to that yet.

Winslow: Steve, I really enjoyed your talk. I have just a couple of minor questions. One is in regard to the question that was just asked about oxygen uptake. Hogan and Wagner showed that VO_2 max in the isolated hind limb of the dog was proportional to the additional convective oxygen transport. That's solid evidence that you are supplying oxygen better. The negative part of that, of course, was that it's all explained by convective and not diffusive oxygen transport. I think that's an answer to Bob Woodson's question.

Flaim: My apologies for ignoring that important paper, thank you.

Winslow: In regard to the clinical trials, you showed us experiments in dogs where I think the dose was 2.7 grams per kilogram. Is that in the same range as you are using in the clinical trials and that you expect to be used clinically?

Flaim: That is presently our current maximum clinical dose that we're pursuing. It could go higher, but that's clinically where we are.

Winslow: And one final question, I wasn't familiar with the concept of "volume-compensated bleed", and I wonder if you'd just explain a little bit what you did there?

Flaim: In those experiments, the blood was removed from the animal and an equal volume of crystalloid, or Hespan, depending on the experiment, was replaced. So the animal was normovolemic despite the fact that it had lost blood.

Winslow: Did you measure blood volume? As you know, blood volume can be very volatile, especially when you are doing crystalloid experiments.

Flaim: In those experiments, we had Swan-Ganz catheters on board all the time to measure pulmonary pressure, so we had a pretty good assessment of what was happening to blood volume.

Winslow: Thank you.

Chapter 7

The Other Blood Substitute: Antigenically Inert Erythrocytes

Mark D. Scott, Ph.D., Kari L. Murad, Ph.D., and John W. Eaton, Ph.D.

ABSTRACT

The effectiveness with which the immune system responds to and destroys heterologous blood cells has been an important driving force for the development of red blood cell (RBC) substitutes. The need for a blood substitute is particularly great in such situations as autoimmune hemolytic diseases, severe trauma in which proper blood typing and matching cannot be carried out quickly enough, or when rare blood types cannot be found. At present, a number of hemoglobin-based solutions are undergoing pre-clinical and clinical testing for use as blood substitutes in the above situations. However, despite substantial activity in this area, serious concerns still exist as to the efficacy, safety, and long-term applicability of these hemoglobin-based blood substitutes. It is our hypothesis that the covalent binding of non-immunogenic materials [*e.g.*, poly(ethylene glycol)] to intact cells may be useful in modulating the antigenicity of the RBC and in the development of a new class of blood substitutes. To this end, PEG-modified RBCs have been produced and found to be structurally and functionally normal while effectively rendering the cell antigenically silent. Furthermore, these non-immunogenic cells have normal *in vitro* and *in vivo* survival when compared to control RBC.

7.1 Introduction and Background

Hemoglobin-based blood substitutes have been an area of intense research and development over the last 10 years for use as clinical alternatives to the antigenically challenged red blood cell (RBC) (Walker *et al.* 1979; Winslow 1992; Chang 1993). Much of this research has necessarily centered on means by which the inherent toxicity of cell-free hemoglobin could be attenuated (Manning *et al.* 1991; McFaul *et al.* 1994; Motterlini *et al.* 1995). While significant advances in decreasing hemoglobins' toxicity/antigenicity have been made (*e.g.*, PEG-hemoglobin; HemAssist), the potential for both short-term and long-term tissue toxicity, due to vascular leakage and iron deposition, are still major concerns (Nho *et al.* 1992; Estep *et al.* 1993; Eaton 1996; Hess, 1996).

In contrast to the infusion of cell-free hemoglobin, the transfusion of matched RBCs is typically without clinical consequence (NIH 1988; Sazama 1990; Institute of Medicine 1996). Only rarely do significant problems arise following even rudimentary typing of the donor and recipients ABO/Rh blood groups. However, the relatively infrequent instances of rare blood types, extreme allosensitization or massive blood loss following trauma have driven research on hemoglobin-based blood substitutes (Beattie and Shafer 1986; Vichinsky *et al.* 1990; Larison and Cook 1994). In large part these studies have focused on purified/modified hemoglobin solutions so as to prevent transfusion reactions, maximize storage potential, and help in ease of use in non-clinical settings (Winslow 1995). Other investigators have focused on the use of liposome-encapsulated purified hemoglobin in an attempt to minimize the potential toxicity of cell-free hemoglobin (Hunt *et al.* 1985; Chang 1993). Unfortunately, even in the latter instance problems have been encountered with stability, extravascular leakage and rapid clearance. Indeed, the rapid rate of clearance is a universal problem for all blood substitutes since none of the existing products come close to the 120-day lifespan of a RBC. Consequently, these products are not suitable as long-term blood replacement therapy (nor have they claimed to be). In addition, these products would likely exacerbate tissue iron loading, and consequent toxicity, in the chronically transfused individual.

Thus, a clear demand still exists for a safe blood substitute. We have approached this problem by acknowledging the wisdom of Mother Nature - hemoglobin belongs in red blood cells. This can, however, cause problems where the major (ABO) blood groups are incompatible or in situations where extreme allosensitization to minor red cell antigens has occurred due to previous transfusions. Thus, some researchers have begun to look at antigenically altered RBCs. Studies by the Goldstein group at the New York Blood Center have focused on the use of selective exoglycosidases to enzymatically remove A or B antigens from RBCs (Goldstein *et al.* 1982; Goldstein 1989; Lenny and Goldstein 1991). While significant success is being met with Type B erythrocytes, Type A RBCs have been more problematic due to sequestered antigenic sites. Furthermore, such treatments will have no effect, and could actually enhance, immunogenicity of other red cell antigens.

Our studies have similarly centered on the intact RBC but have focused on producing antigenically silent RBCs via physical camouflage of the cell surface. This approach is supported by previous studies in which purified proteins were covalently modified with poly(ethylene glycol) [PEG]. In contrast to the unmodified proteins, the PEG-modified proteins were shown to have increased *in vivo* survival and to be non-immunogenic, even with repeated infusions (Abuchowski *et al.* 1977a,b). Indeed, other researchers cognizant of these previous studies have been examining the suitability of PEG-modified hemoglobin and PEG-liposome encapsulated hemoglobin as potential blood substitutes (Nho *et al.* 1992; Senior *et al.* 1991; Maruyama *et al.* 1992; Zalipsky *et al.* 1994). While both of these latter approaches may prove fruitful, our research has explored the hypothesis that the covalent binding of PEG to intact RBCs might sterically mask RBC surface antigens and thereby produce antigenically silent RBCs.

Two significant theoretical/practical issues must be accounted for in producing antigenically silent RBCs via the covalent attachment of non-immunogenic material. First, the attached material must be of sufficient length and have an appreciable zone of exclusion to prevent/minimize the binding of large molecules (antibodies) or interaction with other cells (*e.g.*, macrophages). Second, the derivatization itself cannot significantly impair normal membrane structure or function (*e.g.*, cellular deformability and cation, glucose, or oxygen exchange). Diagrammatically, these issues are demonstrated in Figure 7.1.

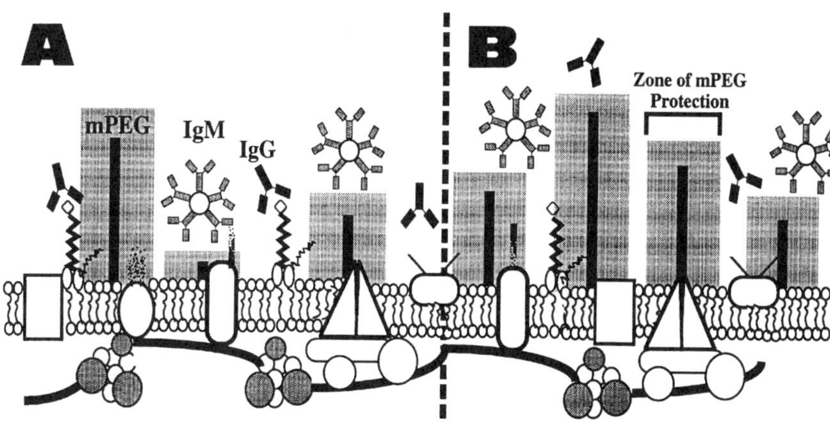

Figure 7.1. Covalent derivatization of the cell surface must take into account both the topography of the cell surface and the exclusion volume of the non-immunogenic material. As shown, insufficient derivatization will result in ineffective exclusion of antibodies and may not prevent cell:cell interaction (**A**). In contrast, more efficient surface derivatization will prevent both antibody binding and cell:cell interaction (**B**).

The potential advantages of a successful implementation of antigenically silent RBCs over either free hemoglobin or liposome-encapsulated blood substitutes are significant: RBC size and function are maintained, hemoglobin is encapsulated and not subject to abnormal extravascular leakage, and hemoglobin is cleared via its physiologically normal route.

Several viable candidates exist for the derivatization of cell surfaces and the generation of antigenically silent RBCs. These include: poly(ethylene glycol), and its derivatives, dextrans, arabinogalactans, and Ficols. However, based on the previous literature, we have concentrated on poly(ethylene glycol) and its derivatives [in a generic sense, PEG can refer to poly(ethylene oxide), poly(oxyethylene), and poly(oxirane)] (Harris *et al.* 1984; Harris 1985; Harris, 1992). The basic chemical structure of PEG is: $HO\text{-}(CH_2CH_2O)_n\text{-}CH_2CH_2OH$. PEG itself is a nontoxic compound approved for internal consumption and, similarly, PEG-conjugated proteins have also been approved by the FDA for clinical use (Fuertges amd Abuchowski 1990; Saifer, Somack and Williams 1994).

It is the physicochemical nature of PEG (in the generic sense) that makes it particularly amenable to biologic use and manipulation. PEG is a polyether polymer having a neutral charge and an extraordinarily wide range of molecular weights. Surprisingly, PEG is soluble in both water and most organic solvents and, of particular interest to this proposal, effectively excludes other polymers from its presence when in an aqueous environment. PEG solubility/partitioning in water or organic phases can be further manipulated by the addition of hydrophobic or hydrophilic tails or by inclusion of segments within the polymer backbone. The terminal hydroxyl groups of PEG provide a site of attachment for other compounds (*e.g.*, linker molecules or proteins). Interestingly, PEG molecules can be made either linear or branched. The variable sizes and shapes of PEG may be of importance in the production of antigenically silent RBCs. It is important to note that a balance must be achieved between antigenic masking and maintenance of protein/cell function. Previous studies have shown that an over-exuberant derivatization of purified proteins will result in loss of enzymatic function (hence, by extrapolation, of cell function and viability). Thus, as shown in Figure 7.2, branched PEGs may have some theoretical advantages over linear molecules. Similarly, longer linear molecules may have greater masking effects than those with shorter chain lengths. Indeed, it is hypothesized that the zone of exclusion is correlated with antigenic masking.

7.2 Experimental Findings

While previous studies and theoretical considerations suggest that PEG might be useful in modifying the antigenicity of intact RBCs (as well as other cell types), experimental evidence of our hypothesis was lacking.

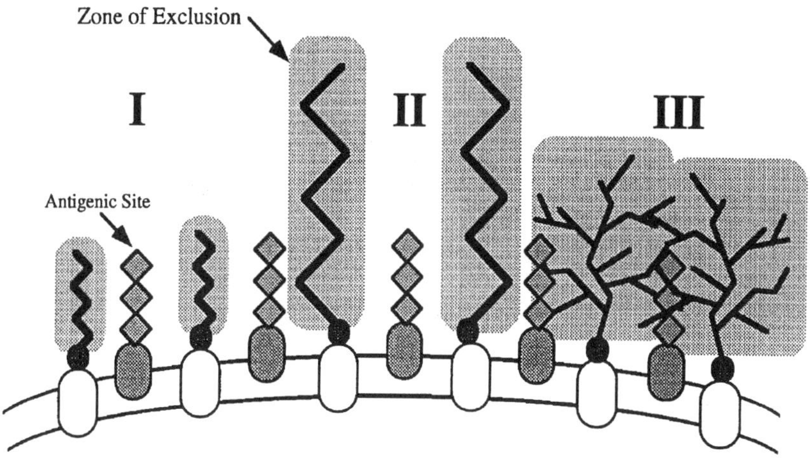

Figure 7.2. The effects of non-immunogenic tails of varying molecular weight and size may differ significantly. (I) Represents a small (5 kDa) linear molecule such as the mPEG discussed in this chapter. (II) Represents a much higher (*e.g.*, 20 kDa) molecular weight linear compound. The longer chain length of (II) might more effectively camouflage the antigenic determinants of the RBC. (III) Represents multi-branched PEG. As indicated by the zone of hydration of the polymer (stippled area), (III) may be the most effective in preventing antigenic recognition.

To test our hypothesis we have derivatized human and mouse RBCs with cyanuric chloride-activated methoxypoly(ethylene glycol) [mPEG; Figure 7.3] (Jackson *et al.* 1987). The activated mPEG (average m.w. of 5 kDa) is added to washed RBCs (12% hematocrit) suspended in isotonic alkaline phosphate buffered saline (PBS; 50 mM K_2HPO_4 and 105 mM NaCl) and incubated at pH 9.2 for 30 minutes at 4°C (Murad *et al.* 1996). Importantly, this derivatization process had no significant effect on RBC lysis (<1% lysis) or, as will be shown, *in vitro* or *in vivo* viability. mPEG concentrations tested to date have ranged from 0 to 50 mg per ml of RBC suspension.

The effects of mPEG derivatization on the antigenicity of control and modified RBCs have been assessed by determining the reactivity of both major (ABO) and minor (Rh and MNS) antigens, direct antibody binding, and by the phagocytic recognition of normal and opsonized control and derivatized RBCs. As demonstrated in Figure 7.4, both ABO and minor antigen reactivities of the mPEG-modified (6 mg/ml) RBCs are significantly decreased (Murad *et al.* 1996). Real time A/B-mediated reactivity in response to appropriate blood typing antisera (Carolina Biological Supply, Burlington, NC) was determined via a novel microagglutination assay using a platelet aggregometer (Chrono-Log, Havertown, PA). Reactivity of selected minor RBC antigens was tested via agglutination assays in the Albany Medical Center Clinical Hematology Laboratory according to established AABB methods and rated on the 4^{+s} system (Vengelen-Tyler 1996). The results of the agglutination assays were fur-

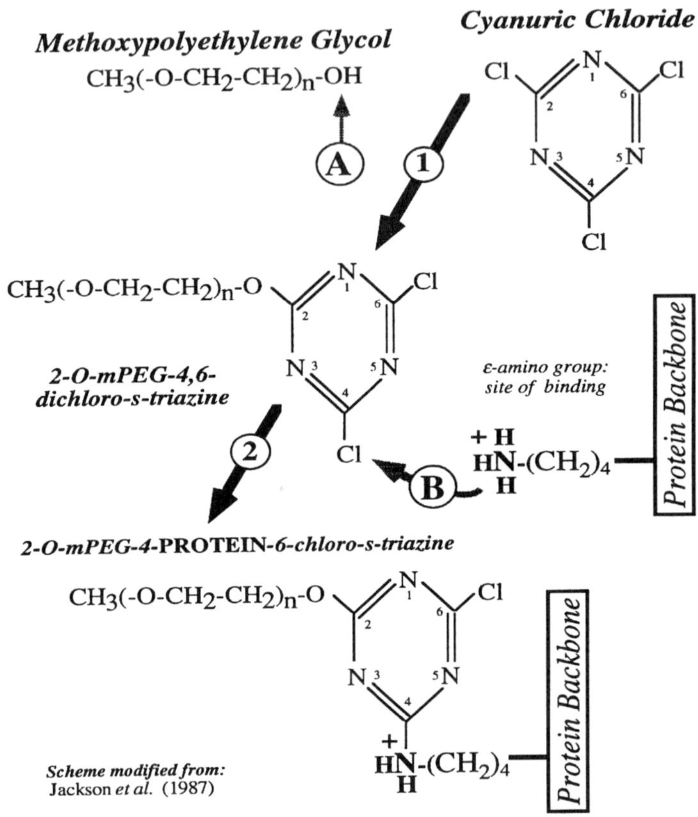

Figure 7.3. Covalent modification of membrane-bound proteins on intact cells. Prior to addition of cells, methoxypoly(ethylene glycol) is activated with cyanuric chloride by incubating the two components at 25°C in anhydrous benzene. The hydroxyl group (A) of the mPEG is a nucleophile and reacts with the alkyl halide of the cyanuric chloride resulting in the release of Cl^- and the formation of activated mPEG (Step 1). Generation of a mPEG-conjugated protein occurs following reaction between a second chloride of the cyanuric chloride linker residue and an available (*i.e.*, surface) amino group (B; primarily lysine, perhaps some arginine) on a protein. This is done in alkaline phosphate buffer (PBS; 50 mM K_2HPO_4 and 105 mM NaCl) at pH 9.2 for 30 minutes (Step 2).

ther confirmed by direct measurement of bound antibodies using an ELISA assay (data not shown; Murad *et al.* 1996). The decrease in antibody binding has an important biologic effect in that mPEG-derivatization significantly decreased phagocytic recognition. This is readily demonstrated by the diminished phagocytosis of control and opsonized sheep RBCs by human peripheral blood mononuclear cells (PBMC). The uptake of these normally detectable sheep RBCs by human PBMC is

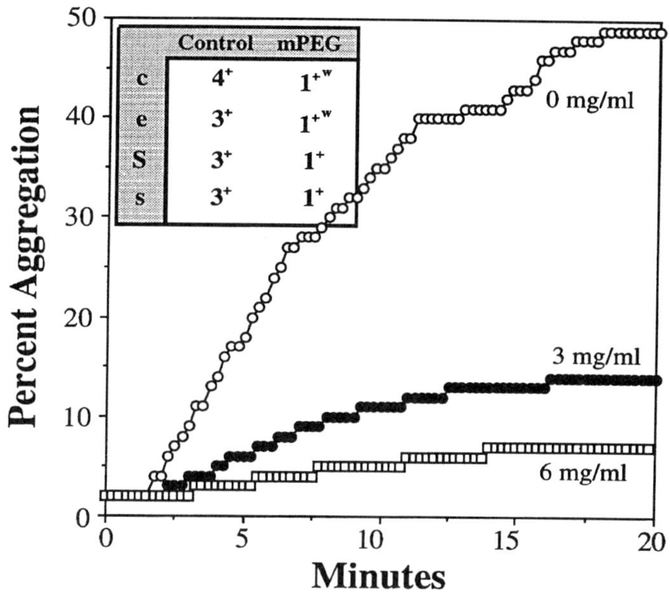

Figure 7.4. ABO recognition by anti-sera can be virtually abolished by mPEG derivatization. ABO reactivity was determined by a microagglutination method developed using a platelet aggregometer (Chrono-Log, Havertown, PA). This method allows us to follow the time-dependent aggregation of stirred RBC suspensions in response to typing sera. TABLE INSERT: Minor antigen reactivity was also substantially decreased following mPEG-modification. The selected minor RBC antigens were tested in the Albany Medical Center Clinical Hematology Laboratory according to established AABB methods and rated on the 4^{+S} system.

decreased in a mPEG-dosage dependent manner as indicated (Figure 7.5). Importantly, addition of *unactivated* mPEG (5 kDa) to intact RBC, followed by washing in saline (3x), has no inhibitory effect on antisera-induced hemagglutination, antibody binding, or phagocytosis.

Despite the dramatic effects of mPEG-derivatization on cellular antigenicity, no significant effects have been observed on either cell structure or function (Murad *et al.* 1996). RBC derivatized with even very high mPEG concentrations (> 30 mg/ml RBC) showed no substantial (*i.e.,* <10%) lysis after 24 hours of further incubation at 37°C. However, very high concentrations of mPEG (>30 mg/ml) did cause significant lysis after an additional 24 hours incubation at 37°C (but not 4°C). Furthermore, the osmotic fragility of the mPEG-modified (6 mg/ml) RBC was unaltered - even after 72 hours incubation at 37°C.

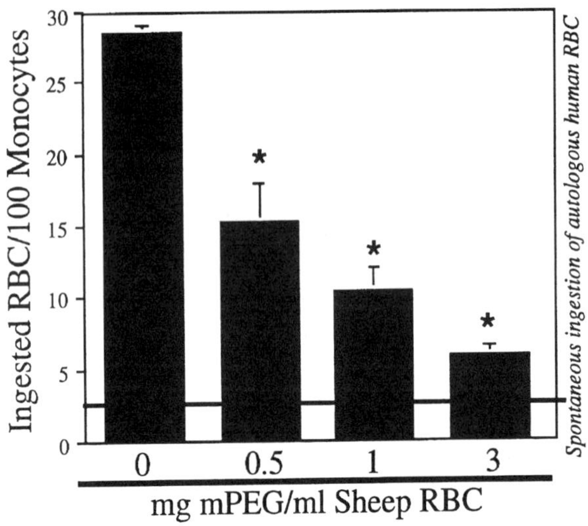

Figure 7.5. The phagocytosis of sheep RBCs by human peripheral blood mononuclear cells (PBMC) is significantly decreased following mPEG modification. PBMC concentration was held constant at 2 x 10^6/ml and a ratio of 10 RBCs per PBMC was used. Following 30 minutes incubation at 37°C the uningested RBCs were removed by hypotonic lysis, and the total number of monocytes and the number of monocytes which had phagocytosed RBCs were counted microscopically. Significance ($p < 0.01$) is denoted by an asterisk (*). The phagocytic index was calculated as the number of monocytes ingesting RBC/total monocyte number.

Morphologically, mPEG-modified (6 mg/ml) RBCs were found to be normal by both light and electron microscopy (Murad *et al.* 1996). The oxygen carrying function of the RBC was also unaffected by mPEG-modification. Finally, the effects of mPEG modification on the hemoglobin oxygen affinity of treated cells were assessed. Oxygen equilibrium curves (obtained using a Hemox-Analyzer; TCS Medical Products, Southampton, PA) revealed that the oxygen affinity of mPEG-treated RBC was within the normal range. Perhaps the most significant indicator of the normality of the mPEG-derivatized RBC, as alluded to in the previous studies, is most dramatically demonstrated by their *in vivo* survival. As shown in Figure 7.6, mPEG-modified (3 mg/ml) mouse RBCs exhibit normal *in vivo* survival as demonstrated in BALB/c mice using fluorescently (PKH-26; Sigma Chemical Co., St. Louis, MO) tagged cells (Schlegel, Lumley-Spanski and Williamson 1992; Murad *et al.* 1996). The labeled RBCs were injected intraperitoneally (*i.p.*) into recipient mice, and cell survival was followed up to 62 days using a Becton-Dickinson Flow Cytometer.

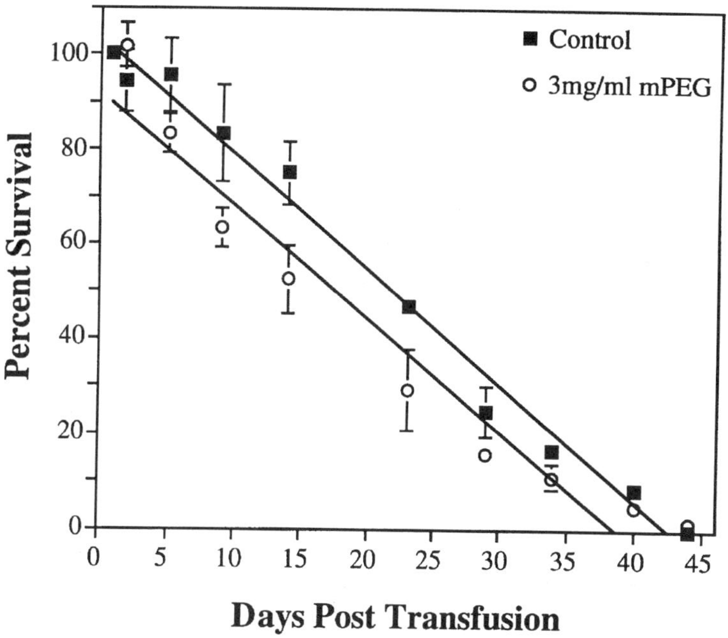

Figure 7.6. *In vivo* survival of mPEG-derivatized mouse RBCs is normal. Each data point represents the mean ± SD of four mice. Survival was followed using a fluorescent fatty acid label (PKH-26; Sigma Chemical Company).

7.3 Conclusions

In summary, we have attempted to produce antigenically-silent RBCs via the covalent attachment of non-immunogenic materials such as mPEG (Figure 7.7). To date our studies indicate that the covalent modification of RBC surfaces with mPEG effectively obscures antigenic determinants, while leaving the RBCs structurally and functionally normal (Murad *et al.* 1996). As a result of these findings, we suggest that RBCs covalently derivatized with mPEG, as well as other non-immunogenic materials, may be an attractive alternative to hemoglobin-based blood substitutes in emergency situations and in chronically transfused patients. These antigenically silent RBCs have significant advantages over hemoglobin-based blood substitutes in that the potentially toxic hemoglobin is compartmentalized, and the cells have normal (at least in mice) *in vivo* survival.

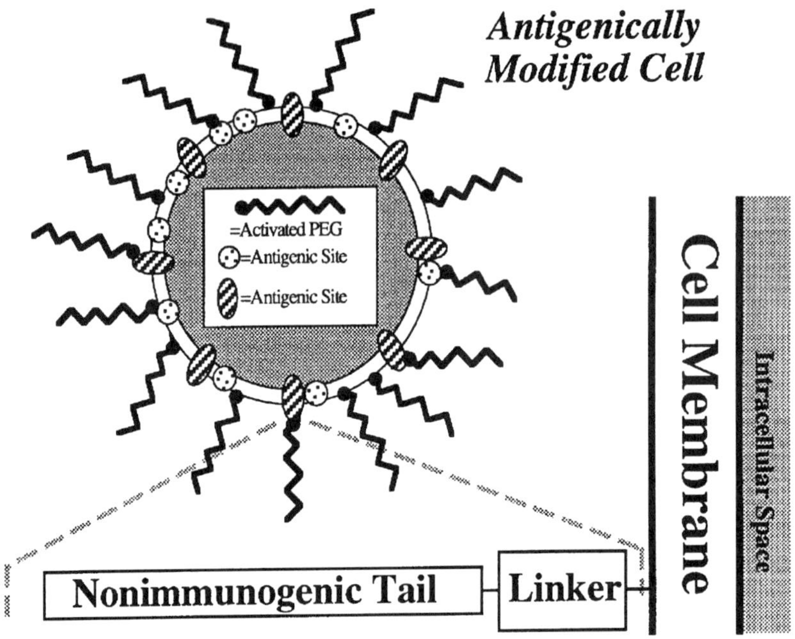

Figure 7.7. Should our hypotheses be validated, these antigenically silent cells may become a clinically useful tool in the armamentarium of transfusion and transplantation medicine as well as a potential alternative to hemoglobin-based blood substitutes in a number of clinical circumstances.

7.4 Acknowledgments

This research was supported by National Institutes of Health grant HL53066.

7.5 References

Abuchowski, A., T. van Es, N.C. Palczuk, and F.F. Davis. Alteration of immunological properties of bovine serum albumin by covalent attachment of poly(ethylene glycol). *J. Biol. Chem.* 252: 3578-3581, 1977a.

Abuchowski, A., J.R. McCoy, N.C. Palczuk, T. van Es, and F.F. Davis. Effect of covalent attachment of poly(ethylene glycol) on immunogenicity and circulating life of bovine liver catalase. *J. Biol. Chem.* 252: 3582-3586, 1977b.

Beattie, K.M., and A.W. Shafer. Broadening the base of a rare donor program by targeting minority populations. *Transfusion* 26: 401-404, 1986.

Chang, T.M.S. Blood substitutes based on modified hemoglobin prepared by encapsulation or crosslinking: an overview. In: *Blood Substitutes and Oxygen Carriers* (T.M.S. Chang, ed.), New York: Marcel Dekker, Inc., 1993, pp. 3-23.

Eaton, J. W. Hemoglobin-based blood substitutes: a dreamlike trade of blood and guile. *J. Lab. Clin. Med.* 127: 416-417, 1996.

Estep, T.N., J. Gonder, I. Bornstein, and F. Aono. Immunogenicity of diaspirin cross-linked human hemoglobin solutions. In: *Blood Substitutes and Oxygen Carriers* (T.M.S. Chang, ed.), New York: Marcel Dekker, Inc., 1993, pp. 396-402.

Fuertges, F., and A. Abuchowski. The clinical efficacy of poly(ethylene glycol)-modified proteins. *J. Controlled Release* 11: 139-148, 1990.

Goldstein, J. Conversion of ABO Blood Groups. *Transf. Med. Rev.* 3: 206-212, 1989.

Goldstein, J., G. Siviglia, R. Hurst, L. Lenny, and L. Reich. Group B erythrocytes enzymatically converted to group O survive in A, B, and O individuals. *Science* 215: 168-170, 1982.

Harris, J.M. Laboratory synthesis of poly(ethylene glycol) derivatives. *JMS-Rev. Macromol Chem. Phys.* C25: 325-373, 1985.

Harris, J.M. Introduction to biotechnical and biomedical applications of poly(ethylene glycol). In: *Poly(ethylene glycol) Chemistry: Biotechnical and Biomedical Applications* (J.M. Harris, ed.) New York: Plenum Press, 1992, pp. 1-14.

Harris, J.M., E.C. Struck, M.G. Case, and M.S. Paley. Synthesis and characterization of poly(ethylene glycol) derivatives. *J. Poly. Sci.* 22: 341-352, 1984.

Hess, J.R. Blood Substitutes. *Semin. Hematol.* 33: 369-378, 1996.

Hunt, C. A., R. R. Burnette, R. D. MacGregor, A. E. Strubbe, D. T. Lau, N. Taylor, and, H. Kawanda. Synthesis and evaluation of a prototypal artificial red cell. *Science* 230: 1165-1168, 1985.

Institute of Medicine Report. HIV and the blood supply. An analysis of crisis decision making. Washington, D.C.: National Academy Press, 1996.

Jackson, C.J., J.L. Charlton, K. Kuzminski, G.M. Lang, and A.H. Sehon. Synthesis, isolation, and characterization of conjugates of ovalbumin with monomethoxypolyethylene glycol using cyanuric chloride as the coupling agent. *Anal. Biochem.* 165: 114-127, 1987.

Larison, P.T., and L.O. Cook. Adverse effects of blood transfusion. In *Modern Blood Banking & Transplantation Practices*, 3rd edition (D. Harmening, ed.) Philadelphia: F.A. Davis Co., 1994, pp. 351-374.

Lenny, L., and J. Goldstein. The production of group O cells. *Biotechnology* 19: 75-100, 1991.

Manning, L.R., S. Morgan, R.C. Beavis, B.T. Chait, J.M. Manning, J.R. Hess, M. Cross, D.L. Currell, M.A. Marini, and R.M. Winslow. Preparation, properties, and plasma retention of human hemoglobin derivatives: comparison of uncrosslinked carboxymethylated hemoglobin with crosslinked tetrameric hemoglobin. *Proc. Nat. Acad. Sci. USA* 88: 3329-3333, 1991.

Maruyama, K., T. Yuda, A. Okamoto, S. Kojima, A. Suginaka, and M. Iwatsuru. Prolonged circulation time *in vivo* of large unilamellar liposomes composed of distearoyl phosphatidylcholine and cholesterol containing amphipathic poly(ethylene glycol). *Biochim. Biophys. Acta* 1128: 44-449, 1992.

McFaul, S.J., P.D. Bowman, V.M. Villa, M.J. Gutierrez-Ibanez, M. Johnson, and D. Smith. Hemoglobin stimulates mononuclear leukocytes to release interlukin 8 and tumor necrosis factor alpha. *Blood* 84: 3175-3181, 1994.

Motterlini, R., R. Foresti, K. Vandegriff, M. Intaglietta, and R.M. Winslow. Oxidative-stress response in vascular endothelial cells exposed to acellular hemoglobin solutions. *Am. J. Physiol.* 269: H648-655, 1995.

Murad, K., F. Koumpouras, M. Talbot, J.W. Eaton, and M.D. Scott. Molecular camouflage of antigenic determinants on intact mammalian cells: possible applications to transfusion medicine. *Blood* 88 (Suppl. 1): 1765, 1996.

Nho, K., D. Glower, S. Bredehoeft, H. Shankar, R. Shorr, and A. Abuchowski. PEG-bovine hemoglobin: safety in a canine dehydrated hypovolemic-hemorrhagic shock model. *Biomat. Artif. Cells Immobil. Biotech.* 20: 511-524, 1992.

NIH Consensus Conference. Perioperative red cell transfusion. *JAMA* 260: 2700-2703, 1988.

Saifer, M.G., R. Somack, and L.D. Williams. Plasma clearance and immunologic properties of long-acting superoxide dismutase prepared using 35,000 to 120,000 dalton poly-ethylene glycol. *Adv. Exp. Med. Biol.* 366: 377-387, 1994.

Sazama, K. Reports of 355 transfusion-associated deaths: 1976-1985. *Transfusion* 30: 583-590, 1990.

Schlegel, R.A., K. Lumley-Sapanski, and P. Williamson. Single cell analysis of factors increasing the survival of resealed erythrocytes in the circulation of mice. *Adv. Exp. Med. Biol.* 326: 133-138, 1992.

Senior, J., C. Delgado, D. Fisher, C. Tilcock, and G. Gregoriadis. Influence of surface hydrophilicity of liposomes on their interaction with plasma and clearance from the circulation: studies with poly(ethylene glycol)-coated vesicles. *Biochim. Biophys. Acta* 1062: 77-82, 1991.

Vengelen-Tyler, V., ed. *AABB Technical Manual, 12th Edition.* Arlington: American Association of Blood Banks, 1996, pp. 609-627.

Vichinsky, E.P., A. Earles, R.A. Johnson, S. Hoag, A. Williams and B. Lubin. Alloimmunization in sickle cell anemia and transfusion of racially unmatched blood. *New Eng. J. Med.* 322: 1617-1621, 1990.

Walker, J.A., R.H. Zaugg, R.Y. Walder, J.M. Steele, and I.M. Klotz. Diaspirins that cross-link ß chains of hemoglobin: bis(3,5-dibromo–salicyl) succinate and bis(3,5-dibromosalicyl) fumarate. *Biochemistry* 18: 4265-4270, 1979.

Winslow, R.M. *Hemoglobin-based Red Cell Substitutes.* Baltimore: John Hopkins University Press, 1992.

Winslow, R.M. Blood substitutes: A moving target. *Nature Med.* 1: 1212-1215, 1995.

Zalipsky, S., E. Brandeis, M.S. Newman, and M.C. Woodle. Long circulating, cationic liposomes containing amino-PEG-phosphatidyl–ethanolamine. *FEBS Lett.* 353: 71-74, 1994.

7.6 Discussion

Meiselman: Mark, I want to congratulate you on that presentation. It brought tears to my eyes, and I was very glad to hear it. For those of you who are not aware, there is a very funny story in which Dr. Armstrong and Dr. Fisher have been working on a very similar approach, pegylating red cells, and only by accident last December did our two groups discover that we are working on parallel paths, but we still hadn't linked together.

Scott: Right. Along with a third and a fourth group as well as it turned out.

Meiselman: That's right, and how dare they without calling me up first, right? I think it's fair to point out that you do reduce cell-cell interaction, you can essentially abolish red-cell aggregation, and therefore, you can drastically lower low-shear blood viscosity. In fact, you turn red cells in plasma into something that looks like red cells in ordinary buffer which means they're nearly Newtonian and have a very low viscosity at low shear rates. So in addition to the antigenicity, or the anti-antigenicity, if you will, you also have a very profound rheological effect. It may well be that the combination of these two has very important long-range implications.

Scott: We have started looking at white cell rolling along the endothelial cells, and we can inhibit that as well. So this goes back to the hyperacute rejection that you can see in tissue transplants as well as a number of other inflammatory states.

Meiselman: It's going to be very interesting because you could even speculate that red-cell adhesion to endothelial cells might be greatly decreased in sickle cell disease or diabetes mellitus. In sickle cell disease, red cell or PMN adhesion is thought to be one of the key factors promoting crisis.

Scott: I agree.

Hearst: It's a wonderful talk. I am puzzled by the fact that you do *in vitro* lysis measurements that show survival of four hours, or 10% lysis in 4 hours...

Scott: Forty-eight hours.

Hearst: Forty-eight hours. And yet you show lifetimes which go out for 40 days. Those two results seem to be totally inconsistent with each other.

Scott: Not really. Mouse red cells are not real happy, first of all, *in vitro*, and even human red cells, which are much more stable *in vitro*, are not real happy when you have them in something as simple as Hank's balanced salt solution with glucose. During this incubation, we don't try to keep the glucose supplemented. What we are trying to do is exacerbate the insult to the cell so that if there is a slight difference, we can pick it up.

Torchilin: Outstanding talk. I like your presentation also very much. I do have a small concern, some small advice and a small question.

Scott: The bad news first, right?

Torchilin: Yes, the bad news first. I personally don't like too much this cyanuric/chloride trichlorotriazine because, you might know that in several cases when it was used to prepare different pharmaceuticals, it was never permitted because of high toxicity. Anyway, it will be degraded in lysosomes or whatever, and cyanuric itself, which is extremely stable in biological conditions, will be released back in circulation and might cause toxic effects. So, I would advise to do something like, for example, SMCC which is very nice stuff; you can do exactly the same chemistry, it disappears without a trace, with no toxicity. You know, cyanuric is not the best stuff to deal with.

Scott: I agree that there is some concern about its potential toxicity. We have looked at some of the other linker molecules, and the problem there is that they're just not as effective.

Torchilin: Another small experimental advice is when you are trying to measure agglutination in your approach, you always have to choose appropriate antibody to agglutinate because you are dealing with different cell types. But we made a similar study of different cells under different circumstances, but it's a very simple approach: we just buy biotinylated cells and then make agglutination with avidin.

It's an absolutely universal reaction; it's very simple to do, and you'll never be confused with different antibodies, with different cell types or whatever. And, the last question I have is the following: you still have your erythrocytes cleared, and probably the mechanism of clearance is the same as for normal erythrocytes. It means that we know how cells are cleared because certain proteins lose the protective coating of neuraminic acid and just some sugar moieties are exposed and recognized by corresponding receptors on the liver cells. It means that by that point you do not have PEG protection if those pieces might be recognized. Might it effect somehow complete lack of antigenicity? But, you know it is early stages, so how will this stuff behave in the later stages?

Scott: The mechanism and the events underlying red-cell clearance are not as clear cut as some people would like to think. For example, if you look at red-cell survival in a SCID, mouse which lacks an immune system, it's still cleared at the same rate as its parental strain; that implies that it's not an antibody mediated event. It has always been my personal bias, and I think Dr. Meiselman might agree with me, that the primary mechanism for red cell clearance is loss of structural deformability, which is going to occur in these red cells at the same rate as a control cell simply because the spectrin and anchyrin and everything else is falling apart, and a red cell cannot replace that. So, I don't think we see increased survival in these cells simply because the real time clock for these cells is not effected, which is just the spontaneous degradation of the cytoskeleton, the metabolic enzymes. We've done a lot on that in thalassemic red cells. For example, thalassemic cells show that loss of glycolysis and deformability precedes the eventual destruction of the red cells - so I think the idea that there are senescence antigens and there are senescent antibodies for red cells is perhaps over exaggerated; it has a role, but I don't think it's the primary mechanism. Again, that's my personal bias.

Intaglietta: I am a little bit unclear as to the logic of this process in the following way: we have heard from Professor Torchilin that the pegylation has a half life of around 48 hours under maximum conditions...

Scott: That's on liposomes.

Intaglietta: Liposomes. Does it have a longer lifetime on red cells?

Scott: I'm not sure he was referring to the PEG itself. He may have been referring to the PEG-liposome particle. So what we're talking about is a normal red blood cell which, in a mouse, survives about 50 days and in a human, 120 days. This is a covalent attachment, and the majority of that PEG is still there at the end of the life span of the red blood cell, though it may also be lost slowly with time. But what we're saying is that the pegylation has no effect on the normal survival of these cells; it doesn't prolong it, and what they're showing with liposomes, which are normally very rapidly cleared, is that the PEG can then prevent some of the mechanisms involved in liposome clearance, but red-cell clearances are a completely different matter.

Intaglietta: But, the statement then is that the pegylation will last the life of the cell?

Scott: I'd like to state that, but I can't as of this time. PEG is, first of all, very, very hard to measure because you can't raise an antibody to it, you can't do a lot of things to it. There are some chemical assays that we're trying to get up and running in the lab, so that is one area that I would say we are trying address as we speak, which is to actually measure the amount of PEG at the start of the *in vivo* survival as well as at the end of the *in vivo* survival, and I think we have a couple of ways of doing that with some fluorescently-labeled PEG and then being able to follow that on a per-cell basis.

Intaglietta: I don't mean to be negative, but I thought you had done that by showing that the sheep cells only last about 72 hours.

Scott: No, we have not measured the PEG on them at the end of that time. Sheep red cells are about the right size for a mouse, but their lipid composition is very foreign. They have no phosphatidylcholine in their membranes. The mouse red cell is about 40-45% phosphatidylcholine in their membrane. So what you have is phosphatidylcholine moving into the sheep red blood and this results in a very detergent-like effect, basically, and a loss of membrane stability and probably lysis of the red cell.

Hess: Let me raise the caveat that just because you can prevent cell-to-cell interaction and the hemagglutination reaction, you may still not be able to prevent immunization. Jack Goldstein has shown that you can reduce the ABO substance from a million copies on a red cell to about 100 and prevent the hemagglutination reaction and even immune clearance of those cells, but they're still immunogenic. People still develop IgG antibodies in response to them, and those antibodies could secondarily cross the placenta and cause some problems.

Scott: That is a concern that we're aware of, and I have to say that we're still at the very early stage on this. We're not going to try these cells on humans tomorrow, and so we're still very early in the process. What we have done to address that are experiments in which mice received multiple injections, whether they be an inbred mouse strain, outbred mouse strain, foreign mouse strains, or sheep red blood cells. Mice are not great for this because they don't have classic transfusion reactions; but in the sheep experiments, for example, which are extraordinarily foreign red blood cells, we can go back two weeks or four weeks later to these sheep and inject either control sheep red cells or the pegylated sheep red cells, and, for example, the ones that had previously received pegylated red cells do not clear the pegylated red cells they receive any faster the second time around. So, it looks like we have prevented any immune sensitization at that point.

Hess: Well that's what Goldstein has done with B cells in O individuals, and the second time you inject them, they still have normal survival, but they are developing IgG antibodies against B.

Scott: I see what you are saying, and we have to look for the development of specific antibodies to these cells, and we will be doing that. We've done a lot, but we haven't done everything.

Hess: The second point is that membrane damage, even in red cells, tends to be a slow event. If you irradiate them, you don't really see the damage for a couple of weeks later, so in 48 hours they may look normal. Two weeks later, they have significantly higher potassium.

Scott: But in this case, we also have *in vivo* survival data which indicate that they have normal red-cell survival over 50-60 days.

Hess: As do radiated red cells.

Scott: We've actually done a fair amount of work on radiated red cells, and I will tell you that unless you get to really high dosages, you don't see membrane damage.

Hess: But you do see much higher potassiums in storage at two weeks.

Scott: Typically when you irradiate red cells clinically, you use 2500-3000 Rads, and that's to kill the white cells. There are reports, and everybody just accepts it, that to do that shortens the storage life of red blood cells from 42 to 28 days. If you look at isolated red blood cells, or even red blood cells with white cells present, before you can detect really significant damage, you're looking at radiation dosages of about 50-fold what's used in the clinical labs. I can show you the literature for that; I may even have it here, I'm not sure.

Hess: Actually, both the Moore study and the Davey study, which are the only two good ones in the literature, would suggest that 3000 is plenty.

Scott: Well, we've looked at it, and we've seen nothing in terms of potassium content or deformability. That's a whole different subject, but as Drs. Fisher, Armstrong, and Meiselman's poster here clearly shows that in terms of mechanical deformability, there's not a problem. We've done storage studies on these cells as well, and they store pretty normally just like control red cells do. I'd be happy to go over this with you. We're aware of a lot of these problems and will try to address them; in some cases, we've made some progress, and in other cases, we just are still at the "hoping-to" stage.

Ten Eyck: I got interested in your description of the way the cells might eventually be cleared. It would appear that what you are hoping is that the pegylation prevents any presentation of antigen during the entire process of breaking up of the cell since your goal here is long-term multiple transfusion cases. Do you think this is likely?

Scott: In part, this "hope" is based on the work with purified proteins. Admittedly, they were looking at a single pegylated protein *versus* red cells, and I've said we don't really care where you've pegylated it as long as it camouflages the antigenic sites. Consequently, we are hoping that the red cells are cleared via a normal pathway, and that as a result of being cleared via that pathway, you do not result in any kind of immune recognition of foreign minor blood group antigens.

Chapter 8

Hemoglobin Encapsulation With Polyethylene Glycol-modified and Unmodified Vesicles: Systemic and Microvascular Hemodynamics at 80% Blood Substitution

Hiromi Sakai, Ph.D., Amy G. Tsai, Ph.D., Marcos Intaglietta, Ph.D., and Eishun Tsuchida, Ph.D.

ABSTRACT

Phospholipid vesicles containing purified hemoglobin (Hb vesicles, HbV) of high stability and uniform size have been developed to provide oxygen carrying capacity to plasma expanders. Their function as a blood replacement was tested in exchange transfusion where 80% of the red blood cell mass was substituted with suspensions of vesicles in 5% human serum albumin (HSA) solution. Vesicles were tested with membranes that were unmodified (HbV) or conjugated with polyethylene glycol (PEG-HbV). Both materials yielded normal systemic hemodynamic conditions at all levels of exchange which could not be achieved with HSA alone. Subcutaneous microvascular studies in awake hamsters showed that PEG-HbV yielded significantly improved microhemodynamic conditions relative to unmodified HbVs. The tissue oxygenation was lower than in the blood-perfused microcirculation. These results highlight the significance of microvascular analysis in the study and design of blood substitutes, while the development and availability of these vesicles provides a unique opportunity to determine the optimal set of parameters needed to design a blood substitute.

8.1 Introduction

Phospholipid or non-phospholipid vesicles containing concentrated hemoglobin (Hb vesicles, HbV) are likely to become industrially produced red cell substitutes (Rudolph 1995, Tsuchida 1995, Rohlfs and Vandegriff 1996), since they replicate the red blood cell membrane function of physically preventing direct contact of hemoglobin with the cellular components of the microcirculation. The desirability of this barrier function is evident in considering the side effects found in the use of acellular hemoglobin solutions, such as chemically-modified Hb and recombinant Hb which are now in clinical trials (Winslow 1995).

The principal systemic side-effect consistently reported in the administration of acellular Hb solutions is a pressor response. The origin of this reaction has been attributed to the nitric oxide (NO) scavenging effect of hemoglobin, due to the intrinsic high affinity of NO to Hb, first described by Palmer, Ferrige and Moncada (1987), a process presumed to lead to vasoconstriction. The hypothesis has also been advanced that due to the high oxygen availability from dissolved Hb, the microcirculation responds according to classic autoregulatory theory and limits oxygen delivery by restricting flow, thus increasing peripheral vascular resistance and blood pressure (Tsai *et al.* 1995, Johnson *et al.* 1995, Vandegriff and Winslow 1995).

NO-scavenging induces platelet activation (Olsen *et al.* 1996), and acellular Hb enhances the biological activity of endotoxins, rendering Hb solutions undesirable in the treatment of septic shock (Kaca *et al.* 1995). Intraperitoneal bleeding has been associated with the use of Hb solutions leading to severe colic. A common cause for these adverse reactions is related to the direct contact of the Hb molecule with the vascular tissue, a problem that in principle is solved by encapsulating Hb. This approach potentially shields the microcirculation from the biological activity or toxicity of Hb and Hb-related products, such as methemoglobin or released heme. Furthermore, the technology allows the co-encapsulation of chemical reagents or enzymes in vesicles and/or their embedding in the lipid bilayer.

Studies of phospholipid vesicles for application to drug delivery system have shown that they present a particular set of problems related to their effects on hemodynamics, saturation of reticuloendothelial system (RES) and complement activation. Polyethylene glycol (PEG) conjugated lipids and glycolipids, such as ganglioside GM_1, have been incorporated into the bilayer membrane to sterically stabilize the vesicles, evade the RES and prolong the circulation time (Allen and Cohn 1987, Woodle and Lasic 1992, Gabizon and Papahadjopoulos 1988). HbV have also been produced including these lipids, particularly GM_1 (Goins, Ligler and Rudolph 1994) however, circulatory retention was not increased probably due to the large dosage, which promptly saturated the RES. HbV incorporating synthetic oligosaccharide lipids had reduced viscosity and cryoprotection (Tsuchida and Takeoka 1995).

HbV with PEG-phosphatidylethanolamine (PEG-PE) exhibited reduced aggregation in the presence of water soluble polymers and had lower viscosity (Yoshioka 1991, Sakai *et al.* 1997). PEG-PE was also found to reduce the immunological responses to infectious challenges and to prolong circulation time (Zheng *et al.* 1993). A PEG-modified HbV (Neo Red Cells) has been produced by Terumo Co., Tokyo, Japan (Takahashi 1995). In general, preclinical tests yield stable cardiovascular systemic parameters and excellent oxygen transport properties when tested in hemorrhagic shock models and extracorporeal circulation (Usuba and Motoki 1995).

Acellular Hb solutions are homogeneous Newtonian fluids that exert physiological oncotic pressures. Conversely, HbV suspensions are non-Newtonian fluids, which like most particle suspensions, lack oncotic properties. Consequently, if HbV suspensions are used in large amounts they must be suspended in a plasma expanders that will provide the necessary oncotic effect. Since HbV interacts with water-soluble polymers, selection of the appropriate plasma expander is important since it will determine viscosity, circulatory fluid balance for the blood-HbV mixture and ultimately oxygen transport properties. In this Chapter we shall therefore discuss preparation technique, rheological characteristics and microhemodynamic behavior of PEG-HbV suspended in the clinically used 5% human serum albumin (HSA) solution in comparison with unmodified HbV.

8.2 Preparation Techniques of PEG-modified Hemoglobin Vesicles

Enclosure of hemoglobin in a lipid vesicle was first devised by Djordjevich and Miller (1980). Tsuchida developed a simplified technique that resolves many of the problems previously encountered in this process, such as Hb purification, particle size polydispersion, and low stability and encapsulation efficiency (Tsuchida and Takeoka 1995). This process uses concentrated stable HbCO and saturated phospholipids as starting materials, extrusion as a method for sizing, and decarbonylation. The characteristics of the resulting PEG-HbV suspension in 5% HSA are summarized in Table 1. Particle diameter is about 250 nm, and the weight ratio of the total amount of Hb to lipids, a parameter indicating the encapsulation efficiency, is 1.9, being the highest value reported for vesicles with a regulated vesicular size. MetHb and HbCO content of the HbV after the ligand exchange reaction is small, and oxygen affinity (P_{50}, pO_2 at which Hb is 50% saturated with oxygen) is controlled by co-encapsulating pyridoxal phosphate (PLP) or inositol hexaphosphate (IHP). MetHb formation is minimized by co-encapsulation of thiol derivatives with active oxygen scavengers and incorporation of tocopherol (Sakai *et al.* 1996, Takeoka *et al.* 1997).

Table 8.1 Chemical characteristics of PEG-HbV suspended in 5% HSA solution in comparison with human blood.

	PEG-HbV/HSA	**human blood**
Diameter (nm)	251± 87	ca. 8000
P_{50} (Torr)	34[a]	28
[Hb] (g/dl)	10	12-17
[Lipid] (g/dl)	5.26	1.8-2.5[b]
[Hb]/[Lipid] (g/g)	1.9	ca. 6.7[c]
MetHb (%)	< 3	< 0.5
HbCO (%)	< 2	< 5
Viscosity (cP at 358 s^{-1})	3.7	3 - 4
Osmolarity (mOsm)	300	ca. 300
Oncotic pressure (Torr)	ca. 20	ca. 25
pH at 37 °C	7.4	7.2 - 7.4
Density (g/cm^3)	1.0336	1.05
Hematocrit (%)	36[d]	40 - 54

[a]PLP/Hb = 3, controllable.
[b]Total cell membrane components.
[c]Weight ratio of Hb to total cell membrane components.
[d]Volume percentage of HbV particles.

Hb denaturation often generates insoluble components leading to increased viscosity and decreased filterability due to obstruction of pores. The purified HbCO solution contains no other proteins, and denaturation is suppressed with carbonylation (Sakai *et al.* 1993), insuring the maintenance of filterability during ultrafiltration up to 45 g/dl and extrusion. The extrusion method using filters with narrowly distributed pore size is used to obtain vesicles with uniform diameter. Although viability of this method for a large-scale production is controversial, it provides homogeneous particles. By contrast, the Microfluidizer process, which is more suitable for large-scale production, yields large amounts of small particles (< 150 nm) with small encapsulation volume and denaturated Hb due to direct exposure to high shear stress and temperatures.

Efficient oxygen transport and minimal side effects from lipids require the encapsulation of large amounts of Hb with a reduced amount of lipids. This is accomplished by exposing the HbV to high, controlled shear stress during extrusion which converts the large multilamellar HbV to smaller sized HbV with fewer lipid bilayers (Takeoka *et al.* 1996). In addition, negatively charged lipids are introduced to reduce the number of bilayers through electrostatic repulsion between bilayers. To accomplish this, the ionic concentration of the Hb solution is kept as low as possible (about 80 mOsm), since the electrostatic interaction is shielded by ionic strength, while the lipid membrane is strong enough to maintain the structure against 300 mOsm in the outer phase.

Hb concentration inside vesicles is determined by the pH of the solution. The isoelectric point (pI) of Hb is 7.0 at 25°C. Hb is negatively charged when pH is above 7.0, and electrostatic repulsion between Hb and the negatively charged bilayer membrane results in a low Hb encapsulation efficiency. Therefore, the solution pH is adjusted to be lower than the pI of the Hb but not much lower to avoid changes in oxygen affinity, Hb denaturation by direct interaction with lipids and metHb formation.

The number of lipid bilayers (lamellarity) decreases with increasing microviscosity of the bilayer membrane. The multilamellar vesicles are converted to smaller sized vesicles with lower lamellarity (1 - 2) by the shear stress during extrusion. When membrane fluidity is high, deformation of vesicles during extrusion occurs more easily even for lipid membranes with a high lamellarity, resulting in maintaining the high lamellarity. Therefore, lipids with a higher phase transition temperature are desirable (*e.g.,* 1,2-distearoyl-*sn*-glycero-3-phosphatidylcholine (DSPC), hydrogenated soy phosphatidylcholine (HSPC)) although this renders extrusion difficult because of the higher shear stress (and therefore higher extrusion pressure) required. These considerations led to the selection of lipids containing 1,2-dipalmitoyl-*sn*-glycero-3-phosphatidylcholine (DPPC) and 1,2-dipalmitoyl-*sn*-glycero-3-phosphatidylglycerol (DPPG).

The surface modifier 1,2-dipalmitoyl-*sn*-glycero-3-phosphatidylethanolamine-*N*-polyethylene glycol$_{5000}$ (PEG-DPPE) in aqueous solution is added to the HbV suspension after filtration sizing to attach PEG chains to the surface of the vesicles, and the hydrophobic fatty acid chains of PEG-DPPE become anchored into the outer surface of the HbV bilayer membrane. The incorporation ratio is more than 90% (Sakai *et al.* 1997) with no change in diameter or leakage of Hb. This allows direct comparison of the effect of surface modification with unmodified HbVs. Finally, using the high quantum yield of HbCO photodissociation, this is converted to HbO_2 by directing visible light onto the HbV liquid membrane under O_2 flow (Chung *et al.* 1995). The osmotic and oncotic pressures are controlled by replacing the outer phase with plasma expanders (HSA, starch, dextran) using ultracentrifugation or dialysis.

8.3 Rheological Properties of PEG-modified Hemoglobin Vesicles

The viscosity of the vesicular suspension of unmodified HbV dispersed in saline is 2.6 cP (Hb: 10 g/dl, Sakai *et al.* 1996). Dispersion in 5% HSA

(Bayer Co., Germany) to adjust colloidal osmotic pressure raises the viscosity of the HbV/HSA to 8.0 cP (measured with an oscillatory capillary rheometer, Anton Parr, Austria, shear rate 358 s^{-1}) with non-Newtonian behavior typical for particle suspensions, and results in remarkably higher viscosities at lower shear rates (Figure 8.1). In the case of the PEG-HbV/HSA, on the other hand, the viscosity is significantly reduced to 3.5 cP and is almost the same as that of human blood (3.7 cP) at all shear rates. The difference between PEG-HbV and the unmodified suspension is due to the formation of aggregates by the unmodified HbVs due to the molecular interaction of HSA with the vesicular surface, leading to increased viscosity. Conversely, surface modification of HbV with PEG chains suppresses HbV aggregation, leading to viscosity values similar to those of human blood. This mechanism was confirmed by optical microscopy showing the presence of flocculated aggregates when HbV was mixed with blood, which were absent in the case of PEG-HbV blood mixtures. Since red blood cells (RBCs) in either case were neither aggregated nor deformed, it appears that HbV and PEG-HbV do not interact with RBCs.

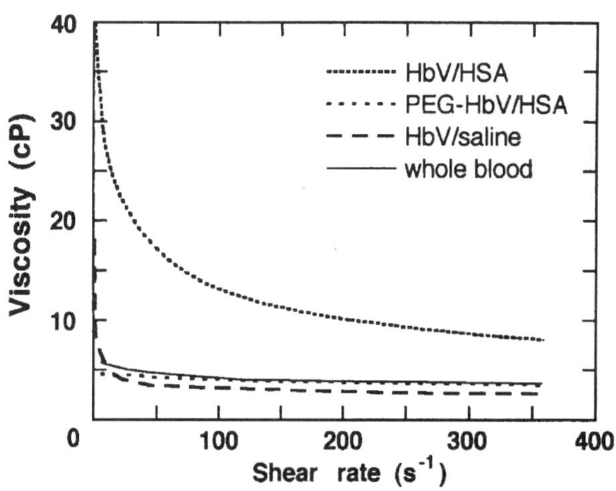

Figure 8.1. Shear rate dependence of the viscosities of PEG-HbV/HSA, HbV/HSA, HbV/saline, and human blood. Measured with a capillary rheometer (Anton Parr Co., *d:* 1.0 mm) at 37°C. Hb concentration of the suspensions (except blood) were adjusted to 10 g/dl.

Both PEG-HbV/HSA and HbV/HSA suspensions passed easily through Nucleopore membrane filters with pore sizes 0.4 - 8.0 μm without changes in vesicular size or Hb leakage. PEG-HbV/HSA permeates faster than unmodified HbV/HSA because PEG-HbV does not aggregate, and even though the HbV/HSA showed aggregation in the optical microscopy, the aggregates dissociated at higher shear rates.

Interaction between vesicles and HSA molecules induced aggregation, whereas quantitative analysis of adsorbed HSA did not indicate significant difference between PEG-HbV and HbV. It is probable that PEG chains prevent intervesicular contact and aggregation rather than HSA adsorption (Klibanov *et al.* 1991). The repulsive interaction between PEG-modified surfaces has been established by measuring the distance between membranes using x-ray diffraction (Needham, McIntosh and Lasic 1992) and steric hindrance was calculated using computer analysis (Torchilin *et al.* 1994). Since PEG chains do not completely cover the surface of the vesicles at the molar composition employed, HSA can pass through the PEG chain layers to the vesicular surface and be adsorbed; however, repulsion between PEG-modified vesicles, which are much larger than HSA, is the preponderant mechanism for overcoming the aggregating effects due to HSA adsorbed on the vesicle surface. This hypothesis is supported by the results of Harasym *et al.* (1995) who found that coupling of avidin onto PEG-modified phospholipid vesicles is not retarded, while aggregation during coupling is suppressed by PEG chains. This steric hindrance is a mechanism effective in preventing aggregation and contact with larger proteins, vesicles, and reticuloendothelial and endothelial cells.

8.4 Systemic and Microcirculatory Hemodynamics at Exchange Transfusion

8.4.1 Exchange transfusion in anesthetized Wistar rats

The oxygen transport capacity of PEG-HbV/HSA in comparison with unmodified HbV/HSA was evaluated by carrying out exchange transfusions to hematocrit (Hct) 5% in anesthetized Wistar rats (Kobayashi *et al.* 1997, Sakai *et al.* 1997). Abdominal aortic blood flow was higher in the PEG-HbV group than in the HbV group. pH and venous pO_2 in the PEG-HbV group tended to be higher than in the HbV group. The mean arterial pressure showed a slight transient increase at the first stage of hemodilution, which may be due to some form of immunological reaction related to phospholipid vesicle injection. Simultaneous thrombocytopenia was observed irrespective of PEG modification. This is explained as accumulation of platelet and vesicles in lung after complement activation (Miyamoto *et al.* 1988, Loughley *et al.* 1990, Rudolph 1995). The PEG-HbV group showed a significantly higher blood flow rate in the abdominal aorta ($\approx$ +50%) and lower total peripheral resistance with ($\approx$ -20%) than in the HbV group, effects attributed to the lower viscosity of the PEG-HbV/HSA. The HbV group was slightly hypoxic, while mixed venous pO_2 in the PEG-HbV group was significantly higher than in the HbV group. Tissue oxygen tensions measured by oxygen electrodes in the renal cortex and skeletal muscle for both groups decreased by about 70% from initial values and were significantly lower than control, although they were significantly higher than in animals who received only HSA.

8.4.2 Microcirculatory effects in conscious hamster dorsal skin-fold chamber

The microvascular effects of exchange transfusing PEG-HbV/HSA to 7% Hct were studied in conscious hamsters fitted with a dorsal skin-fold chamber. Microvascular hemodynamics and pO_2 in vessels and tissue were evaluated on-line using conventional microvascular methodology for the measurement of microscopic vessel hemodynamic parameters (Intaglietta and Tompkins 1973, Intaglietta, Silverman and Tompkins 1975, Torres Filho and Intaglietta 1993).

Male Syrian golden hamsters (55 - 85 g body weight [b.w.]) fitted with a dorsal skin-fold chamber were used in these investigations. Animals were anesthetized with sodium pentobarbital (50 mg/kg b.w., i.p.) prior to chamber implantation. The carotid artery and jugular vein were cannulated two or three days later using the same anesthesia. All experiments were performed after a recovery period of at least 24 hours. Preparations with signs of inflammation, edema, bleeding spots and no-flow states were excluded from further investigations. Inclusion criteria for systemic parameters were mean arterial blood pressure >85 mm Hg, hematocrit >45%, heart rate >350 beats/min, and systemic pO_2 >60 mm Hg.

Three groups of animals were exchange transfused with HSA, HbV/HSA, or PEG-HbV/HSA. Exchanges were carried out to 30%, 60% and 80% removal of the red blood cell mass. Five or eight animals were studied at each exchange level and transfusion group. All groups tolerated the exchanges and survived the experiments.

The HSA-transfused group showed a decrease in blood pressure and heart rate. The HbV groups had slightly higher values and a transient abnormal high value accompanied with arrhythmia, probably due to the higher flow resistance due to high viscosity. Normal blood pressure and blood gas parameters were observed for the PEG-HbV animals, including the group with 80% exchange (Figure 8.2). There was no vasoconstriction of arterioles in either vesicle group, while arterioles in the HSA-exchanged group constricted significantly. Microvascular flow decreased in all groups, the effect being particularly severe for both the HbV and HSA groups at 80% exchange. This effect is probably due to blood redistribution from the skin to vital organs consequent to vasoactivity in larger vessels not evident in this preparation.

All groups maintained functional capillary density (FCD) up to the 60% exchange. At the 80% exchange, the HSA group exhibited pathologically low values of FCD and microvascular blood flow velocity, probably due to wide spread vasoconstriction not reflected in the skin microcirculation. By contrast the PEG-HbV group showed the highest values for these parameters after exchange transfusion. Tissue pO_2 was lower than control for all groups, although the PEG-HbV group was consistently higher than the other groups.

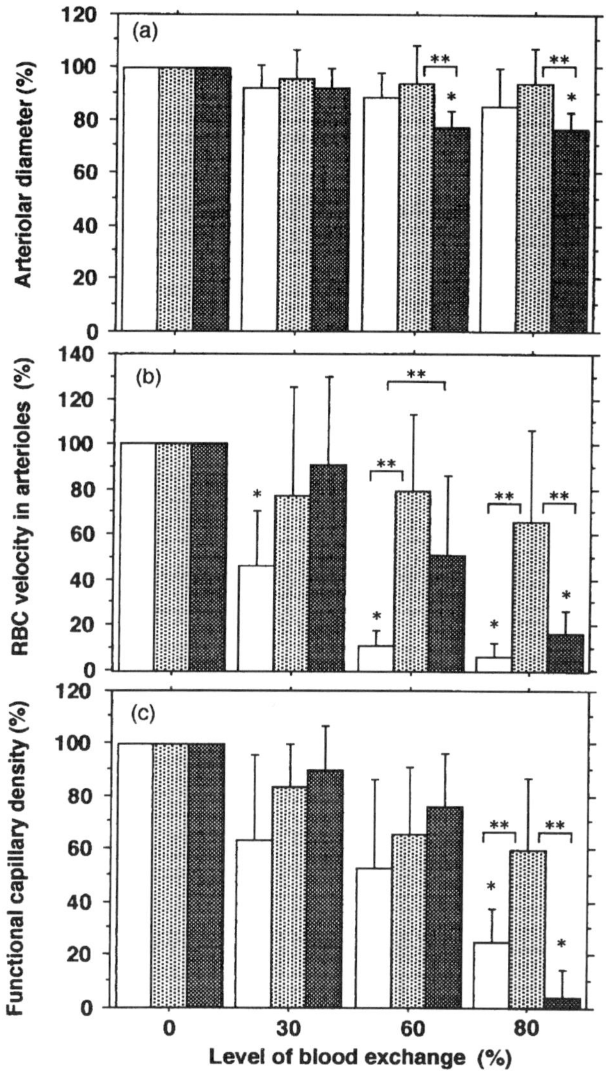

Figure 8.2. Representative microcirculatory parameters at each level of exchange transfusion with (white bar) HbV/HSA, (grey bar) PEG-HbV/HSA, and (black bar) HSA, using Syrian golden hamsters (n=5-8) fitted with dorsal skin-fold chambers. (a) changes in diameters of precapillary arterioles 40 - 60 μm in diameter; (b): changes in red blood cell velocities in the same arterioles; (c): changes in functional capillary densities. All the values are expressed as percentages of the initial values. *Statistical difference from the initial value ($p<0.05$) **Statistical difference within the groups ($p< 0.05$).

8.5 Summary and Assessment

These findings show that PEG modification significantly improves the performance of HbV. This result, not evident from the analysis of systemic parameters, showing stable hemodynamic conditions for both the PEG-modified and unmodified groups, becomes apparent when analyzing the corresponding microvascular responses.

Although exchange transfusion with PEG-HbV produces better microvascular conditions than unmodified HbV, the overall microvascular responses are not fully satisfactory since tissue oxygenation is deficient for both materials. This result may be related to rheological effects and autoregulatory responses. Unmodified HbV exhibit higher viscosity due to the formation of aggregates, which may hinder capillary perfusion leading to low tissue pO_2. Conversely, low viscosity associated with the PEG-modified vesicles probably causes a decrease of shear stress and the consequent reduction in the release of endothelial relaxing factors (Malek and Izumo 1995), inducing vasoconstriction, decreased capillary density and tissue pO_2.

These effects may in part be magnified by autoregulatory responses due to the greater availability of oxygen from vesicles when compared to RBCs. Furthermore, although oxygen affinity of both types of HbVs is nearly the same as for blood, the HbVs should show a faster oxygen uptake and release due to their smaller particle size (Vandegriff and Winslow 1995). Paradoxically, high oxygen availability at the arteriolar level may engage mechanisms designed to maintain arteriolar pO_2 at a preset level, a process leading to vasoconstriction superposed to the responses to non-optimal rheological properties.

In summary, PEG-HbV particles have been developed with stable and uniform characteristics that show improved microvascular responses to exchange transfusion when compared with unmodified vesicles. The availability of this material provides a unique opportunity for exploring, in a systematic basis, variables such as viscosity, oxygen carrying capacity, and oxygen affinity that are critical in the design of oxygen carrying blood replacement fluids (Tsai, Kerger and Intaglietta 1995, 1996, Intaglietta, Johnson and Winslow 1996) that support tissue oxygenation.

8.6 Acknowledgments

This work has been supported in part by USPHS/NHLBI Program project No. HL48018 and Grants-in-Aid for Scientific Research from the Ministry of Education, Science, Sport and Culture, Japan (No. 07508005). H. Sakai is an Overseas Research Fellow of the Japan Society for the Promotion of Science.

8.7 References

Allen, T.M., and A. Cohn. Large unilamellar liposomes with low uptake into the reticuloendothelial system. *FEBS Lett.* 223: 42-46, 1987.

Chung, J.E., K. Hamada, H. Sakai, S. Takeoka, and E. Tsuchida. Ligand exchange reaction of carbonylhemoglobin to oxyhemoglobin in a hemoglobin liquid membrane. *Nippon Kagaku Kaishi* 2: 123-127, 1995.

Djordjevich, L., and I.F. Miller. Synthetic erythrocytes from lipid encapsulated hemoglobin. *Exp. Hemat.* 8: 584-592, 1980.

Gabizon, A., and D. Papahadjopoulos. Liposome formulations with prolonged circulation time in blood and enhanced uptake by tumors. *Proc. Natl. Acad. Sci. USA* 85: 6949-6953, 1988.

Goins, B., F.S. Ligler, and A.S. Rudolph. Inclusion of ganglioside GM_1 into liposome encapsulated hemoglobin does not extend circulation persistence at clinically relevant doses. *Artif. Cells, Blood Substitutes, Immobil. Biotech.* 22: 9-25, 1994.

Harasym, T.O., P. Tardi, S.A. Longman, S.M. Ansell, M.B. Bally, R.P. Cullis, and L.S. Choi. Poly(ethylene glycol)-modified phospholipid prevent aggregation during covalent conjugation of proteins to liposomes. *Bioconjugate Chem.* 6: 1043-1802, 1995.

Intaglietta, M., P.C. Johnson, and R.M. Winslow. Microvascular and tissue oxygen distribution. *Cardiovasc. Res.* 32: 632-643, 1996.

Intaglietta, M., N.R. Silverman, and W.R. Tompkins. Capillary flow velocity measurements *in vivo* and *in situ* by television methods. *Microvasc. Res.* 10: 165-179, 1975.

Intaglietta, M., and W.R. Tompkins. Microvascular measurements by video image shearing and splitting. *Microvasc. Res.* 5: 309-312, 1973.

Johnson, P.C., K. Richmond, R.D. Shonat, A. Toth, M. Pal, M.E. Tischler, and R.M. Lynch. Oxygen delivery regulation: Implications for blood substitutes. In *Blood Substitutes: Physiological Basis of Efficacy* (R.M. Winslow, K.D. Vandegriff, and M. Intaglietta, eds.). Boston: Birkhäuser, 1995, pp. 175-186.

Kaca, W., R.I. Roth, K.D. Vandegriff, G.C. Chen, F.A. Kuypers, R.M. Winslow, and J. Levin. Effects of bacterial endotoxin on human cross-linked and native hemoglobins. *Biochemistry* 34: 11186-11185, 1995.

Klibanov, A., K. Maruyama, A.M. Beckerleg, V.P. Torchilin, and L. Huang. Activity of amphipathic poly(ethylene glycol) 5000 to prolong the circulation time of liposomes depends on the liposome size and its unfavorable for immunoliposome binding to target. *Biochim. Biophys. Acta* 1062: 142-148, 1991.

Kobayashi, K., Y. Izumi, A. Yoshizu, H. Horinouchi, S.I. Park, H. Sakai, S. Takeoka, H. Nishide, and E. Tsuchida. The oxygen carrying capability of hemoglobin vesicles evaluated in rat exchange transfusion models. *Artif. Cells, Blood Substitutes, Immobil. Biotech.* 1997 (in press).

Loughley, H.C., M.B. Bally, L.W. Reihish, and P.R. Cullis. The binding of phosphatidylglycerol liposomes to rat platelets is mediated by complement. *Thromb. Haemostas.* 64: 172-176, 1990.

Malek, A.M., and S. Izumo. Control of endothelial cell gene expression by flow. *J. Biomechanics.* 28: 1515-1528, 1995.

Miyamoto, K., E. Schultz, T. Heath, M.D. Mitchell, K.H. Albertine, and N.C. Staub. Pulmonary intravascular macrophages and hemodynamic effects of liposomes in sheep. *J. Appl. Physiol.* 64: 1143-1152, 1988.

Palmer, R.M.J., A.G. Ferrige, and S. Moncada. Nitric oxide release accounts for the biological activity of endothelium-derived relaxing factor, *Nature* 327: 524-526, 1987.

Needham, D., T.J. McIntosh, and D.D. Lasic. Repulsive interactions and mechanical stability of polymer-grafted lipid membranes. *Biochem. Biophys. Acta* 1108: 40-48, 1992.

Olsen, S.B., D.B. Tang, M.R. Jackson, E.R. Gomez, B. Ayala, and B.M. Alving. Enhancement of platelet deposition by cross-linked hemoglobin in a rat carotid endarterectomy model. *Circulation* 93: 327-332, 1996.

Rohlfs, R.J., and K.D. Vandegriff. Non-phospholipid liposomes: a novel method for the preparation of hemoglobin containing lipid vesicles. In *Blood Substitutes: New Challenges* (R.M. Winslow, K.D. Vandegriff, and M. Intaglietta, eds.). Boston: Birkhäuser, 1996, pp. 163-184.

Rudolph, A.S. Encapsulation of hemoglobin in liposomes. In *Blood Substitutes: Physiological Basis of Efficacy* (R.M. Winslow, K.D. Vandegriff, and M. Intaglietta, eds.). Boston: Birkhäuser, 1995, pp. 90-104.

Sakai, H., K. Hamada, S. Takeoka, H. Nishide, and E. Tsuchida. Physical characteristics of hemoglobin vesicles as red cell substitutes. *Biotechnol. Progress* 12: 119-125, 1996.

Sakai, H., S. Takeoka, S.I. Park, T. Kose, Y. Izumi, A. Yoshizu, H. Nishide, K. Kobayashi, and E. Tsuchida. Surface-modification of hemoglobin vesicles with polyethyleneglycol and effects on aggregation, viscosity, and blood flow during 90%-exchange transfusion in anesthetized rats. *Bioconjugate Chem.* 8: 23-30, 1997.

Sakai, H., S. Takeoka, H. Yokohama, Y. Seino, H. Nishide, and E. Tsuchida. Purification of concentrated hemoglobin using organic solvent and heat treatment. *Protein Expression Purif.* 4: 563-569, 1993.

Takahashi, A. Characterization of neo red cells (NRCs), their function safety *in vivo* tests. *Artif. Cells, Blood Substit., Immobil. Biotech.* 23: 347-254, 1995.

Takeoka, S., T. Ohgushi, T. Ohmori, K. Terase, H. Nishide, and E. Tsuchida. Layer controlled hemoglobin vesicles by interaction of hemoglobin with phospholipid assembly. *Langmuir* 12: 119-125, 1996.

Takeoka, S., T. Ohgushi, H. Sakai, T. Kose, H. Nishide, E. Tsuchida. Construction of artificial methemoglobin reduction systems in Hb vesicles. *Artif. Cells, Blood Substit., Immobil. Biotech.* 25: 31-41, 1997.

Torchilin, V.P., V.G. Omelyaneko, M.I. Papisov, A.A. Bogdanov Jr, V.S. Trubetskoy, J.N. Herron, and C.A. Gentry. Poly(ethylene glycol) on the liposome surface: on the mechanism of polymer-coated liposome longevity. *Biochim. Biophys. Acta* 1195: 11-20, 1994.

Torres Filho, I.P., M. Intaglietta. Microvascular PO_2 measurements by phosphorescence decay method. *Am. J. Physiol.* 265*(Heart. Circ. Physiol.* 34*)*: H1434-H1438, 1993.

Tsai, A. G., H. Kerger, and M. Intaglietta. Microcirculatory consequences of blood substitution with αα-hemoglobin. In *Blood Substitutes: Physiological Basis of Efficacy* (R.M. Winslow, K.D. Vandegriff, and M. Intaglietta, eds.). Boston: Birkhäuser, 1995, pp. 155-174.

Tsai, A. G., H. Kerger, and M. Intaglietta. Microvascular oxygen distribution: effects due to free hemoglobin in plasma. In *Blood Substitutes: New Challenges* (R.M. Winslow, K.D. Vandegriff, and M. Intaglietta, eds.). Boston: Birkhäuser, 1996, pp. 124-131.

Tsuchida, E. Introduction: overview and perspective. In *Artificial Red Cells* (E. Tsuchida, ed.). New York: John Wiley and Sons, 1995, pp. 1-20.

Tsuchida, E., and S. Takeoka. Stabilized hemoglobin vesicles. In *Artificial Red Cells* (E. Tsuchida, ed.). New York: John Wiley and Sons, 1995, pp. 35-64.

Usuba, A., and R. Motoki. Safety and efficacy of encapsulated hemoglobin in hemorrhagic shock. In *Artificial Red Cells* (E. Tsuchida, ed.). New York: John Wiley and Sons, 1995, pp. 65-92.

Vandegriff, K.D., and R.M. Winslow. A theoretical analysis of oxygen transport: a new strategy for the design of hemoglobin-based red cell substitutes. In *Blood Substitutes: Physiological Basis of Efficacy* (R.M. Winslow, K.D. Vandegriff, and M. Intaglietta, eds.) Boston: Birkhäuser, 1995, pp. 143-154.

Winslow, R.M. Blood substitutes: a moving target. *Nature Med.* 1: 1212-1215, 1995.

Woodle, M.C., and D.D. Lasic. Sterically stabilized liposomes. *Biochim. Biophys. Acta* 1113: 171-199, 1992.

Yoshioka, H. Surface modification of haemoglobin-containing liposomes with polyethylene glycol prevents liposome aggregation in blood plasma. *Biomaterials* 12: 861-864, 1991.

Zheng, S., R. Beissinger, R.L. Sherwood, D.L. McCormick, D.D. Lasic, and F.J. Martin. Liposome-encapsulated hemoglobin: a red blood cell substitute. *J. Liposome Res.* 3: 575-588, 1993.

8.8 Discussion

Cokelet: This is a tremendous amount of work, and I'd hate to see any information that you've worked so hard to get to be lost, so I'd like to ask a few questions. Have you determined the heterogeneity of things such as red-cell flux or hematocrit distribution in A4 vessels as a function of whether or not you have the pegylated vesicles *versus* control blood?

Sakai: Up to A4, it's difficult to measure the hematocrit, so I don't observe it, but in the capillaries, it is quite obvious that some capillaries are rich in the red blood cells, some are not. So there is a distribution of the red blood cells.

Cokelet: Have you quantified the heterogeneity in the capillaries? That would be very useful to know for a lot of different reasons. I think you have the data.

Torchilin: So you showed the very nice differences between pegylated and non-pegylated stuff. I do have several small experimental questions. Many people are trying to incorporate PEG-PE into prepared liposomes; they never succeeded because the transfer of PEG from micelles to liposomes is very low. The only mechanism how something can be incorporated into liposomes from outside is so-called free vacancy mechanism, and the free vacancy is very rare especially for liposomes which are around 200 nm. It might exist in very small liposomes which lie below 70 nm because of very high tension in the inner bilayer and cracks which appear in the outer bilayer. This was shown by Lee Huang that there is incorporation of stuff into these cracks, but for 200 nm, people were unable to incorporate PEG-PE from outside. So my question No. 1 is what was the ratio between liposomes and PEG which you incubated in the same solution? What was the molar ratio?

Sakai: About the incorporation ratio, you mean?

Torchilin: No, but first, how you incorporated it. You had liposomes, and then you added to the same solution PEG with a folded tail, so how much polymer was there per mole of lipids, approximately?

Sakai: This reaction is very simple, and we just mixed the polyethylene glycol lipid with the HbV suspension.

Torchilin: Yes, this is what confused me. If you just mix, it doesn't work, and this was a problem which really exists all those times. This is why people always add PEG-PE into the lipid mixture before the liposome preparation.

Sakai: Yes. We have to encapsulate a large amount of hemoglobin, and if there is crowding of the PEG chains, and if it is present inside the vesicles, the volume of the inside is minimized. So, our concept is just to modify the outer surface of the vesicle; it is very important. And, we add a certain amount of PEG lipid, and more than 90% of PEG lipid is completely inserted into the bilayer membrane.

Torchilin: But you know this from NMR studies. My question is (and I did it, so I know it), if you just mix PEG-PE micelles the liposomes make and the NMR spectrum, you'll get the same picture like you get. How do you differentiate between the polymer which is in micelle and in liposome?

Sakai: After the mixture, we washed. There may be some that are not incorporated, but they are washed out.

Torchilin: Ah ha. Still you have some stuff not incorporated, and you washed it away?

Sakai: Yes.

Torchilin: Okay, thank you.

Phillips: So, you're just using 1% PEG incorporated. Is there any reason that you haven't tried larger amounts of PEG to possibly increase the circulation longer?

Sakai: Of course, we can control the PEG modification, and we decided this value from the rheological point of view. Maybe there is optimal conditions, for example, for the prevention of complement activation, or something else. We just decided on this value. And this was found by Dr. Takeoka that we can minimize PEG modification to obtain the same viscosity. So from the rheological point of view, we can minimize the PEG modification.

Phillips: And, what's your osmotic pressure?

Sakai: We have never measured the osmotic pressure of the vesicle itself, but it is suspended in HSA, so maybe you can imagine the oncotic pressure. And the total concentration of PEG chain in the suspension is less than 1%, so the contribution of the PEG chain to oncotic pressure is very small I think.

Osmotic pressure may be very important as you suggested. Some studies done by the Navy have shown that hypertonic saline makes liposome-encapsulated hemoglobin effective in the microcirculation.

The advantage of our product is that we can control the outer suspending media, so we can regulate the oncotic pressure at any value, so the PEG modification is not there.

Phillips: Yes, it's not difficult, but that's something that we have to do.

Chapter 9

Hemoglobin Oxygen Affinity and the Design of Red Cell Substitutes

Robert M. Winslow, M.D and Kim D. Vandegriff, Ph.D.

ABSTRACT

A model is described for evaluating a number of properties of cell-free oxygen carriers with regard to their potential to produce autoregulatory vasoactivity in arterioles. The model is based on the Krogh cylinder, an idealized segment of vessel. It is unique because it "maps" the regulatory region of the arterioles - the precapillary segment which senses O_2 supply and controls local vascular tone. Through a detailed analysis of the shape and position of oxygen equilibrium curves, the amount of O_2 delivered to this sensitive region is analyzed as a function of diffusion, hemoglobin concentration, and P50. The results support the emerging general theory that cell-free oxygen carriers may overcome a diffusive limitation to O_2 delivery to tissue, resulting in an over-supply of O_2 to regulatory arterioles, leading to local vasoactivity. The model predicts that two potential strategies to overcome this limitation are to lower P50 and to lower the oxygen carrying capacity of the blood.

9.1 Introduction

9.1.1 Physiological importance of blood oxygen affinity

Reduced oxygen affinity is a goal of chemical modification of hemoglobin so deeply ingrained in the design of a "blood substitute" that it is hardly questioned (Winslow 1992). The source of this nearly universal assumption is, oddly enough, the high mountains. In 1944 Alberto Hurtado and his colleagues published a report from Morococha, Peru (4,300 m), in which they claimed that the oxygen equilibrium curve of blood samples collected from the miners was shifted to the right (lower oxygen affinity, higher P50) compared to sea level controls (Aste-Salezar and Hurtado 1944). This finding made its way into such prestigious publications as the Handbook of Physiology (Hurtado 1964) and has become a staple of physiology textbooks since that time.

High altitude natives seem an excellent population in which to study the importance of the apparently tightly regulated P50 value since classical physiology has assigned an adaptive role to P50 in such subjects. In a personal conversation with Dr. Hurtado in Lima shortly before his death in 1978, he described the tedious process of collecting samples of blood in Morococha, transporting them to Lima by car, and then performing analyses using the van Slyke apparatus (the studies were done before the advent of the Clark glass oxygen electrode). The work was also done before the appreciation of the role of intracellular 2,3-DPG in the modulation of oxygen affinity, and, in particular, of the fact that intracellular metabolites change rapidly in the minutes and hours after blood is taken from the body. Hurtado described 14 different assumptions which led to "corrections" applied to the data in order to arrive at what he called a "standard" OEC. By his definition, a standard OEC is one measured at pH 7.4, PCO_2 40 Torr, and 37°C. He reported a mean P50 at Morococha of 26.91 ± 0.23 mm Hg (n=30) and at sea level 24.6 ± 0.15 mm Hg, a net right-shift in the high altitude natives of 2.24 mm Hg (Hurtado 1964).

These results were important for Peruvian as well as international science in the 1940's. Hurtado's work had been funded by the U.S. Air Force and he and his colleagues were eager to provide information that would be useful to the war effort but, even more than that, information that would place Peru squarely on the map in regard to high altitude and oxygen transport physiology. Thus it was very important to perpetuate the notion that high altitude natives were specially "adapted" to their high altitude environment and, furthermore, that much more research would need to be done to understand the full mechanisms and implications of this adaptation.

In fact, Hurtado's findings ran counter to predominant physiologic thinking of the time. For example, Joseph Barcroft, after a visit to Morococha, observed that the human fetus exists essentially on the summit of Mt. Everest, since its blood PO_2 is reduced to about the same level (Barcroft *et al.* 1923). He knew that fetal blood has increased oxygen affinity (reduced P50) and assumed that this was essential in promoting the efficient transport of O_2 across the placenta. Barcroft extrapolated the concepts to the high altitude environment and speculated that higher affinity, not lower, would be advantageous when oxygen is in short supply.

The discovery of the interaction of 2,3-DPG with hemoglobin further strengthened the Hurtado position. Chanutin and Curnish (1967) and Benesch and Benesch (1969) reported the strong allosteric interaction of 2,3-DPG with hemoglobin. A number of workers, including Lenfant and his colleagues (1971), then showed that intracellular 2,3-DPG rises with progressive altitude in natives and the picture seemed complete: 2,3-

DPG shifts the OEC to the right, facilitating tissue oxygenation. The 2,3-DPG data also completed the analysis of the mechanisms that shift the OEC from its position for pure hemoglobin to its position within the red blood cell: there are only three effectors, H^+, CO_2, and 2,3-DPG (all other effectors, such as ATP, in aggregate play a very small additional role).

Our own studies in Morococha were done in 1978-1980 in the same laboratory in which Hurtado had worked earlier. However, by 1978 it was possible to install modern equipment in the laboratory, including a blood gas instrument, a microprocessor-based computer, and a new instrument that was capable of recording the whole blood OEC at controlled pH, PCO_2 and temperature within minutes of obtaining the sample using a modern glass PO_2 electrode. We also moved a sophisticated Zeiss spectrophotometer to the mountain laboratory for assays of red cell 2,3-DPG. We made such measurements in over 50 residents of Morococha (4,300 m altitude) and later in an additional 100 subjects of Cerro de Pasco (4,200 m altitude) (Winslow and Monge 1987). We found that, indeed, 2,3-DPG is elevated in the blood of natives, shifting Hurtado's "standard" OEC to the right. But analysis of arterial samples taken from the same subjects showed them to be in a state of chronic respiratory alkalosis: pH values were high and PCO_2 low compared to sea-level controls (Figure 9.1). The mean *in vivo* P50 at Morococha is significantly higher than in sea level controls ($P < 0.005$), but the range of values is

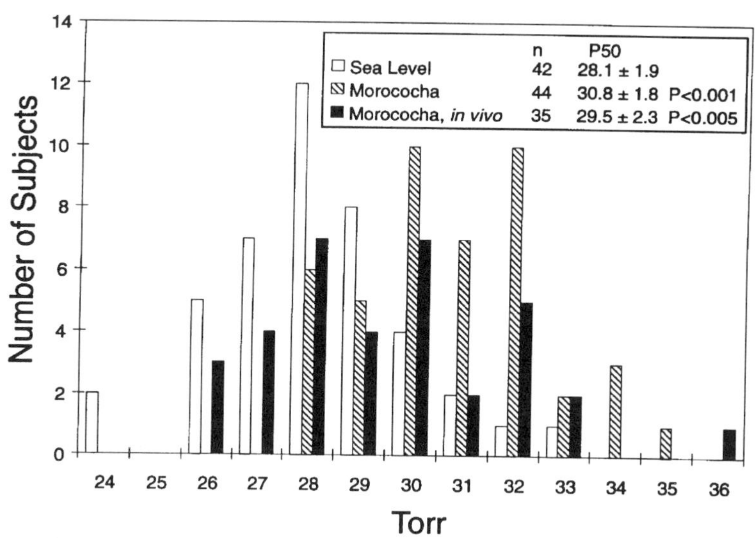

Figure 9.1. Distribution of "*in vivo*" P50 values in sea level and high altitude natives. Note that there is considerable overlap. Only 2 of 35 altitude residents have P50's above the sea level range, and only 7 of the sea level values falls below the altitude range. The mean of the in vivo values for the altitude residents is significantly lower than the mean of the uncorrected P50's because the high-altitude natives had pCO_2's lower and pH's higher than the sea level controls.

broad: only 2/35 Morococha residents had P50's that fell above the sea level range. Similarly, only 7/42 sea level residents had P50 values which fell below the Morococha *in vivo* range. Our conclusion was that P50 is probably not a major component of adaptation in high altitude natives.

The range of P50 values, both at sea level and altitude, was an unanticipated result, but the instrument we had developed jointly at the NIH and the University of Milan was highly accurate and reproducible (Winslow *et al.* 1977). We found, for example, that "normal" sea level P50's ranged from 24 to 33 Torr and "normal" altitude P50's from 26 to 36 Torr (Figure 9.1). We speculated, therefore, that individuals at either end of the P50 spectrum might be advantaged or disadvantaged in some subtle way in regard to oxygen transport. We initiated a series of tests, again in high altitude natives, to assess oxygen transport function under the stress of cycle ergometry to see if there was a difference in performance between subjects with high *versus* low P50 (Winslow and Monge 1987). In the end, there was no discernible difference. In fact, there was no significant difference between subjects with high or low hemoglobin concentrations or between subjects native to the Andes *versus* Himalayas in regard to blood P50. We carried out additional studies on animals native to either sea level or altitude and found examples in which the P50 is lower at altitude and ones in which it is higher. We studied sheep and goats especially carefully because these animals have a genetic mechanism whereby hypoxia induces a structurally different hemoglobin β chain to be produced. Conventional thinking (Huisman and Kitchens 1968) had suggested that this event reduced oxygen affinity, a presumed beneficial effect. In fact, our studies showed that *in vivo*, the P50 did not change much when this switch occurred, but that there was a significant difference in CO_2 transport (Winslow *et al.* 1989).

If a P50 shift is not an adaptive mechanism in altitude natives, perhaps it plays a more important role in sojourners - sea level residents acutely exposed to altitude. West and Wagner (1981) had shown that uptake of oxygen in the lung could be limited by diffusion when alveolar PO_2 is low or when pulmonary blood flow (cardiac output) is high. Based on our work with human blood under physiological conditions, it was possible to calculate the magnitude of the effect a shift in P50 would have on pulmonary O_2 uptake (Figure 9.2). Our prediction was that under extremely low ambient PO_2, lower P50 would facilitate O_2 uptake in the lung, as had been predicted by Barcroft, and that as the work level increases ($\dot{V}O_2$), this effect would become even more important (Winslow 1988) .

The predictions were confirmed in 1981 when we set up a laboratory above the Khumbu ice fall below the summit of Mt. Everest at approximately 6,300 m above sea level. There we collected blood samples from climbers on their way to and, in one case, just after reaching the summit at 8,800 m. We also collected blood samples from the same subjects at intermediate altitudes. We found that up to an altitude of approximately 5,400 m the rise in 2,3-DPG and respiratory alkalosis are essentially offsetting, in agreement with our previous studies in the Andes (Table 9.1).

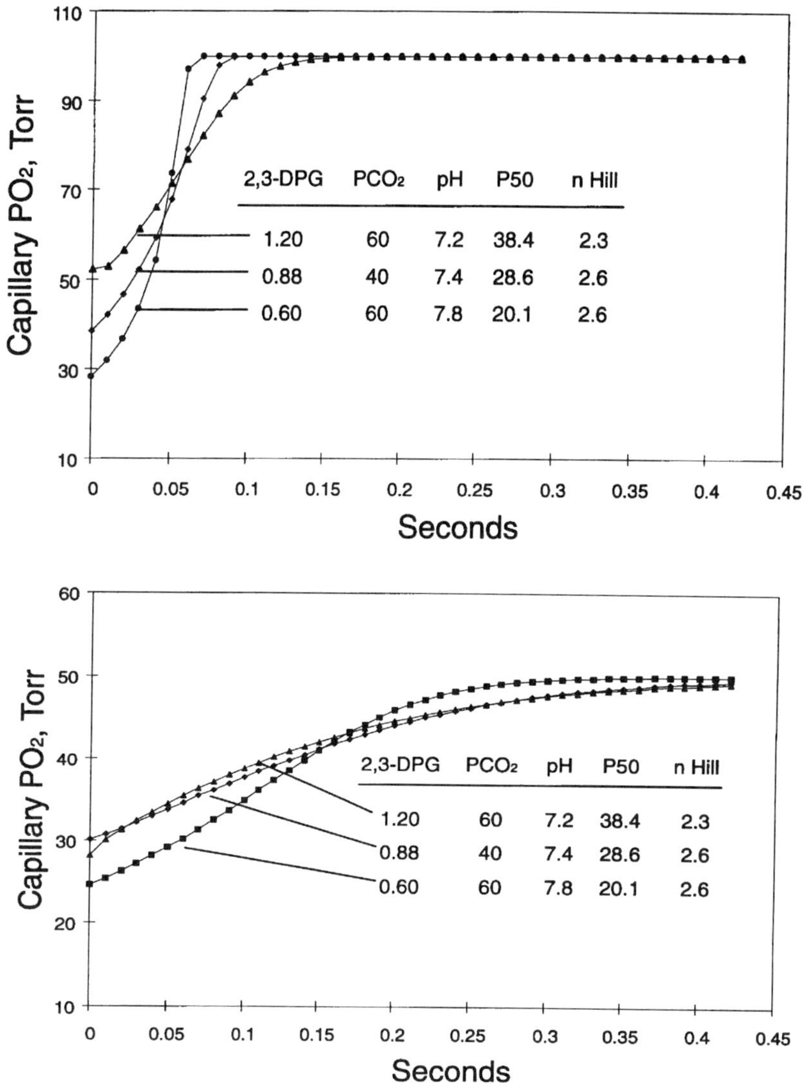

Figure 9.2. The effect of P50 shifts on uptake of O_2 in the lung. (A), normal sea level alveolar PO_2; (B), alveolar PO_2 corresponding to approximately 15,000 feet above sea level. At sea level, a rise in P50 is predicted to raise mixed venous PO_2 but increase the time required to oxygenate in the lung. Lower P50 decreases the mixed venous PO_2 but shortens the time for oxygenation. At altitude, increasing P50 has almost no effect, while decreasing the P50 again lowers mixed venous PO_2 but provides a higher end-capillary PO_2.

Table 9.1 Blood oxygen affinity at altitude

Location	pH	no. subjects	2,3-DPG/Hb M/M	$PaCO_2$ Torr	PaO_2 Torr	$P50_{7.4}$ Torr	$P50_{in\ vivo}$ Torr	SaO_2
Sea Level	7.399	18	0.84	40.0	90.0	28.1	28.1	0.95
6,300 m	7.467	14	1.04	18.4	39.1	29.8	27.6	0.71
8,050 m	7.552	2	1.18	12.8		29.6	24.9	
8,848 m	7.780	1		7.7	28.0	27.4	19.4	0.72

Adapted from Winslow, Samaja and West (1984).

However, above that altitude, the rise in 2,3-DPG is less significant than alkalosis. The net result is that at extreme altitude the P50 actually drops to about 19 Torr (a striking finding, since it is exactly the P50 of fetal blood - thus the relevance of Barcroft's remark). Analysis of these data by West and his colleagues has shown that without this marked increase in oxygen affinity, because pulmonary oxygen uptake is severely diffusion-limited, Everest would never have been climbed without supplemental oxygen (West *et al.* 1983).

All of the studies summarized above led to the general conclusion that the O_2 transport process is highly autoregulated. That is, changes in any of the links in the oxygen transport chain (ventilation, diffusion, hemoglobin concentration, oxygen affinity, cardiac output, or perfusion) can be compensated by changes in one or more of the other links. The net result is that autoregulation makes estimation of the relative importance of any one of the components of O_2 transport difficult.

9.1.2 Autoregulation of tissue oxygen supply

Autoregulation is the process whereby the delivery of O_2 to tissues is matched to demand. Thus, autoregulation can be considered to be a balance between blood flow and O_2 extraction (Shepherd *et al.* 1973) (Figure 9.3). The mechanisms which ensure autoregulation involve both central nervous and peripheral components. The central nervous mechanisms are comprised of the control of ventilation, hypoxic ventilatory responses, and carotid body reflexes. Peripheral mechanisms are the result of local metabolic controls and have been studied extensively in denervated animals. In such preparations when blood pressure is decreased, oxygen extraction increases. The oxygen extraction ratio (OER) is the fraction of O_2 that is removed from blood on a passage from the arterial to venous circulation and is defined as

$$1. \quad OER = \frac{C(a-v)O_2}{CaO_2}$$

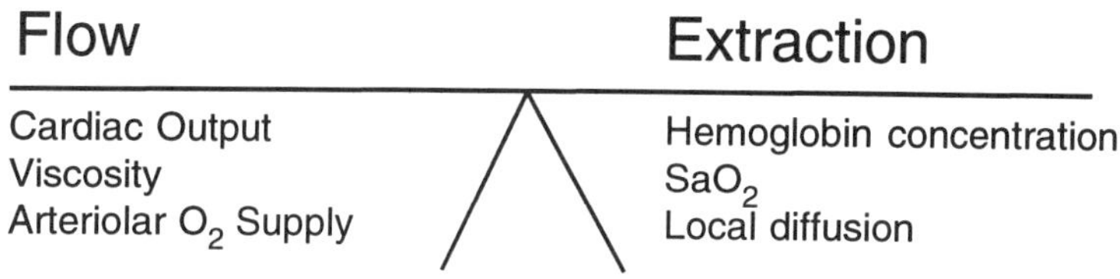

Figure 9.3. Autoregulation is a balance between blood flow and extraction of oxygen. The major determinants of each are shown.

Arterial O_2 content (CaO_2), venous O_2 content (CvO_2) and their difference ($C(a\text{-}v)O_2$) are determined predominantly by the product of the hemoglobin concentration and fractional saturation, because normally approximately 97% of blood O_2 is carried bound to hemoglobin, the remaining O_2 being physically dissolved in plasma.

As an example of an autoregulation experiment. Shepherd *et al.* (1973) studied decapitated dogs in which blood pressure was maintained by infusion of epinephrine. When the blood pressure was lowered by either decreasing the epinephrine infusion or reducing the level of venous blood return to the heart, cardiac output fell precipitously to about 60% of its control value. At the same time, the extraction of O_2 in the circulation increased by a comparable amount, so that tissue oxygen consumption ($\dot{V}O_2$) was preserved. The authors concluded that this response could not have been mediated by any nervous reflex and therefore must have a metabolic basis, presumably linked to the supply of oxygen.

The subject of autoregulation was reviewed recently by Johnson *et al.* in a previous chapter in this series (1995). These authors pointed out that local regulatory mechanisms are in place to sense both too little and too much oxygen delivery to tissues and that vasoconstriction could result from excessive local oxygen supply. The exact mechanisms for this control are still not completely understood but could be mediated by the release of vasoactive substances such as prostaglandins (Messina . Johnson *et al.* stressed that blood substitutes that elevate O_2 availability at the arteriolar level could cause vasoconstriction, reduce blood flow, and, paradoxically, decrease oxygen delivery to tissue.

Recently, Tsai, Kerger and Intaglietta (1996) have suggested that the A2/A3 arterioles are the likely site of control of local flow in the microcirculation of the hamster skin-fold preparation (see Figure 9.4). The vessels at this level are richly innervated, and direct PO_2 measurements have shown values of approximately 35 to 45 Torr. Interestingly, blood oxygen equilibrium curve which steepens significantly as O_2 is unloaded to tissues (Figure 9.4, lower panel). This combination of a discreet segment of arterioles and a steep slope of the OEC suggests a sensitive control mechanism: small changes in PO_2 could result in important changes in local blood flow.

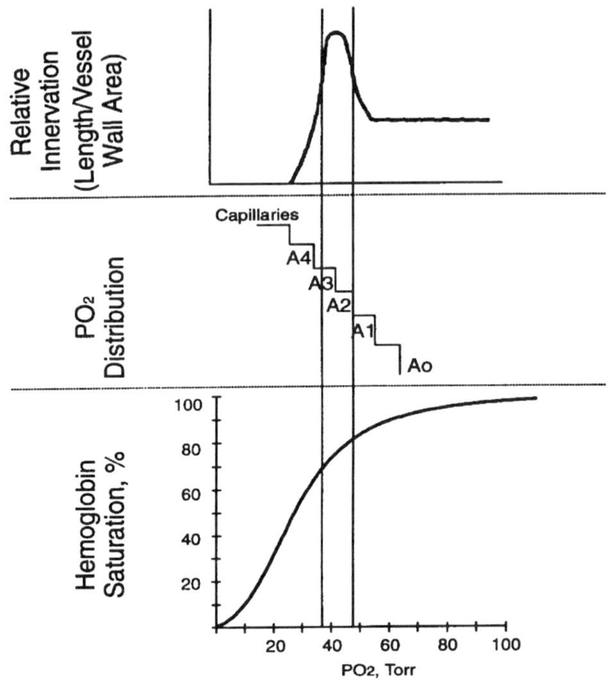

Figure 9.4. The location of the oxygen regulatory segments in the arteriolar vessels. The greatest innervation occurs at the A2/A3 level, corresponding to PO_2 between 35 and 45 Torr (Tsai, Kerger and Intaglietta 1996).

This hypothesis becomes more intriguing when one considers the proposal by Homer, Weathersby and Kiesow (1981) and Federspiel and Popel (1986) that the presence of cell-free hemoglobin could augment the delivery of oxygen to tissues because of improved local diffusion of oxygen. That is, because the distance for diffusion from hemoglobin to tissue sites and the surface area for diffusion are both increased, O_2 availability could be increased. We have previously proposed that this combination of events could, paradoxically, lead to decreased tissue oxygenation (Vandegriff and Winslow 1995) and that the rational design of a cell-free oxygen carrier must take such considerations into account.

Intaglietta and his coworkers have discussed this new hypothesis from the standpoint of the rheologic properties of cell-free oxygen carriers, suggesting that if O_2 availability is increased, increasing viscosity or decreasing oxygen capacity is necessary to offset the potential vasoconstrictive effect that would result (Tsai, Kerger and Intaglietta 1996). In this chapter, we wish to examine the theoretical consequences of altering of the shape and position of the hemoglobin oxygen dissociation curve on local O_2 supply.

9.2 A model for the role of O_2 affinity in tissue oxygenation

The ability to model the detailed shape of the OEC (Winslow, Samaja and West 1984) and the recent description of the distribution of PO_2 in the microcirculation (Tsai, Kerger and Intaglietta 1996) provide the basis for useful calculations of the role of P50 and other parameters of O_2 delivery on local tissue oxygenation.

9.2.1 Krogh cylinder

The familiar Krogh cylinder is shown in Figure 9.5, where blood flow is from left to right. Oxygen enters and exits by convection (flow) and also by diffusion. The model will not consider entry of O_2 into the cylinder by diffusion from vessels with higher PO_2, but this is known to occur (Ellsworth and Pittman 1990). Thus, the mass balance calculations to be presented consider only input by convection and exit of O_2 by convection and diffusion.

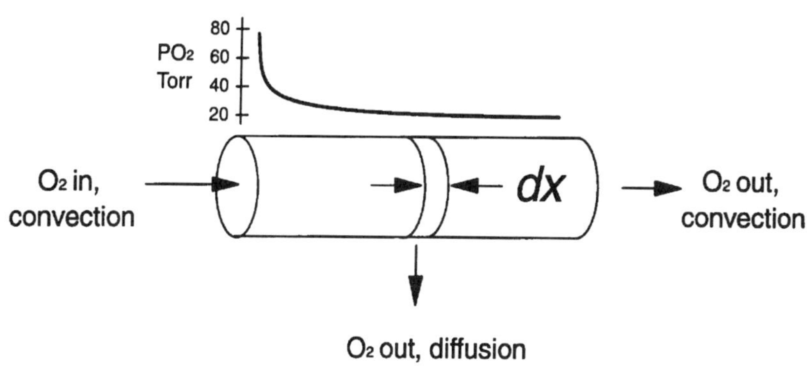

$$\frac{dO_2}{dx} = \frac{k\,(PcO_2 - PtO_2)\,\pi\, r^2}{Q}$$

Figure 9.5. The Krogh cylinder model. Mass balance of oxygen is determined by an equivalence between the O_2 that is delivered to the cylinder by convection and that which is lost by both convection and diffusion.

The amount of oxygen that enters the cylinder is the product of the oxygen content and the blood flow. The oxygen content (CaO_2),

$$2. \quad CaO_2 = Y x\,[Hb] \times 1.34 + \alpha\, PO_2$$

is determined by hemoglobin concentration [*Hb*] and fractional saturation with oxygen (*Y*), which is related to PO_2 by the oxygen equilibrium curve (OEC). An additional small amount of O_2 is carried as dissolved O_2 and is given as the product of the PO_2 and the solubility coefficient for O_2, α. The constant 1.34 in Equation 2 is the amount of O_2 bound to 1 g/dl of oxyhemoglobin. The blood flow (*Q*) is related to the blood pressure (mean arterial pressure, *MAP*) and resistance (systemic vascular resistance, *SVR*),

$$3. \quad Q = \frac{MAP}{SVR}$$

which can also be expressed in terms of the flow through a segment *dx* in Figure 9.5,

$$4. \quad Q = \frac{dx\,\pi\, r^2}{dt}$$

where *dx* is the length of a segment of the cylinder, *r* is its radius, and *dt* is the time required to transit the segment.

The amount of O_2 that leaves the cylinder by convection is the amount that enters less the amount lost by diffusion. The diffusive loss of O_2 is given by the Fick diffusion equation,

$$5. \quad \frac{dO_2}{dt} = k \times (PcO_2 - PtO_2)$$

in which the rate of O_2 loss is determined by the gradient between capillary and tissue PO_2, $(PcO_2 - PtO_2)$ and a diffusion constant, *k*, which includes the permeability and solubility of O_2 in plasma and tissues, as well as the effective distance and surface area for diffusion. Equations 4 and 5 can be used to calculate the amount of O_2 lost by diffusion in the segment *dx*,

$$6. \quad \frac{dO_2}{dx} = \frac{k(PcO_2 - PtO_2)\,\pi\, r^2}{Q}$$

Figure 9.5 shows the decrease of PO_2 along the cylinder, perfused with normal blood, calculated using equation 6. Inspection of the Fick equation (Equation 6) shows that the amount of O_2 transferred over the segment dx is inversely dependent on the flow rate, Q. Thus, the faster the flow rate, the less O_2 will be lost to the segment by diffusion, and *vice versa*.

9.2.2 Calculation algorithm

The algorithm used for the calculations is shown in Figure 9.6. Constants are first entered, including hemoglobin concentration (Hb, g/dl), initial PO_2 of the blood, 2,3-DPG/hemoglobin molar ratio, pH and PCO_2. Tissue PO_2 (PtO_2, Torr), mean arterial pressure (*MAP*, mm Hg) and systemic vascular resistance are also entered. Finally, relative values for viscosity, μ, and a relative diffusion constant, k, are entered. The program first defines a total length of the cylinder, L (200 relative units), and computes a flow rate (Q) from Equation 3. Next, the relative "dwell"

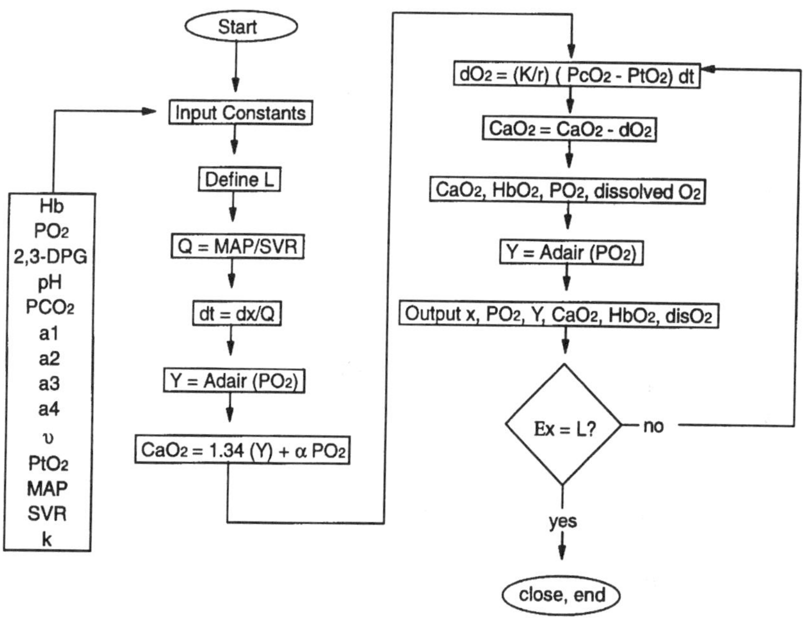

Figure 9.6. The algorithm used to calculate O_2 progress curves in the Krogh cylinder.

time (dt) for each segment, dx, is calculated as dx/Q. The hemoglobin saturation (Y) is calculated from the PO_2 and the Adair constants (Winslow and Samaja 1981), and total O_2 content (CaO_2) is calculated from Equation 2. Now for each dx, the amount of O_2 unloaded is calculated from the Fick equation (Equation 6), using the empirical diffusion constant, k, the PO_2 gradient (PcO_2-PtO_2), the "dwell" time, dt, and the total

O_2 is decremented by that amount. This total O_2 must now be distributed between the two oxygen compartments, HbO_2 and dissolved O_2, by an iterative procedure, assuming the position of the OEC has not changed. Data for each segment are saved, and if the end of the cylinder has been reached, the program ends. Programs were written in Microsoft Fortran and executed on a Pentium 90 microcomputer.

9.2.3 Map of the capillary

Using the normal OEC (i.e., P50 = 28.1, Winslow *et al.* 1977), the Krogh cylinder model was used to compute the distribution of O_2 between dissolved (PO_2) and hemoglobin-bound (HBO_2) in the capillary. Figure 9.7 is a plot of PO_2 in the cylinder as a function of axial position. This figure should be compared with Figure 9.4, which shows that under normal conditions the PO_2 in the A2/A3 arterioles is between 35 and 45 Torr. Thus, Figure 9.7 represents a physical transformation map of the PO_2 data, placing the regulatory arterioles in the model cylinder between 10 and 25 arbitrary units.

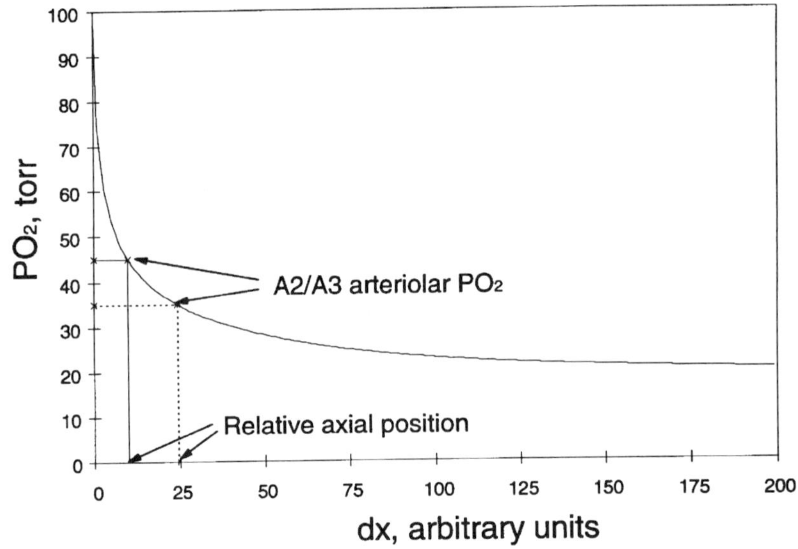

Figure 9.7. A physical "map" of the Krogh cylinder. Using the PO_2 values from Figure 9.4, we can assign a region between 15 and 25 arbitrary units in the Krogh cylinder model to the regulatory region.

9.2.4 Example OEC's

To illustrate the usefulness of the model, oxygen equilibrium curves with three different P50's were chosen. In order to perform the calculations according to the algorithm in Figure 9.6, Adair parameters for the OEC's were calculated according to Winslow and Samaja (1981). The parameters are given in Table 9.2, and the OEC's are plotted in Figure 9.8. The boundaries of the A2/A3 arteriolar PO_2 are indicated in the figure. Figure 9.9 plots the amount of O_2 given up to A2/A3 arterioles by blood with the three OEC's shown in Figure 9.8. A right-shift (higher P50) of the OEC increases the O_2 delivered to this segment, and a left-shift (lower P50) reduces the O_2 supplied. This simple illustration shows that shifts of P50 can have profound effects on the O_2 supplied to the A2/A3 arterioles.

Table 9.2 Parameters for OEC simulations

Affinity	low	normal	high
2,3-DPG/Hb, M/M	1.32	0.88	0.44
pH	7.0	7.2	7.8
pCO_2, Torr	60	40	20
a_1	8.30×10^{-3}	1.53×10^{-2}	2.56×10^{-2}
a_2	8.33×10^{-4}	1.10×10^{-3}	2.53×10^{-3}
a_3	2.43×10^{-11}	1.24×10^{-7}	1.17×10^{-4}
a_4	2.45×10^{-7}	1.82×10^{-6}	9.42×10^{-6}
P50, Torr	47.0	28.6	14.9
Hill's n	2.07	2.62	2.29

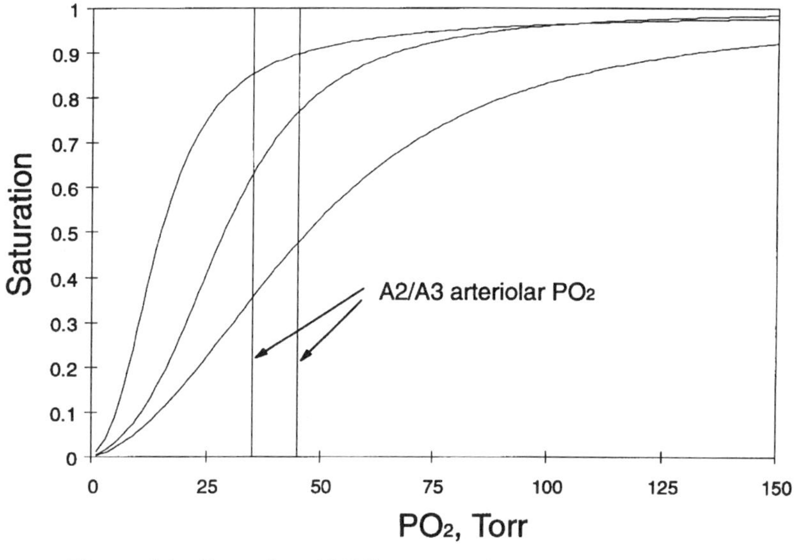

Figure 9.8. Examples of OEC's computed using the parameters in Table 9.2.

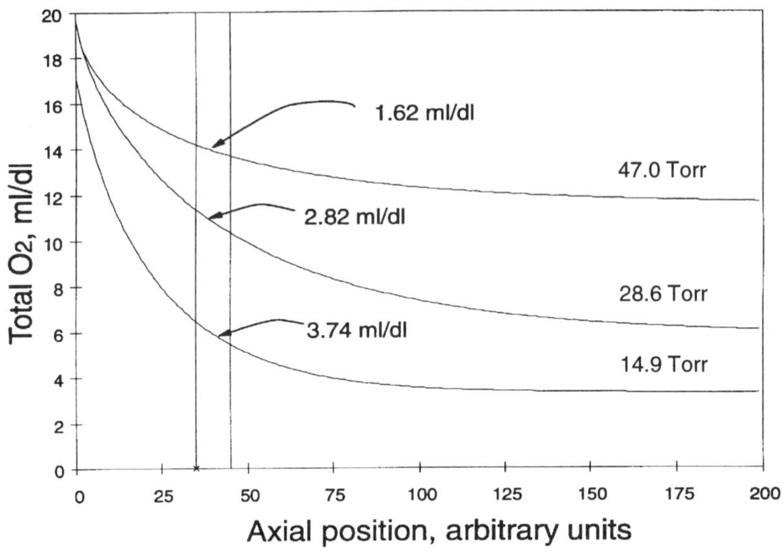

Figure 9.9. The distribution of O_2 supplied to the Krogh cylinder. The three curves correspond to the curves in Figure 9.8. The P50's are indicated. The amount of O_2 given up to the region corresponding to the A2/A3 arterioles is indicated.

9.2.5 Effect of P50 on arteriolar O_2 supply

In order to further estimate the effect of varying the P50 on arteriolar O_2 supply, families of OECs were generated with P50 values from approximately 15 to 45 Torr. For each curve, the amount of O_2 supplied between 10 and 24 arbitrary units in the Krogh cylinder model was calculated. Thus, plots of O_2 supplied *versus* P50 were drawn (see Figure 9.10).

Figure 9.10 makes a number of important points. Under "normal" conditions (k=0.01, [Hb]=15 g/dl, P50=28.1 Torr), approximately 2.81 ml/dl of O_2 are supplied to the A2/A3 arterioles. When the only change in the calculations is to increase k to 0.02, such as would occur by decreasing the diffusion distance in half, nearly 3.5 ml/dl of O_2 is supplied to the same region. Such a change would induce autoregulatory constriction of the arterioles, increasing the O_2 consumption by this tissue, decreasing functional capillary density, and could decrease the net transfer of O_2 to tissue. With this increase in diffusion, Figure 9.10 indicates that compensation could occur if the P50 is lowered to approximately 24 Torr. A second interesting observation from Figure 9.10 is that this situation could also be compensated by decreasing the hemoglobin concentration: in this case, decreasing from 15 to 12.5 g/dl results in a return of O_2 delivered to A2/A3 arterioles to about 2.8 ml/dl at a P50 of 28.1 Torr. Finally, Figure 9.10 shows that when diffusion is increased, regardless of hemoglobin concentration, the O_2 delivered to arterioles decreases when P50 rises above 35-40 Torr. The reason for this is that curves with these high P50's do not fully saturate, effectively reducing the O_2 capacity, at 100 Torr.

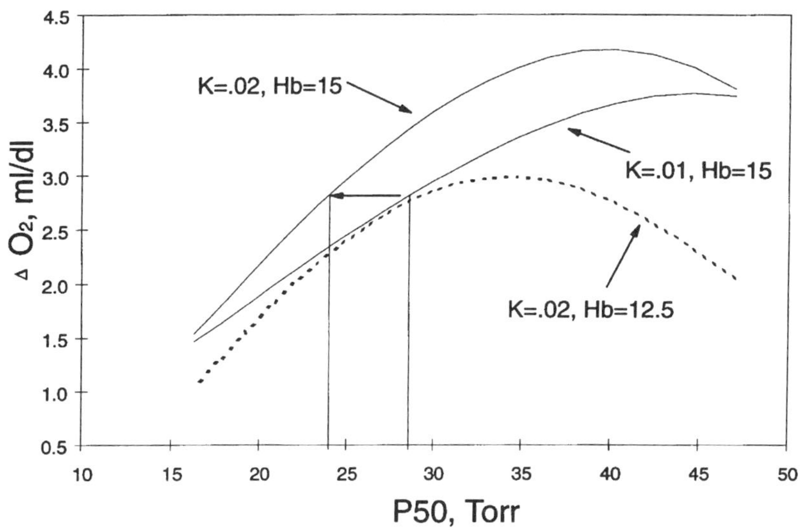

Figure 9.10. Oxygen supplied to A2/A3 arterioles ($\Delta\ O_2$) as a function of P50. The upper curve results from doubling the diffusion constant, *k* (equation 6), which results in an increase of O_2 supplied to the arterioles. One way this could be compensated would be to reduce the P50 to approximately 24 Torr, as indicated.

9.3 Discussion

Creation of models such as the one described here is a very instructive exercise. Whether or not the model accurately reflects the actual *in vivo* situation is not the entire point: quantitation of concepts allows them to be tested more accurately by experimentation. This model predicts that when an oxygen carrier is placed in the plasma space, autoregulatory vasoconstriction may be mitigated by altering the properties of the solutions. These could include raising the oxygen affinity or lowering the hemoglobin concentration. Intaglietta has further suggested that vasoconstriction will increase flow velocity, decreasing tissue oxygenation and that this effect may be prevented by increasing viscosity (Intaglietta, Johnson and Winslow 1996). Other variables are also important, such as pressure and flow (cardiac output), but not enough data are available to model these at present. A major concern with the present model is whether the "map" created in Figure 9.7 is valid. That is, if hemoglobin, for example, is placed in the plasma space, will the A2/A3 arterioles "reset" to a different point of regulation? This is not known, but it would not be surprising if this does occur over a period of time.

Previous studies have shown that arteriolar diameter is dependent on, among other factors, the availability of oxygen (Gorczynski and Duling 1978, Arfors, etc.)

Our theoretical conclusions are very similar to the results of Stein and Ellsworth (1993) who were able to show that increased red cell oxygen affinity in hamsters provided an advantage for oxygen exchange in capillary beds when oxygen supply was severely limited by hemodilution and hypoxia. We suggest further, however, that a consequence of overcoming this diffusion limitation by cell-free hemoglobin is an autoregulatory constriction of precapillary arterioles which will decrease capillary perfusion and increase capillary blood flow, both effects that will predictably decrease tissue oxygenation.

Attempts to demonstrate increased diffusive transport of O_2 by cell-free oxygen carriers have been disappointing (Hogan *et al.* 1994, Biro *et al.* 1991). Our results suggest that the increased diffusive O_2 transport by cell-free carriers is offset by autoregulatory vasoconstriction. This would not be surprising in view of the complex systems that are apparently in place to ensure even, constant supply of O_2 to tissues (autoregulation). A possible explanation for the disappointing results with hemoglobin-based oxygen carriers has been that most are vasoactive. The nature of the vasoactivity is not known, either with regard to its etiology, its location in the circulation, or its differential effects in different oxygen beds. The known affinity of Hb for NO may provide a part of the explanation, but not all observations can be explained by this mechanism (see Rohlfs *et al.*, this volume). Autoregulation, mediated by O_2 supply, may be an alternative or perhaps an additional mechanism to explain vasoactivity (Vandegriff and Winslow 1995, Tsai, Kerger and Intaglietta 1996).

A quantitative approach to tissue oxygenation is much more complex than the description of O_2 uptake in the lung (Winslow 1984). This is because in the lung, all uptake occurs in capillaries where the PaO_2 is constant, and the PCO_2 and pH relationships are relatively straightforward. Furthermore, the adequacy of pulmonary models can readily be checked by analysis of inspired and expired gas. Nevertheless, the laws governing gas exchange in the tissues are the same as those in the lung, even if all of the constants are not defined, and the precise gradients are not known. Furthermore, we do not yet have detailed information on Bohr effects and other allosteric effects for most of the cell-free hemoglobins. Thus, exact modeling of these materials is not yet as feasible as those using red blood cells only.

So far, there is little direct evidence to support a link between P50 and vasoactivity. Vandegriff and Rohlfs presented preliminary data, comparing the hypertensive effects of hemoglobins which were very well matched in physical properties except for P50 (Vandegriff *et al.* 1996, Rohlfs *et al.* 1996). They found a significantly more persistent rise in mean arterial pressure in exchange-transfused rats who had received high-P50 hemoglobin compared to low P50 hemoglobin. Clearly, more studies of various types are needed in order to test these new ideas. Preclinical animal models of hemodilution and shock/resuscitation should be chosen carefully, and the dosage of oxygen carriers must be tailored to individual properties, not only of toxicity, but by their potential to enter into autoregulation of O_2 delivery to tissues.

It should be noted that models of hemodilution and reperfusion might not be comparable with regard to efficacy of hemoglobin-based oxygen carriers. In the hemodilution model, the oxygen carrier is injected into an animal with a "normal" state of vascular tone. In the other, shock/reperfusion, the oxygen carrier is injected into an animal with already constricted vascular beds. Effects under both circumstances might be different and difficult to predict without further data in each model.

It is premature to speculate from our analysis on the question of which cell-free oxygen carrier is likely to be most successful. The product that the U.S. Army chose to develop as a model, ααHb, however, would not seem to be optimal, because it has a P50 close to that of normal blood. Our model predicts that this product will lead to local vasoconstriction (indeed, it regularly causes hypertension in animals), and therefore the potential advantages of its ability to perfuse under-perfused tissues might be offset by vasoconstriction. In fact, one of the reasons for choosing this product was that its P50 was similar to that of blood. Other workers had considered the question (Gould *et al.* 1982), and one manufacturer even assumed that higher P50 would be superior to a normal value, and built a mutation into its recombinant product that would accomplish this goal (Looker *et al.* 1992). Our conclusions from high altitude, of course, were influenced by oxygen limitation. When oxygen can be supplied on the arterial side, it is still possible that a higher P50 might have beneficial effects. In fact, studies by a number of groups with IHP-loaded red blood cells seem to suggest that if arterial *blood* can be loaded with oxygen satisfactorily, then oxygen extraction might be greater in the tissue, lowering the requirement for higher blood flow. In other words, a higher extraction could lessen the burden on the heart to maintain its output. The concepts must now be tested in appropriate animal models. The calculations described here have provided our group a useful framework on which to design and interpret such experiments.

9.4 Acknowledgments

This work was supported by a grant from the National Heart, Lung and Blood Institute of the National Institutes of Health (P01 HL48018).

9.5 References

Aste-Salazar, H., and A. Hurtado. The affinity of hemoglobin for oxygen at sea level and high altitudes. *Am. J. Cardiol.* 142: 733-743, 1944.

Barcroft, J., C.A. Binger, A.V. Bock, J.H. Doggart, H.S. Forbes, G. Harrop, J.C. Meakins, and A.C. Redfield. Observations upon the effect of high altitude on the physiological processes of the human body carrried out in the Peruvian Andes chiefly at Cerro de Pasco. *Philos. Trans. R. Soc. London. Ser. B.* 211: 351-480, 1923.

Benesch, R., and R.E. Benesch. Intracellular organic phosphates as regulators of oxygen release by haemoglobin. *Nature* 221: 618-622, 1969.

Biro, G. P., P.J. Anderson, S.E. Curtis, and S.M. Cain. Stroma-free hemoglobin: its presence in plasma does not improve oxygen supply to the resting hindlimb vascular bed of hemodiluted dogs. *Can. J. Physiol. Pharmacol.* 69: 1656-1662, 1991.

Chanutin, A., and R.R. Curnish. Effect of organic and inorganic phosphates on the oxygen equilibrium curve of human erythrocyte. *Arch. Biochem. Biophys.* 121: 96-102, 1967.

Ellsworth, M.L., and R.N. Pittman. Arterioles supply oxygen to capillaries by diffusion as well as by convection. *Am. J. Physiol.* 258: H1240-H1243, 1990.

Federspiel, W.J., and A.S. Popel. A theoretical analysis of the effect of the particulate nature of blood on oxygen release in capillaries. *Microvasc. Res.* 32: 164-189, 1986.

Gorczynski, R.J., and B.R. Duling. Role of oxygen in arteriolar functional vasodilation in hamster striated muscle. *Am. J. Physiol.* 235(5): H505-H515, 1978.

Gould, S.A., L.R. Sehgal, A.L. Rosen, H.L. Sehgal, H.D. Levine, C.L. Rice, and G.S. Moss. Hemoglobin solution: is a normal [Hb] or P50 more important? *J. Surg. Res.* 33: 189-193, 1982.

Hogan, M. C., S.S. Kurdak, R.S Richardson, and P.D. Wagner. Partial substitution of red blood cells with free hemoglobin does not improve O_2 uptake of working *in situ* dog muscle. Adv. Exp. Med. Biol. 361:375-378, 1994.

Hogan, M.C., D.C. Wilford, P.E. Keipert, N.S. Faithfull, and P.D. Wagner. Increased plasma O_2 solubility improves O_2 uptake of *in situ* dog muscle working maximally. *J. Appl. Physiol.* 361:2470-5, 1992.

Homer, L.D., P.K. Weathersby, and L.A. Kiesow. Oxygen gradients between red blood cells in the microcirculation. *Microvasc. Res.* 22: 308-323, 1981.

Huisman, T.H.J., and J. Kitchens. Oxygen equilibria studies of the hemoglobins from normal and anemic sheep and goats. *Am. J. Physiol.* 214: 140-146, 1968.

Hurtado, A. Animals in high altitudes: Resident man. In *Handbook of Physiology*. Adaptation to the environment (D.B. Dill, Ed.). Washington, D.C.: Am. Physiol. Soc., 1964, pp. 843-860.

Intaglietta, M., P.C. Johnson, and R.M. Winslow. Microvascular and tissue oxygen distribution. Cardiovasc. Res. 32: 632-643, 1996.

Johnson, J.C., K. Richmond, R.D. Shonat, A. Toth, M. Pal, M.E. Tischler, and R.M. Lynch. Oxygen delivery regulation: Implications for blood substitutes. In *Blood Substitutes: Physiological Basis of Efficacy* (R.M. Winslow, K.D. Vandegriff and M. Intaglietta, Eds.). Boston: Birkhäuser, 1995, pp. 175-186.

Lenfant, D., J.D. Torrance, and C. Reynafarje. Shift of the O_2-dissociation curve at altitude: mechanism and effect. *J. Appl. Physiol.* 30(5): 625-631, 1971.

Looker, D., D. Abbott-Brown, P. Cozart, S. Durfee, S. Hoffman, A. J. Mathews, J. Miller-Roehrich, S. Shoemaker, S. Trimble, G. Fermi, N.H. Komiyama, K. Nagai, and G.L. Stetler. A human recombinant haemoglobin designed for use as a blood substitute. *Nature* 356: 258-260, 1992.

Messina, E.J., D. Sun, A. Koller, M.S. Wolin, and G. Kaley. Increases in oxygen tension evoke arteriolar constriction by inhibiting endothelial prostaglandin synthesis. *Microvasc. Res.* 8:151-160, 1994.

Rohlfs, R.J., A. Gonzales, M.L. Gonzales, D. Baker, M. McCarthy, M.D. Magde Jr., K.D. Vandegriff, J.G. Adamson, and R.M. Winslow. Effect of altering O_2 binding properties of cell free hemoglobin on pCO_2 and lactate levels during exponential hemorrhage following 50% exchange transfusion. VIth International Symposium on Blood Substitutes, Montreal, Quebec, Canada, 1996.

Shepherd, A.P., H.J. Granger, E.E. Smith, and A.C. Guyton. Local control of tissue oxygen delivery and its contribution to the regulation of cardiac output. Am. J. Physiol. 225: 747-755, 1973.

Stein, J.C., and M.L. Ellsworth. Capillary oxygen transport during severe hypoxia: Role of hemoglobin oxygen affinity. *J. Appl Physiol.* 75: 1601-1607, 1993.

Tsai, A., H. Kerger, and M. Intaglietta. Microcirculatory consequences of blood substitution. In *Blood Substitutes: Physiological Basis of Efficacy* (R.M. Winslow, K.D. Vandegriff and M. Intaglietta, Eds.). Boston: Birkhäuser, 1995, pp. 155-174.

Vandegriff, K.D., and R.M. Winslow. A theoretical analysis of oxygen transport: A new strategy for the design of hemoglobin-based red cell substitutes. In *Blood Substitutes: Physiological Basis of Efficacy* (R.M. Winslow, K.D. Vandegriff and M. Intaglietta, Eds.). Boston: Birkhäuser, 1995, pp. 143-154.

Vandegriff, K.D., R.J. Rohlfs, A. Gonzales, M.L. Gonzales, M. McCarthy, M.D. Magde Jr., J.G. Adamson, and R.M. Winslow. Effect of O2 binding properties of cell free hemoglobins on mean arterial pressure following 50% exchange transfusion. [abstract] VIth International Symposium on Blood Substitutes, Montreal, Quebec, Canada, 1996.

Wagner, P.D., and J.B. West. Effects of diffusion impairment on O_2 and CO_2 time courses in pulmonary capillaries. *J. Appl. Physiol.* 33: 62-71, 1972.

West, J.B., P.H. Hackett, K.H. Maret, J.S. Milledge, R.M. Peters, C.J. Pizzo, and R.M. Winslow. Pulmonary gas exchange on the summit of Mt..Everest. *J. Appl. Physiol.* 55: 678-687, 1983.

West, J.B., and P.D. Wagner. Predicted gas exchange on the summit of Mt. Everest. *Resp. Physiol.* 42: 1-16, 1981.

Winslow, R.M. A model for red cell O_2 uptake. Int. J. Clin. Monit. Comp. 2:81-93, 1985.

Winslow, R.M. Optimal hematologic variables for oxygen transport, including P50, hemoglobin cooperativity, hematocrit, acid-base status and cardiac function. *Biomat., Art. Cells, Art. Org.* 16: 149-171, 1988.

Winslow, R.M. *Hemoglobin-based Red Cell Substitutes*. Baltimore: Johns Hopkins University Press, 1992.

Winslow, R.M., and C.C. Monge. *Hypoxia, Polycythemia, and Chronic Mountain Sickness*. Baltimore: Johns Hopkins University Press, 1987.

Winslow, R.M., C.C. Monge, N.J. Statham, C.G. Gibson, S. Charache, J. Whittembury, O. Moran, and R.L. Berger. Variability of oxgyen affinity of blood: Human subjects native to high altitude. *J. Appl. Physiol.* 51: 1411-1416, 1981.

Winslow, R.M., J.M. Morrissey, R.L. Berger, P.D. Smith, and C.G. Gibson. Variability of oxygen affinity of normal blood: An automated method of measurement. *J. Appl. Physiol.* 45: 289-297, 1978.

Winslow, R.M., M. Samaja, and J B. West. Red cell function at extreme altitude on Mount Everest. *J. Appl. Physiol.* 56: 109-116, 1984.

Winslow, R.M., M. Samaja, N.J. Winslow, L. Rossi-Bernardi, and R.I. Shrager. Simulation of the continuous O_2 equilibrium curve over physiologic range of pH, 2,3-diphosphoglycerate, and pCO_2. *J. Appl. Physiol.* 54(2):524-529, 1983.

Winslow, R.M., M.L. Swenberg, R.L. Berger, R.I. Shrager, M.Luzzana, M. Samaja, and L. Rossi-Bernardi. Oxygen equilibrium curve of normal human blood and its evaluation by Adair's equation. *J. Biol. Chem.* 252: 2331-2337, 1977.

Winslow, R.M., M-L. Swenberg, J. Benson, M. Perrella, L. Benazzi. Gas exchange properties of goat hemoglobins A and C. *J. Biol. Chem.* 264: 4812-4817, 1989.

9.6 Discussion

Hearst: I think to make the model work you have to have some kind of mechanism that senses oxygen, or senses the oxygen uptake and gives you a feedback that vasoconstricts or whatever. Is there anything known about the biochemistry of that oxygen-sensing event in the bloodstream?

Winslow: There are different oxygen sensors - certainly in the erythropoietin system, in the carotid body as well as in arterioles in general. The biochemical basis for the sensors is not very clear in each case. We talked about one possibility, which is the regulation of endothelial nitric oxygen synthase, an oxygen dependent enzyme. There are others as well which could involve prostacyclin synthesis, for example. It seems the challenge is to figure out the biochemical link between the supply of oxygen and vasoactivity.

Hearst: For many years, I've been involved in the molecular biology of photosynthetic bacteria, and there's a man by the name of Carl Bauer at the University of Indiana who has just discovered in *Rhodobacter encapsulatis* the oxygen-sensing mechanism by which the bacteria changes from a respiratory organism into a photosynthetic organism. Basically, it does this by sensing oxygen pressure. I'm curious as to whether there might be some linkage, genetic linkage, between these.

Winslow: Do you know what the biochemical basis for that is?

Hearst: I would have to go to the literature. I don't remember well enough to expound on it, but I would be happy to get you the information.

Winslow: As you know, there are many heme-containing proteins and enzymes which are candidates for this kind of thing. Thank you for your comment.

Johnson: As a followup to that very interesting question, there is quite a literature in microcirculation showing that the arterioles in fact are very sensitive to changes in oxygen levels. If you elevate the perfusate oxygen level over a microcirculatory bed, you can, in some instances, actually stop flow, but certainly, you see kind of a uniform vasoconstriction among all levels of arterioles. So, it's a very potent phenomenon, and in some instances, it seems that NO is involved, and in other instances, perhaps it's prostaglandins, and recently cytochrome P-450 metabolites have been shown to be involved, so there are several mechanisms there that apparently are responsible. This is an area of active investigation. I'd like to point out the interesting implications that come up in this model, and that is at one in the same time you have an exchange network that is a flow regulation network, and I think that's a formidable problem, but it's interesting to see this analysis.

Winslow: I didn't emphasize that the model is sensitive to flow because the higher the flow the less oxygen is transferred in any given segment.

And so, by altering flow properties, you can also change the overall gas exchange in the arteriole.

Mailett: I find it curious that you've not mentioned the work of Page and Hellums who have obtained experimental data for oxygen transport by red cell and red cells mixed with hemoglobin solutions in an artificial *in vitro* capillary. My specific question is does your model, based on oxygen equilibrium curves, account for intraluminal resistances to diffusion of oxygen in the arteriole?

Winslow: To answer the second question first, no, it doesn't break down specific resistances. It uses a lumped diffusion constant, and we have no experimental basis to do that. To answer the first question, in my talk yesterday - maybe you missed it - I talked extensively about the Page and Hellums work, and I showed some of their data. It is a strong component in our thinking.

Levin: Bob, you didn't say anything about the erythropoietin response today. What stimulates my question is a report that erythropoietin levels can change in patients who get cancer chemotherapy before their hematocrit falls, and I realize this is potentially a tangent, but that clearly is another variable here.

Winslow: The linkage between erythropoietin and oxygen sensing is still not totally understood even though there's a lot of work going on that. I'm sorry I can't give you an answer to your question.

Wong: In your autoregulation, there's a vasoconstriction component, and there's been a lot of discussion about blood substitutes and blood pressure. Can you conceive of the oxygen tension affecting blood pressure in some way that is relevant to this response of blood substitutes?

Winslow: This has been a question that we've asked too: Is it possible that this kind of microcirculatory vasoconstriction can produce systemic hypertension? Maybe Marcos would like to comment on that.

Intaglietta: Well, there is very strong evidence that peripheral vascular resistance is essentially regulated at the level of the arterioles; that is, the active regulatory component of mean arterial blood pressure. Therefore, if vasoconstriction is induced, in principle, mean arterial blood pressure should be elevated; I say in principle because this is a very highly compartmentalized response, and different organs might respond in different ways, but there is a direct linkage between the constriction of arterioles and the regulation of blood pressure. Maybe Paul Johnson would like to supplement this comment.

Johnson: Because of the baroreceptor mechanism, any increase would be modulated, and blood pressure, I think, should be maintained unless there's an overwhelming effect here which is sustained for a long period of time.

Chapter 10

The Mechanism of Tissue Oxygenation and the Design of Oxygen Carrying Plasma Expanders

Amy G. Tsai, Ph.D., Barbara Friensenecker, M.D., Hiromi Sakai, Ph.D., Heinz Kerger, M.D. and Marcos Intaglietta, Ph.D.

ABSTRACT

The development of an oxygen carrying plasma expander requires the understanding of their behavior in the microcirculation. New methodology for the measurement of blood and tissue pO_2 used in conjunction with classical methods for the analysis of the transport properties of blood and the microvessels provides an experimental basis for establishing an analytical framework with which to assess the consequences of altering the physical properties of blood, in particular blood viscosity, oxygen carrying capacity and the metabolism of the cellular components of the microcirculation. Use of optical techniques to assess flow and oxygen delivery in the microcirculation of the hamster skin-fold model has provided a new conceptual framework for understanding how oxygen is delivered and used by the tissues. Central to this new formulation is the consumption of oxygen by the microvessel wall, which is shown to play a significant role in determining tissue oxygenation. Hemoglobin-based plasma expanders tend to increase the metabolism of the cellular components of the vessel wall as a consequence of energy consuming vasoconstrictor effects. Furthermore, the viscosity of the mixture of blood and an oxygen carrying plasma expander must be matched to the remainder of the physical properties of the circulating mixture in order to achieve tissue oxygenation, since low blood viscosity is not necessarily beneficial for the maintenance of tissue oxygenation. The new information on how oxygen is managed at the microcirculatory level coupled with analytic methods and microvascular data, allows implementation hypothesis-driven design of oxygen carrying plasma expanders.

10.1 Introduction

The design of a plasma expander that works in synergy with blood requires the simultaneous solution of biological and transport problems operational at the level of microscopic blood vessels, i.e., the microcirculation, where blood and tissue interact, and diffusional processes and convective transport become superposed. The ideal replacement of blood is a fluid with identical physical and biological properties, however the cellular nature of blood renders this goal of difficult realization. Specification of the characteristics of an effectual plasma expander was until recently also hampered by the imperfect knowledge of the mechanisms that control tissue oxygenation, particularly the metabolic activity of the endothelium and smooth muscle, and the role that this oxygen sink plays in setting tissue pO_2.

Our understanding about oxygen delivery by the microcirculation has been dominated by the so-called Krogh cylinder formulation (Krogh 1918) which focuses on how oxygen is transported from blood to tissue by single capillaries, tissue oxygenation being extrapolated from the behavior of the unitary components. A critical assumption underlying this analysis is the historical perception that capillaries are the suppliers of oxygen to the tissue, where they function in a role that is a mirror image from that in the lung, where they were first observed.

The finding that significant amounts of oxygen exit the arteriolar network challenges the traditional view of the role of capillaries in tissue oxygenation, and recent studies (Intaglietta, Johnson and Winslow 1996) demonstrate that in fact most of the oxygen, at least in some tissues, is delivered by the arteriolar network. The presence of the substantial longitudinal oxygen gradient (direction of blood vessel axis) in the past could not be explained under the assumption that the oxygen gradients across the vessel wall are negligible. It has become recently apparent that the vessel wall is an important site of biological activity, which results in the presence of large oxygen gradients within the arteriolar walls. These large oxygen gradients may be due to either a large diffusional resistance within the wall (Hellums *et al.* 1996) or an enhanced metabolic rate, leading respectively to a small or large rate of oxygen exit from the blood vessels, the difference being about an order of magnitude (factor of 10). Mass balance measurements show conclusively that the rate of oxygen exit is large and commensurate with the existence of a large oxygen sink within the vessel wall.

In terms of plasma expanders, we find that their presence in blood modifies vessel wall metabolism, thus introducing an additional variable that must be factored into the design of oxygen carrying blood replacement.

10.2 The Vessel Wall Oxygen Gradient

The significance of arterioles in tissue oxygenation was first demonstrated by Duling and Berne 1970, who found that a relatively large amount of oxygen exits the arteriolar network. Kuo and Pittman 1988, determined that this rate of exit was about 10-times that which could be accounted for under the assumption that the oxygen gradients across the vessel wall are of the same order as those predicted by the level of oxygen consumption of parenchymal tissue, leading to the hypothesis that diffusion in the vessel wall tissue is an order of magnitude higher than in other tissues (Popel, Pittman and Ellsworth 1988). These conclusions were in part due to the lack of information on the pO_2 gradients in the vicinity of blood vessels and within the vessel wall, since there was no methodology that could reliably measure simultaneously blood and tissue pO_2 at the microscopic level.

An optical method for measuring pO_2 in blood and tissue (Torres Filho and Intaglietta 1993) is now available which is based on the injection of a palladium-porphyrin dye bound to albumin and measuring the decay of light-flash excited phosphorescence (Vanderkooi *et al.* 1987). The rate of decay of the phosphorescence is independent of both the concentration of the compound and the intensity of excitation light, but is a function of the amount of oxygen surrounding the dye, which quenches light emission. This allows measurements of intravascular pO_2 in single microvessels and in microscopic regions of the tissue to be obtained simultaneously to other microvascular parameters like diameter and blood flow.

Results obtained with this methodology provide a view that differs from the traditional perceptions of tissue oxygenation. Tissue pO_2 is found to be essentially uniform within a resolution of 20 μm (Toth *et al.* 1996), tissue oxygen availability at arterial and venous capillary sites being essentially the same at a scale of 20 μm diameter areas. Furthermore, in the tissues presently studied, the only detectable pO_2 gradients are in the immediate vicinity of arterioles and venules. Thus, resulting tissue oxygenation is determined by the arteriolar diffusion and consumption (metabolism) of the arteriolar wall and oxygen shunting to the venous exit according to the distribution shown in Figure 10.1. The capillaries, interposed between the arteriolar supply and the venous exit, provide a relatively small amount of oxygen to the tissue, whose function being also that of smoothing out tissue pO_2 heterogeneity.

The presence of significant pO_2 gradients in the immediate vicinity of the vessel wall was already indicated by Duling, Kushinsky and Whal 1979, who found differences as large as 27 mm Hg across the microvascular wall. Groebe and Thews (1990) arrived at similar conclusions on the basis of model calculations. Torres Filho *et al.* (1994), utilizing the phosphorescence decay technique in the skin fold of SCID mice, obtained evidence for the presence of large gradients at the vessel wall.

The measurement and interpretation of the vessel wall gradient in a three dimensional tissue is technically complicated because of the cylindrical geometry and the potential contribution of optical signals from over and underlying tissue. To circumvent this problem, we carried out measurements in the rat mesentery in a configuration where the blood vessels became linear sources of oxygen that deliver oxygen to a two-dimensional tissue region sandwiched between transparent, impermeable barriers. This system also revealed a steep gradient in the immediate vicinity of the vessel wall.

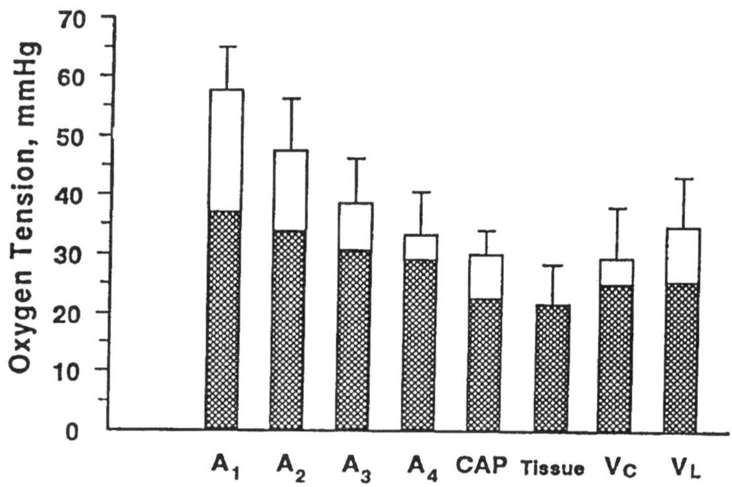

Figure 10.1. Distribution of oxygen tension in the subcutaneous connective tissue of the hamster skin fold in the awake animal. Bars are blood pO_2 in each of the arteriolar vessels types classified according to their diameter from A_1, 50 - 70 μm diameter, to A_4, terminal arterioles. CAP: capillaries. Tissue comprises measurements in locations void of capillaries and larger vessels. V_c: collecting venules, and V_l: large venules. The hatched portion of the bar is the measurement of pO_2 for each vessel order outside of the vessel wall. The white area in the bar represents the vessel wall pO_2 gradient. Note the comparatively small contribution of capillaries to tissue oxygenation once the utilization of oxygen by the vessel wall is taken into account.

The large consumption of oxygen by the endothelium-smooth muscle sink may be a consequence of the extensive metabolic activity of these cellular species. Evidence for the correspondingly large oxygen consumption is only recently emerging from studies where the oxygen consumption of the tissue mass is measured with and without the endothelium (Curtis *et al.* 1995). In terms of oxygen carrying plasma expanders based on the use of natural or modified hemoglobin molecules, vessel wall gradients are a factor because their presence may significantly increases vessel wall metabolism, negatively affecting tissue oxygenation as oxygen from the arteriolar supply is intercepted by the enhanced consumption of the vessel wall.

The link between hemoglobin and vessel wall metabolism is not presently established. Experiments from our laboratory show that vasoconstriction is directly associated with increased wall gradients, and most hemoglobin-based plasma expanders have been found to be hypertensive. This reaction may in part be due to scavenging of the endothelial derived vasodilator NO by hemoglobin (Rees, Palmer and Moncada 1989), however NO production by the endothelium should be directly transmitted to the underlying smooth muscle with little possibility for being captured by the blood borne hemoglobin molecule.

Tsai, Kerger and Intaglietta (1996) developed a model of the pO_2 distribution in the microcirculation when the physical parameters of the blood plasma expander mixture are used to predict tissue pO_2. In this model, hemodilution with a non-oxygen carrying colloid yields the same drop in oxygen tension along the circulation, and therefore the same level of capillary/tissue oxygenation because the ratio of viscosity/intrinsic oxygen carrying capacity remains constant. In contrast, while hemodilution with an oxygen carrying plasma expander also causes viscosity to decrease, oxygen carrying capacity of the blood/expander mixture is maintained, increasing the delivery of oxygen to the microcirculation. Paradoxically excess oxygen engages autoregulation, causing vasoconstriction (Prewitt and Johnson 1976). Superposed to oxygen autoregulation is also flow-dependent regulation (Smieško, Lang and Johnson 1989). In this control system, lower shear stress resulting from decreased viscosity that is not compensated by a proportional increase in flow velocity, diminishes the production of endothelium-derived vasodilators (Frangos *et al.* 1985), further potentiating the vasoconstrictor stimulus. Thus, in view of the link between vasoconstriction and vessel wall metabolism, we may expect that most hemoglobin-based plasma expanders will cause some degree of vessel wall metabolism increase.

10.3 Hypothesis-driven Design of Plasma Expanders

Plasma expanders and blood substitutes appear to have evolved from empirical formulations rather than a deliberate attempt to design a fluid that fulfills a hypothesis oriented criterion. This is in part the consequence of the lack of a full understanding of the relationship between the physical parameters that determine the transport function of blood. Tsai, Kerger and Intaglietta (1996) provided a preliminary framework for the formulation of a hypothesis-driven design, which can now be expanded to fully account for the mechanisms of tissue oxygenation, incorporating the effects of tissue wall metabolism.

A quantitative formulation that expresses the relationship between the variables that determine oxygen distribution in the microvascular network necessary to achieve a given level of tissue oxygenation according to the scheme shown in Figure 10.2 was derived by conventional mathematical means (Intaglietta 1997). Such a model was previously devel-

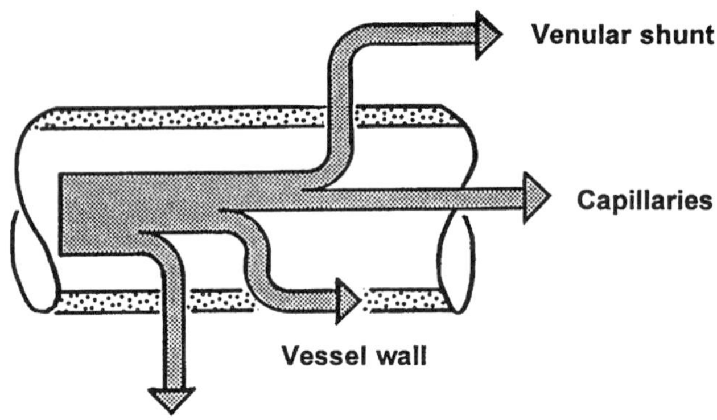

Figure 10.2. Partition of oxygen fluxes between compartments in the subcutaneous connective tissue of the hamster skin fold in the awake animal. Capillaries account for a comparatively small fraction of the oxygen supply in blood. Tissue oxygenation is the resultant of the combined input from the arterioles and the capillaries, however, the arteriolar supply is filtered by the consumption of oxygen by the vessel wall.

oped for the case in which oxygen exited the microcirculation by a diffusion process void of metabolic oxygen consumption in the medium (Tsai, Kerger and Intaglietta 1996). This model predicted capillary pO_2 under the assumption that these vessels, according to the present interpretation of tissue oxygen distribution, are essentially in equilibrium with tissue pO_2. Following the same procedure based on mass balance considerations for a segment of any microscopic blood vessel (Mirhashemi, Messmer and Intaglietta 1987, Torres Filho, Kerger and Intaglietta 1996, Kerger *et al.* 1995, Intaglietta *et al.* 1996), a model is developed for a cylindrical segment of a blood microvessel of length dx of branching order i where the rate of oxygen entering the upstream cross section at x is m_i given by:

$$(1) \quad m_i = Q_i[S_{o,i} + n_i pO_{2,i}]\, F(Hb)$$

where Q_i is the volumetric flow rate and F represents the intrinsic oxygen carrying capacity of blood related to the hemoglobin concentration $Htc \approx F(Hb)$. $S_{0,i} + n_i pO_{2,i}$ is the linearized relationship between blood oxygen and the prevailing partial pressure of oxygen $pO_{2,i}$ that approximates the hemoglobin oxygen dissociation curve in the branch i of length L_i ($S_{0,i}$ is saturation at zero pO_2 for each segment i, and n_i is the linearized slope of the dissociation curve for that segment). Blood oxygen content decreases along the vessel in proportion to oxygen exit across the vessel wall $m_{diffusion}$. Rate of oxygen exit is determined by the oxygen diffusion coefficient, D, the surface area of the vessel $\pi d_i dx$ (d_i: inside vessel diameter), g_o the rate of oxygen consumption in the vessel wall, and the gradient of oxygen tension at the blood/tissue interface. The vessel wall is assumed to be thin, allowing the use of linear (rather than cylindrical) geometry for diffusion in this region. Solution of the diffusion equation in a consuming medium is obtained in Cartesian geometry (r = direction of diffusion, equivalent to the Cartesian coordinate and not the cylindrical coordinates variable) yields the concentration profile:

$$(2) \quad c(r) = \frac{g_o}{D} r^2 + \alpha pO_{2,i}$$

where α is the oxygen solubility in tissue and δ is the distance from the blood tissue interface at which all the delivered oxygen has been consumed given by:

$$(3) \quad \delta = \sqrt{\frac{2D\alpha pO_{2,i}}{g_o}}$$

The concentration gradient at the blood/tissue interface is given by:

$$(4) \quad \frac{dc}{dr}\Big|_{r=0} \sim -\sqrt{\frac{2g_o pO_{2,i}}{D}}$$

leading to a rate of oxygen exit per unit vessel length dx given by:

$$(5) \quad m_{diffusion} = \pi d_i \sqrt{2Dg_o\alpha pO_{2,i}}\, dx$$

Oxygen partial pressure is the variable of choice since in a gas it is proportional to oxygen concentration. In blood, oxygen concentration is related to pO_2 through the oxygen saturation curve, which describes the oxygen held in chemical binding. In this system it is practical to express mass balance as a function of partial pressures rather than concentrations (molecule per unit volume) because of the changes present at the blood/vessel wall interface.

The mass balance for oxygen in vessel segment i is obtained from equations 1 and 5 whereby:

$$(6) \quad m_i = m_i + \frac{\partial m_i}{\partial x} dx + m_{diffusion}$$

and combining equations 1, 5 and 6 we obtain the differential equation describing oxygen distribution for a blood vessel cylinder of length dx and order i:

$$(7) \quad \frac{dpO_{2,i}}{dx} = \pi d_i \frac{\sqrt{2g_o \alpha pO_{2,i}}}{Q_i n_i (Hb)}$$

Integration of equation 4 over the extent of the vascular segment L_i yields:

$$(8) \quad pO_{2,i}^{1/2} = pO_{2,i-1}^{1/2} - k_i \text{ where } k_i = \frac{\pi d_i L_i}{n_i Q_i (Hb)} \sqrt{2g_o \alpha D}$$

which indicates that if we know pO_2 at the beginning of the vascular segment, i.e., the end of the previous segment i - 1, we can calculate pO_2 for the end of the ith segment. Knowing pO_2 at i = 0, i.e., central oxygen tension, allows prediction of pO_2 at any subsequent order of vascular branching according to:

$$(9) \quad pO_{2,i}^{1/2} = pO_{2,i}^{1/2} - \sum_1^n k_i$$

Blood flow in any segment is given by Poiseuille's equation:

$$(10) \quad Q_i = \frac{\pi d_i^4 \Delta P_i}{128 \mu L_i}$$

where μ is blood viscosity. Introducing this expression into equation (8) and rearranging the summation we obtain:

$$(11) \quad K_n = \sum K_i = \frac{128 \mu}{(Hb)} \sqrt{2g_o \alpha D} \sum_1^n \frac{L_i^2}{n_i d_i^3 \Delta P_i}$$

Equation 11 shows two distinct group of terms. One group is common to all vessel segments and includes blood viscosity, hematocrit or blood oxygen carrying capacity and vessel wall metabolism. The second group is a summation where each term is specific to each vascular segment. The combination of these terms allows the prediction of the outcome in terms of capillary blood pO_2 of given changes in the physical properties of blood. It should be noted that in terms of the methodologies developed and in the context of experimental studies, each of the parameters given in equation 11 can be measured by means of commercially available instruments in experimental preparations.

The derived expressions show that, solely on the basis of the prevailing transport phenomena, better oxygenation results from lowering viscosity. The factor g_o represents the vessel wall metabolism, which was not previously taken into consideration as a component in the management of oxygen distribution. The significance of this factor is that metabolism of the vessel wall, is directly affected by the composition of blood and flow velocity. Furthermore g_o has a basal value representative of the baseline activity necessary for the living processes of the tissue in the microvessel wall and alteration of this activity such as an inflammatory process or increased tone leads to the increase in tissue metabolism and, therefore, lowering of tissue oxygenation (since the increase in K_n lowers capillary pO_2).

10.4 The Role of Autoregulation

The delivery of oxygen to the tissue, which we define as the resulting capillary blood oxygen tension, is regulated by related active and passive mechanisms (Johnson and Intaglietta 1976, Johnson 1986). As shown by the foregoing analysis, the physical properties of blood play a key role in setting the passive component of regulation through the interaction between blood viscosity, oxygen carrying capacity and position within the microvascular network of the dissociation curve for hemoglobin (i.e., the value of n at each segment i). The existence of this coupling has only recently come under scrutiny and is of importance for blood substitutes, since their use decreases the concentration of red blood cells, the major determinant of blood viscosity. Altering blood viscosity changes blood flow velocity, whereby lowering viscosity increases flow velocity, which lowers diffusional oxygen exit from the arterioles and increases their oxygen tension (Mirhashemi, Messmer and Intaglietta 1987, Mirashemi *et al.* 1988).

Superposed to the passive delivery of oxygen determined by the physical properties of microcirculation is a process of active blood flow regulation and oxygen delivery that insures that parenchymal cells receive an adequate supply of oxygen to satisfy oxidative metabolism. Furthermore, blood flow regulatory mechanisms also prevent an over-abundance of oxygen delivery to the tissues. The hypothesis in explaining the linkage between blood supply and oxygen demand assumes the existence of chemical vasodilator signals transmitted from parenchymal cells to the resistance vessels, reducing tone of these vessels and allowing blood flow to increase when tissue oxygen tension falls below critical levels. Conversely, increasing blood oxygen tension over normal levels elicits vasoconstriction (Detar and Bohr 1968).

The prevailing assumption is that both passive and active flow regulation are focused on insuring that capillaries receive an appropriate supply of oxygenated blood. The parameter that characterizes the role of capillaries as a system for oxygenating blood is functional capillary density defined as the number of capillaries that possess red blood cell transit (Tsai, Friesenecker and Intaglietta 1995). This parameter is subject to a physiological variability that is directly related to oxygenation and local hydrostatic blood pressure. Over-oxygenation and hypotension lower functional capillary density with the consequence that tissue oxygen decreases.

There is a component of autoregulation that is directly linked to flow which is sensed by the endothelium. The mechanism relates blood viscosity, μ, and flow velocity v, which determine shear stress τ_{wall} at the blood vessel wall ($\tau_{wall} \approx \mu v$). Production of the vasodilator prostacyclin by the endothelium is a direct function of the shear stress generated by blood at the vascular wall (Frangos *et al.* 1985). Consequently, lowered blood viscosity is beneficial only if blood flow velocity increases in proportion so that τ_{wall} remains constant; otherwise, if flow velocity does not increase to the required level, the net effect of lowered viscosity in terms of autacoid regulation is vasoconstriction.

The implication of these considerations is that cell free oxygen carriers may perform their task of substituting red blood cells in oxygen delivery, however, their transport properties must be combined in prescribed ways so that the consequent physiological reactions do not negate the intended function. This becomes apparent in predicting the consequences of substituting blood with stroma-free hemoglobin solutions, which is the current direction of the technology for artificial blood.

10.5 Microcirculatory Effect of Hemoglobin Solutions as Artificial Blood

When our analytical results are used to predict the outcome of changing blood physical properties in the microcirculation, we find that many of the expected benefits are not obtained. Similar results are found in experimental studies of the change of systemic parameters in large animals subjected to isovolemic exchanges with oxygen carrying plasma expanders (Lee *et al.* 1995). According to equation 11, hemodilution with a non-oxygen carrying colloid will yield the same drop in oxygen tension along the circulation, and, therefore, the same level of capillary/tissue oxygenation, because the ratio viscosity/hematocrit remains constant. In contrast, when hemodilution is carried out with an oxygen carrying plasma expander, viscosity decreases, but the oxygen carrying capacity of the blood/expander mixture is maintained, therefore more oxygen arrives to the microcirculation. Paradoxically, excess oxygen engages autoregulation, causing vasoconstriction, which as shown in equations 10 and 11 has a fundamental effect on oxygenation due to the exponential dependence on diameter.

These effects are fully predicted from the previous analytical development. Furthermore, they are also found in experimental animal models subjected to blood exchanges with hemoglobin-based blood substitutes when the exchange is carried out to a level that is beyond the self-regulating capacity of the circulation for compensating for variability in the factors given by equation 11. If we assume that blood viscosity is directly proportional to blood hematocrit, equation 11 predicts that capillary oxygenation is independent of the concentration of red blood cells. However, since blood viscosity is approximately dependent on hematocrit squared, it is apparent that hemodilution with a low-viscosity colloid such as dextran (70,000 MW) or starch will tend to over-oxygenate the tissue. It is generally accepted that iso-oncotic, isovolemic hemodilution has no vasoactive effects, however, it is also well established that halving blood viscosity through the reduction of hematocrit does not double cardiac output, an effect that should be a direct consequence of vasoconstriction as suggested by considerations of autoregulation and our analytical development.

To test our analysis of oxygen exchange in the presence of molecular oxygen carrying plasma expanders in solution, we carried out isovolemic exchanges in the hamster skin-fold preparation. This model has been utilized in our laboratory for over a decade (Papenfuss *et al.* 1979). It allows systemic and microvascular data to be obtained in the awake condition, particularly tissue pO_2 in the intercapillary region. In these experiments we reduced systemic hematocrit by replacing blood with different hemoglobin-based blood substitutes (Tsai, Kerger and Intaglietta 1995b). Our general finding is that up to substitutions of 50% of the red cell mass, hemoglobin solutions of different types, dextran, starch and saline yield the same level of tissue oxygenation (Intaglietta and Winslow 1995). In other words, the systemic circulation and the microcirculation have sufficient reserve oxygen carrying capacity for compensating the loss of red blood cells.

When the hematocrit reduction is in excess of 80%, hemoglobin solutions do not yield expected results. At 10-12% hematocrit, blood viscosity, even with the added molecular suspension, is about one-third of normal, but cardiac output is about normal. This causes a severe reduction of functional capillary density caused by the vasoconstriction implicit to maintenance of normal peripheral vascular resistance in the presence of significantly reduced blood viscosity. Furthermore, the drop of pO_2 within the vessel wall virtually doubles and consequently tissue pO_2 falls (Tsai, Kerger and Intaglietta 1996). Our analysis suggests that these phenomena could be corrected by raising blood viscosity as shown by Waschke *et al.* 1994.

10.6 Summary and Assessment

Artificial blood can now be designed utilizing analytical techniques that show the relationship between the factors that regulate tissue pO_2. Application of this methodology is practical also because a comprehensive theory on the management of oxygen by the microcirculation is now available. This theory shows that there is no single factor that is responsible to insure that a given oxygen carrying formulation will oxygenate tissue. In particular, it shows that lower viscosity and increased oxygen carrying capacity (or delivery capacity), a common feature of most oxygen carrying plasma expanders, may actually hinder oxygen delivery by the microcirculation. Current analytical developments based on microvascular experimental data show that viscosity, oxygen carrying capacity and availability, slope of the oxygen dissociation curve for hemoglobin, and vessel wall metabolism must combine in a prescribed way to obtain the desired results.

10.7 Acknowledgments

This work was supported by USPHS Program Project HL48018.

10.8 References

Curtis, S.E., B. Vallet, M.J. Winn, J.B. Caufield, C.E. King, C.K. Chapler, and S.M. Cain. Role of vascular endothelium in O_2 extraction during progressive ischemia in canine skeletal muscle. *J. Appl. Physiol.* 79: 1351-1360, 1995.

Detar, R., and D.F. Bohr. Oxygen and vascular smooth muscle contraction. *Am. J. Physiol.* 214: 241-244, 1968.

Duling B.R., and R.M. Berne. Longitudinal gradients in periarteriolar oxygen tension. A possible mechanism for the participation of oxygen in the local regulation of blood flow. *Circ. Research* 27: 669-678, 1970.

Duling B.R., W. Kushinsky, and M. Whal. Measurement of perivascular pO_2 in the vicinity of pial vessels in the cat. *Pflügers Arch.* 383: 29-34, 1979.

Frangos, J.A., S.G. Eskin, L.V. McIntire, and C.L. Ives. Flow effects on prostacyclin production in cultured human endothelial cells. *Science* 227: 1477-1479, 1985.

Groebe, K., and G. Thews. Calculated intra- and extracellular pO_2 gradients in heavily working red muscle. *Am. J. Physiol.* 259*(Heart Circ. Physiol.* 28*)*: H84-H92, 1990.

Hellums, J.D., P.K. Nair, N.S. Huang and N. Oshima. Simulation of intraluminal gas transport processes in the microcirculation. *Ann. Biomed. Eng.* 24: 1-24, 1996.

Intaglietta, M. Whitaker Lecture 1996: Microcirculation, biomedical engineering and artificial blood. *Ann. Biomed. Eng.*, in press, 1997.

Intaglietta, M., P.C. Johnson, and R.M. Winslow. Microvascular and tissue oxygen distribution. *Cardiovasc. Res.* 32: 632-643, 1996.

Intaglietta, M., and R.M. Winslow. Artificial blood. In: *The Biomedical Engineering Handbook* (J.D. Bronzino, ed.) Boca Raton: CRC Press & IEEE Press, 1995, pp. 2011-2022.

Kerger, H., I.P. Torres Filho, M. Rivas, R.M. Winslow, and M. Intaglietta. Systemic and subcutaneous microvascular oxygen tension in conscious Syrian golden hamsters. *Am. J. Physiol.* 267*(Heart. Circ. Physiol.* 37*)*: H802-810, 1995.

Krogh, A. The number and distribution of capillaries in muscle with the calculation of the oxygen pressure necessary for supplying the tissue. *J. Physiol.* 52: 409-515, 1918.

Kuo, L., and R.N. Pittman. Effect of hemodilution on oxygen transport in arteriolar networks of hamster striated muscle. *Am. J. Physiol.* 254*(Heart. Circ. Physiol.* 23*)*: H331-H339, 1988.

Johnson, P.C. Brief Review: Autoregulation of blood flow. *Circ. Research* 59: 483-495, 1986.

Johnson, P.C., and M. Intaglietta. Contributions of pressure and flow sensitivity to autoregulation in mesenteric arterioles. *Am. J. Physiol.* 231*(Heart. Circ. Physiol.* 6*)*: 1686-1698, 1976.

Lee R., K. Neya, T.A. Svizzero, and G.J. Vlahakes. Limitations of the efficacy of hemoglobin-based oxygen-carrying solutions. *J. Appl. Physiol.* 70: 236-242, 1995.

Mirhashemi, S., G.A. Breit, R.H. Chávez, and M. Intaglietta. Effects of hemodilution on skin microcirculation. *Am. J. Physiol.* 254*(Heart. Circ. Physiol.* 23*)*: H411-H416, 1988.

Mirhashemi, S., K. Messmer, and M. Intaglietta. Tissue perfusion during normovolemic hemodilution investigated by a hydraulic model of the cardiovascular system. *Int. J. Microcirc.: Clin. Exp.* 6: 123-136, 1987.

Papenfuss, H.D., J.F. Gross, M. Intaglietta, and F.A. Treese. A transparent access chamber for the rat dorsal skin fold. *Microvasc. Res.* 18: 311-318, 1979.

Popel, A.S., Pittman, R.N., and M.L. Ellsworth. Rate of oxygen loss from arterioles is an order of magnitude than expected. *Am. J. Physiol.* 256*(Heart. Circ. Physiol.* 25*)*: H921-H924, 1988.

Prewitt, R.L., and P.C. Johnson. The effect of oxygen on arteriolar red cell velocity and capillary density in rat cremaster muscle. *Microvasc. Res.* 12: 59-70, 1976.

Rees, D.D., Palmer, R.M.J., and S. Moncada. Role of endothelium derived nitric oxide in the regulation of blood pressure. *Proc. Natl. Acad. Sci. USA* 86: 3375-3378, 1989.

Smieško, V., D.J. Lang, and P.C. Johnson. Dilator response of rat mesenteric arcading acterioles to incresaed blood flow. *Am. J. Physiol.* 257*(Heart. Circ. Physiol.* 26*)*: H1958-H1965, 1989.

Torres Filho, I.P., Y. Fan, M. Intaglietta, and R.K. Jain. Noninvasive measurement of microvascular and interstitial oxygen profiles in a human tumor in SCID mice. *Proc. Natl. Acad. Sci. USA* 91: 2081-2085, 1994.

Torres Filho, I.P., and M. Intaglietta. Microvessel pO_2 measurements by phosphorescence decay method". *Am. J. Physiol.* 265*(Heart. Circ. Physiol.* 34*)*: H1434-H1438, 1993.

Torres Filho, I.P., H. Kerger, and M. Intaglietta. pO_2 measurements in arteriolar networks. *Microvasc. Res.* 51: 202-212, 1996.

Toth, A., M. Pal, M.E. Tischler, and P.C. Johnson. Are there oxygen deficient regions in skeletal muscle? *Am. J. Physiol.* 270*(Heart Circ Physiol.* 39*)*: H193-H1939, 1996.

Tsai, A.G., B. Friesenecker, and M. Intaglietta. Capillary flow impairment and functional capillary density. *Int. J. Microcirc.: Clin. Exp.* 15(suppl. 5): 238-243, 1995a.

Tsai, A.G., H. Kerger, and M. Intaglietta. Microcirculatory consequences of blood substitution with αα-hemoglobin. In: *Blood Substitutes. Physiological Basis of Efficacy* (R.M. Winslow, K.D. Vandegriff, M. Intaglietta eds.). Boston: Birkhäuser, 1995b, pp. 155-174.

Tsai, A.G., H. Kerger, and M. Intaglietta. Microvascular oxygen distribution: Effects due to free hemoglobin in plasma. In: *Blood Substitutes. New Challenges* (R.M. Winslow, K.D. Vandegriff, M. Intaglietta, eds.), Boston: Birkhäuser, 1996, pp. 124-131.

Vanderkooi J.M., G. Maniara, T.J. Green, and D.F. Wilson. An optical method for measurement of dioxygen concentration based upon quenching of phosphorescence. *J. Biol. Chem.* 252: 5476-5482, 1987.

Waschke, K.F., Krieter, H., Hagen, G., Albrecht, D.M., Van Ackern, K., and W. Kushinscky. Lack of dependance of cerebral blood flow on blood flow viscosity after blood exchange with Newtonian O_2 carrier. *J. Cer. Blood Flow and Met.* 14: 871-876, 1994.

10.9 Discussion

Meiselman: Mesmerized is perhaps a better word than stunned. Marcos, what basis do you have to claim that just because there's a large oxygen tension gradient across the wall of the blood vessel that the blood vessel is consuming a great deal of oxygen? Why not the alternative which is that it's conductivity, if you will, for oxygen is low and, therefore, just like insulation in a wall, you can have a large temperature gradient across the wall if it's insulated, but the flux of heat will be reduced.

Intaglietta: The basis for that is that if you have a high insulation in the wall, as you very aptly illustrate, then very little oxygen can go out. If it were heat, for instance, if you have very high insulation in the wall, very little heat could escape. And so, the trick is to essentially measure how much oxygen, or heat, goes out. We have done that; the mass balance indicates that it is not a barrier for the diffusivity of oxygen that causes the large gradient but is the sink of oxygen, the consumption there, that causes the drop of oxygen. Many people throughout the last 10 or 15 years have tried to explain this measured, validated, very large loss of oxygen in the blood vessels by various assumptions. For instance, they increased the diffusivity by a factor of 10.

But, really it is not physically practical to assume a high diffusivity because there is no mechanism by which we can increase the diffusivity of oxygen in an aqueous medium by a factor of 10. A remaining explanation is high consumption at that point.

Wong: Your advice in your punch line is to have viscosity close to that of blood, but blood, of course, is non-Newtonian. Do you mean that we should try to approach the high shear rate of blood viscosity?

Intaglietta: Yes. The suggestion of these studies is that in those vessels, particularly the arterioles, where the hematocrit is still high, we should attempt to maintain a shear stress at the wall which is in the same range as that for normal blood. This cannot be done with fluids that lower viscosity significantly by a factor of 2 or 3.

Keipert: Marcos, this is a fascinating story, and I tend to certainly agree with the importance of viscosity. If I think back to the days when I was doing exchange transfusions with hemoglobins way back as a graduate student I was always troubled by the fact that I could get much better survival with highly polymerized solutions than I could with non-polymerized solutions even if oxygen contents and whatnot were very similar, and the P50s were also similar. You can polymerize to the point where the P50 drops.

To what extent do you think the viscosity of the drug itself is important in more clinically relevant situations in the 30-50% exchange region in terms of actual doses? And then the second question is related to the tissue pO_2 measurements. The polarographic electrodes that are traditionally used consume oxygen; they either poke holes, and you get some bleeding around the electrodes, or, with the surface electrodes, they tend to have a large catch in volume; they tend to look at a large area of tissue. Could you define with a palladium porphyrin technique what is the actual diameter - what is the spot of light, if you will - that you can look at and obtain a pO_2 measurement from, and how much oxygen is actually consumed with the Xenon flash?

Intaglietta: Let me answer the first question of what is relevant at the clinical exchange of 50%. Well, I am not a clinician, and I will give you an answer which is probably not satisfactory. I think that saline would work just as well because at 50% exchange, everything works as far as I can tell in this experimental procedure. Of course, a doctor will never do that for very good reasons. But, in doing that in a clinical setting, one is really ignoring this tremendous capacity for adaptation that the circulation has which was addressed very well in Professor Winslow's lecture. Does viscosity have significance at a 50% exchange? I think so, but it is probably a very reversible effect. It is at these very high levels of exchange where the effects essentially become nonreversible. Once functional capillary densities drop below 60%, they don't come back up, and eventually are lethal to a tissue, at least in the tissue where it happened.

Now, in terms of the palladium porphyrin technique. We have measured in various ways the comparison between the microelectrodes, polarographic microelectrodes, and the palladium porphyrin, and for a microelectrode with a tip of roughly 4 or 5 microns like Donald Buerk used, the oxygen consumption appears to be not significant for the microelectrode. Likewise for the oxygen technique because we can interrogate in an area of about, let us say, 20-30 microns long and about 5 microns wide. We always look at rectangles to get more signal. We can interrogate this area repeatedly, for instance, with 30, 100, or 300 flashes. In extreme cases like 300 flashes, we will see drops in the partial pressure of oxygen of 1 or 2 mm Hg, things like this.

So, on our estimations, and we have fairly well documented work on this, it is not a consideration how much oxygen is used by light. The technique uses oxygen but not in a significant way for our measurements.

Unidentified: So, then the actual are you're looking at is roughly 5 x 25 microns in area.

Intaglietta: Yes, exactly.

Unidentified: The only reason is—and I'm not a clinician either—the only reason I brought up the more moderate levels of hemodilution was thinking about the clinical situation. I agree. If you do a 30, 40, 50% exchange in an animal, those animals all do fine. Clinically, in patients who are coming out of surgery with hemoglobins of 7 or 8, which is half of their starting level, you see incidents of silent ischemia and myocardial ischemic events happening post-surgically. So some of the tissues may be fine, but some tissues, like the heart, the gut, may not be fine, and these drugs may still provide some antihypoxic protection to certain tissues under those conditions. I just wanted to know whether you felt that the viscosity would still play a role in that type of situation.

Intaglietta: It will play a role if that hemoglobin is not red cells. If half of that hemoglobin, for instance, is red cells and the other half is a molecular solution, then suddenly you have a viscosity that is really very low, and then, I think, at that point it becomes critical because those capillaries as far as we can tell will shut down in many of the tissues.

Meiselman: Well, let's see. I tried once, Marcos, let me try again. Actually, believe it or not, I think there's some validity in your argument that viscosity election might be helped, and that comes from the engineering field of secondary oil recovery where you're trying to get oil out of porous rock, and the way to prevent fingering of your chasing fluid, which is usually an aqueous fluid, is to increase its viscosity, and therefore, you minimize fingering which would be preferential or shunting of fluid in only a few channels.

So, maybe via the analogy to this technique, you would then have flow through a large number of capillaries, and preferential channels in the microcirculation would be less likely. But, I am at a loss to understand how simply elevating viscosity would lead necessarily to an increased wall shear stress. Yet you'd need an increased wall shear stress for prostacyclin and NO release. I understand that relationship, but, you know, we're talking about the product of flow times viscosity being proportional to shear stress. You've got one going up and the other conceivably going down, where do you gain?

Intaglietta: What the data show is that with the higher viscosities - but higher always with a caveat, I'm not speaking higher than blood - it's a relationship between very low viscosities and not-so-low viscosities, blood flow is significantly higher with the higher viscosity. So, therefore, the product that you are alluding to is much higher because now you have the combination of flow and viscosity, and therefore, the shear stress is much higher. That is where the gain comes. Now, the exact mechanism might be not so obvious but the experimental basis definitely supports this. There is nothing more startling than to look at microcirculation - and we do this in the laboratory all the time - introducing this very high viscosity materials, making exchanges with them, and to see how flow suddenly begins at rates that were not present even under controlled conditions.

So, that is the experimental observation, and the only mechanism to the present that we can evoke is through the shear stress dependent release of prostacyclin and NO which is fairly well documented.

Johnson: This discussion about viscosity and so on makes me think, too, about the effects a blood substitute might have in instances of peripheral vascular disease where the problem really is in the larger vessels which have high viscosity, and their downstream vessels probably are completely dilated already. In those vessels typically the blood has low viscosity. It seems to me that if you used the blood substitute with low viscosity, it might actually improve the circulation in that situation because you're reducing viscosity in the region of high resistance, and you're not changing it much in the region of downstream low resistance. Would you agree with that reasoning?

Intaglietta: I fully agree with that, Paul, but I want to shift the focus on the situation at hand here where we have these very deep exchanges. Where our red cells are really no longer a factor, they cannot contribute a viscosity component, and it is at that point where essentially the viscosity of the circulating fluid is the viscosity of water where the organism gets into problems.

Keipert: I have one other thing I'd like to get your opinion on. Several years ago when I first went to one of these two-day meetings on nitric oxide, I first learned about the shear component involved in releasing nitric oxide and dilating vessels, etc., and one of the things that we never see in our preclinicals with perflubron emulsion is vasoconstriction. We sometimes see, or we see indications of it, would be some potentially regional mild vasodilatation, some improvement of the microcirculation in certain capillary beds. We've always been intrigued by that. When I came back after that meeting, I said, "I know the answer!" - the perflubron emulsion particles in the blood are causing additional shear on that endothelium and improving locally some vasodilatation. It's not enough that you ever see it systemically, but locally in those tissue beds. Based on everything you've learned now, do you think that could be a possible explanation why we see improved microcirculation, we see what appears to be decreases in heterogeneity of flow, and that's part of the additional enhancement in tissue oxygenation that we see in a lot of these tissue beds?

Intaglietta: Yes, I would agree with that. That would be probably the first conclusion that I would come to, but I would not underestimate the mechanism that was illustrated by Kim Vandegriff which is the high oncotic pressure. I think that when we go down to these very deep exchanges which, I'm sure, do not correspond to the experiments you are alluding to, it is the very high oncotic pressure that contributes to keep those capillaries open. That helps because of a combination of two factors: The lack of a vasoconstrictor stimulus and the high oncotic pressure essentially dehydrates the endothelium, a mechanism that has been used for the groups that are interested in the hyperosmotic resuscitation, but this is outside of what you were asking. I would say yes, that indeed, the increase of viscosity introduced by your compounds could be lead to an increase of perfusion.

Chapter 11

Colloid Osmotic Effects of Hemoglobin-based Oxygen Carriers

Kim D. Vandegriff, Ph.D., Ronald J. Rohlfs, Ph.D., and Robert M. Winslow, M.D.

ABSTRACT

The solution properties of hemoglobin-based oxygen carriers have important implications on their effectiveness for blood substitution and blood-volume restitution. The introduction of acellular hemoglobin solutions into the plasma space will effect fluid shifts between intravascular and interstitial compartments based on Starling's Law of transcapillary fluid balance. Colloid osmotic pressures as a function of protein concentration have been measured for several hemoglobins, including unmodified, cross-linked, polymerized, and surface-conjugated. Thermodynamic analyses of these data provide a simple method to determine the proteins' average molecular weights and reveal important information about their solution properties. The tetrameric and polymerized hemoglobins exhibit nearly ideal solution behavior. In contrast, hemoglobins modified at their surface with synthetic polymers of polyethylene glycol have higher oncotic activity and evident solution non-ideality. According to this analysis, the surface-modified hemoglobins have markedly increased effective volumes and molecular sizes in solution. These properties may have important implications in optimal formulations of hemoglobin-based oxygen carriers.

11.1 Introduction

Cell-free, hemoglobin-based oxygen carriers (HBOCs) are being developed for clinical use to avoid risks associated with whole blood or red blood cell transfusions (Winslow 1992). To be effective, these products must sustain oxygen-carrying capacity and restore intravascular volume during blood loss or hemodilution procedures. An important consideration is the large dose that will be required of these cell-free solutions for clinical utility, because this intravenous influx of protein solution will change the solution properties of blood, including viscosity and/or colloid osmotic (oncotic) pressure (COP). In this chapter, physical measurements and theoretical analyses of the COP of HBOC solutions are discussed. Theoretical effects of changes in viscosity were addressed in an earlier chapter in this series (Tsai, Kerger and Intaglietta 1996).

Colloid osmotic pressure, being a colligative property, depends upon the concentration of protein exerting the force. Typically, HBOC solutions are formulated iso-oncotically: the underlying assumption being that the properties of cell-free HBOC solutions should approximate those of blood. The physiological consequences of changing the oncotic properties of blood are not well defined. The kidney reacts to shifts in fluid balance by adjusting the filtration and reabsorption of water (Guyton 1986), but since most HBOC studies have been carried out with iso-oncotic solutions, there is little information about the potential problems or benefits of altering blood COP.

One study that did vary from the iso-oncotic paradigm used a hyperoncotic HBOC; however, the reasoning behind this was to introduce the oxygen carrier as rapidly as possible in an exchange-transfusion protocol, rather than to test specifically for the physiological effects of higher protein activity (Hess, Wade and Winslow 1991). The authors reported an increase in blood volume based on calculations of the mass balance of red blood cell and plasma hemoglobin. They concluded that the intravascular expansion provided hemodynamic stability by counteracting decreasing blood viscosity and loss of hemoglobin from the vascular space.

In general, studies specifically directed to measure the effects of different HBOC oncotic pressures on blood volume, vascular retention time, oxygen delivery, fluid shifts, and/or blood flow have not been designed to focus on optimal formulations for clinical use, even though the success of these products will depend in large part on these physiological responses.

11.2 Body Fluid Compartments

In healthy animals, the total volume of body water is tightly regulated. In humans, it remains constant to within ±1% of body weight per day. About one-third of body water is extracellular, residing in intravascular and extravascular compartments. Approximately 25% of this extracellular fluid is in the blood plasma; the remaining 75% is in the interstitial space. Volume regulation in these compartments depends upon forces that redistribute the fluid between the blood and the interstitium. The balance of these forces is determined by two pressures exerted in each compartment: hydrostatic and colloid osmotic. Hydrostatic pressure is hydraulic, the result of the physical resistance offered when fluid is forced through an opening such as a blood vessel. Colloid osmotic pressure depends, on the other hand, on the molecular components dissolved in the fluid and, in particular, on their solution properties.

11.2.1 The plasma compartment

Proteins make up the majority of solids in plasma at about 7-7.5 g/dl. These proteins are typically divided into three groups: albumin, fibrinogen, and globulin. They do not readily move into the interstitium; thus there is normally a higher protein concentration in the intravascular than in the extravascular space. This creates an oncotic pressure gradient that tends to hold fluid within the circulation. In the situation we are studying in which red blood cells are replaced by a hemoglobin solution, the HBOC becomes an additional plasma protein that will contribute to the total oncotic pressure in plasma (as long as the HBOC remains in the intravascular compartment). The total COP of blood after HBOC infusion will depend on the concentration and solution properties of the HBOC and on the amount of blood protein lost during hemorrhage or hemodilution.

11.2.2 The interstitial compartment

The interstitium is defined as the space between vascular walls and extravascular cells. The structure of the interstitium is similar in all tissues. It is made up of a salt solution containing dissolved proteins (derived from plasma) and a fibrous network of collagen, which has a gel phase of glycosaminoglycans, providing the interstitial structure. Adhesion receptors called β-integrins anchor connective tissue cells to the structural interstitial fiber network (Reed, Woie and Rubin 1997). The interstitial proteins exert an oncotic pressure in opposition to that in the vascular space.

11.2.3 Oncotic pressures in extracellular fluid spaces

Human plasma contains approximately 4.5 g/dl albumin (COP ~22 mm Hg), approximately 2.5 g/dl globulin (COP ~6.0 mm Hg), and approximately 0.3 g/dl fibrinogen (COP ~0.2 mm Hg), exerting a total COP in human plasma of approximately 28 mm Hg (Guyton, Taylor and Granger 1975). The protein concentration is normally less in the interstitium, but interstitial glycosaminoglycans, especially hyaluronan, have high exclusion volumes because of their random-coil structure (the physical basis underlying this property will be discussed in more detail in section 11.4.3). The high exclusion volume raises interstitial COP. However, interstitial COP is still typically 8-12 mm Hg lower than plasma COP. A secondary factor that controls interstitial COP is the rate of protein removal by the lymphatic system. For example, if proteins were not removed by lymphatic flow, the interstitial protein concentration would continue to rise until it equaled that in plasma.

11.3 Transcapillary Protein and Fluid Movement

The concentration of plasma proteins in tissues depends on several factors, including the permeability of the capillary wall to proteins, the leakage rate of proteins across the capillary wall due to hydrostatic pressure, and the ability of the lymphatic system to return proteins to the vascular system. Because of the high surface area of capillary beds, microcirculatory vessels are the primary components responsible for protein and fluid exchange between intra- and extravascular compartments. The capillary wall is a thin membrane of endothelial cells that are semipermeable to plasma proteins. Substances move from the microcirculation into the interstitium by one of three pathways: (1) through junctions between endothelial cells, (2) by transport inside vesicles across the endothelium (transcytosis), or (3) if the substances are lipid soluble, by simple diffusion through the hydrophobic endothelial cell membranes.

The lymphatic system drains fluid and proteins from the interstitium back into the venous circulation, and the constant circulation of fluid and proteins between extracellular compartments maintains the fluid balance between intravascular and extravascular volumes. If the oncotic force exerted by proteins on either vascular side is altered, this balance will be disrupted, and, depending on the direction of fluid flow, the result will be either edema, in which case tissue becomes over-hydrated, or tissue dehydration.

11.3.1 Starling forces

The rate of filtration across a capillary wall depends upon a balance of factors called the Starling forces. The Starling forces are: (1) the filtration pressure, which is the hydrostatic pressure in the blood vessel minus the hydrostatic pressure in the interstitium (P_p - P_i), and (2) the osmotic pressure, which is the colloid osmotic pressure in the plasma minus the colloid osmotic pressure in the interstitial fluid (π_p - π_i). These forces oppose each other as shown in the Starling equation (Starling 1896, Landis 1927),

$$(1)\ J = K_c (P_p - P_i) - \sigma (\pi_p - \pi_i)$$

which gives the rate of fluid flux, J, where K_c and σ are membrane parameters. K_c is a filtration coefficient of the capillary wall that characterizes the ability of solvent to flow across the wall, and σ is the osmotic reflection coefficient of the capillary wall that is a relative measure of the selective permeability of the wall to proteins (*i.e.*, $\sigma = 1$ when the capillary wall is completely impermeable to the protein, and $\sigma = 0$ when the wall is freely permeable to the protein).

11.3.1.1 Hydrostatic pressures

Hydrostatic pressure is directly proportional to blood flow (Q), such that if Q increases but venous pressure does not change, hydrostatic pressure will increase. By extension, precapillary vasoconstriction will decrease capillary hydrostatic pressure. Capillary hydrostatic pressures (P_p) are higher at the arterial supply end of the circulation (~30 mm Hg) and lower at the venous end (~15 mm Hg). Interstitial hydrostatic pressures (P_i) vary from organ to organ: from subatmospheric in subcutaneous tissue, to positive in the liver and kidney, and even relatively higher pressure in the brain (Ganong 1983).

11.3.1.2 Colloid osmotic pressures

The oncotic pressure generated by proteins opposes hydrostatic pressures in plasma and interstitial spaces, and the balance of these forces determines the overall direction of fluid movement between vascular and extravascular compartments. At the arterial end of the capillary where filtration pressure across the vessel wall exceeds intravascular oncotic pressure, fluid moves into the interstitial space. At the venular end of the capillary where intravascular oncotic pressure exceeds filtration pressure, fluid moves back into the capillary. This feature allows movement of nutrients from blood to tissue and waste products from tissue to blood.

11.3.1.3 Fluid-shift pathology

An interesting aspect of the Starling Equation (Equation 1) is that it can describe, in mathematical terms, effects of capillary endothelial damage. When endothelium is damaged, the filtration coefficient (K_c) will increase and the permeability factor (σ) will decrease. As K_c rises, the hydrostatic pressure term in Equation 1 increases. As σ decreases, the capillary wall becomes more permeable to proteins, increasing π_i and decreasing π_p. All of these factors contribute to an acceleration of fluid movement into tissue, creating the pathological state of tissue edema. This is particularly critical in the lung, in which pulmonary edema increases the distance for oxygen diffusion across alveolar membranes (West 1985).

11.3.2 COP and HBOC design

The effects of Starling forces on transcapillary fluid movement introduces COP as a factor to be considered in HBOC design. *In vivo* fluid shifts following HBOC infusions have been studied only minimally. The problem arises because modifications to the hemoglobin molecule can alter the protein's colloid osmotic properties, with different types of modifications causing different effects on COP. Since COP is directly related to the physical attributes of the protein, rational design of a HBOC formulation must take the properties of the protein solution into account. These solution properties are described by thermodynamic equations relating the interaction between solvents and solutes.

11.4 Solution Thermodynamics

The underlying basis of colloid osmotic pressure is defined by the thermodynamic properties of solutions. A simple description of a macromolecule in solution is based on the partial molar free energy (*i.e.*, the chemical potential) of the solvent, μ_1,

$$(2)\ \mu_1 = \mu_1^o + RT\,ln(X_1 f_1)$$

where μ_1^o is the chemical potential of pure solvent, X_1 is the mole fraction of solvent, and f_1 is a solvent activity coefficient. *The basic principle is that the chemical potential of a solvent is reduced by the presence of a solute.* This is described as follows: the mole fraction of solvent is equal to $(1 - X_2)$, where X_2 is the mole fraction of a solute, so when calculated as a series, $\ln(1 - X_2) \approx -X_2 - X_2^2/2 \ldots$ (note: for parameters, subscripted 1 refers to solvent and subscripted 2 to solute),

$$(3)\ \mu_1 = \mu_1^o - RT(X_2 + \ldots) + RT\,ln\,f_1$$

Thus, μ_1 is decreased by a factor related to the contribution of solute, $RT(X_2 + \ldots)$. The mole fraction of solute can be expressed in terms of solute concentration (C_2) as,

$$(4)\ X_2 \approx \frac{C_2 V_1^o}{M_2}$$

where V_1^0 is the molar volume of pure solvent, and M_2 is the molecular weight of solute. For the last term in Equation 3, the factor f_1 will be less than 1, because at any given concentration of solute, solvent activity will be reduced. As a result, $(\ln f_1)$ can be represented by a negative power series in C_2, starting with C_2^2,

$$(5)\quad \ln f_1 = -(aC_2^2 + bC_2^3 + \ldots)$$

where a, b, *etc*. are constants. Then

$$(6)\quad \mu_1 = \mu_1^o - RTV_1^o\left(\frac{C_2}{M_2} + BC_2^2 + \ldots\right)$$

where $B = a/V_1^0$.

The quantities $1/M_2$ and B are called the first and second virial coefficients, respectively. From Equation 6, the higher the molecular weight (M_2), the lower the reduction in chemical potential (μ_1). Conversely, the greater the magnitude of the second virial coefficient, B, the greater the reduction in μ_1.

The second virial coefficient, B, is important because it provides a measure of solution ideality, a concept defined such that in an ideal solution, there is no interaction between solvent and solute molecules. Conversely, in a non-ideal solution, solvent and solute molecules interact, and the more interaction that takes place between solvent and solute, the more non-ideal the solution becomes. Solution non-ideality can be estimated by the expression (van Holde 1985),

$$(7)\quad S_i = (1 + BM_2C_2)$$

such that when $S_i = 1$, the solution is perfectly ideal, and as the value of S_i increases above 1, the solution becomes more non-ideal. However, considering Equation 6, even for a perfectly ideal solution (where $B = 0$), the chemical potential of solvent will still be reduced by the addition of solute, as determined then, independently, by the first virial coefficient,

$$(8)\quad \mu = \mu_1^o - RTV_1^o\left(\frac{C_2}{M_2}\right)$$

This relationship shows that the higher the molecular weight of solute, the lower the reduction in the chemical potential of solvent. For non-ideal solutions, the reduction in μ_1 will be determined by both M_2 and B.

11.4.1 Equilibrium across a membrane and osmotic pressure

In a two-compartment system (with sides **A** and **B**) separated by a semi-permeable membrane through which the solvent but not the solute can pass, pure solvent will diffuse across the membrane in both directions simultaneously, but the rate of its flow will be greater toward the side containing solute to maintain chemical equilibrium. For example, if solute molecules are restricted to side **A**, then the presence of solute lowers the chemical potential of the solvent in compartment **A**, such that at the same temperature and pressure,

$$(9)\quad \mu_1^A < \mu_1^B$$

To attain equilibrium across this membrane, the difference in chemical potential between compartments **A** and **B** must be balanced by a force exerted in compartment **A**. Since there is no barrier to temperature equilibration across the membrane, pressure provides the compensating force. The pressure difference required to attain equilibrium in chemical potential is called the *osmotic pressure* (π). It is measured experimentally in an osmometer as the hydrostatic pressure difference required to stop flow of solvent across a membrane.

Thermodynamically, the change in chemical potential with pressure at constant temperature (T) is given by

$$(10)\quad \left(\frac{\partial \mu_1}{\partial P}\right)_T = V_1$$

where V_1 is the partial molar volume of solvent. Assuming that $V_1 = V_1^0$ = a constant, the osmotic force needed to balance the chemical potential across the membrane is given by

$$(11)\quad \pi = RT\left(\frac{C_2}{M_2} + BC_2^2 + \ldots\right)$$

By rearranging Equation 11 and ignoring the higher order terms, we arrive at the linear equation,

$$(12)\quad \frac{\pi}{C_2} = \frac{RT}{M_2} + RTBC_2$$

which is useful because it allows the first and second virial coefficients, M_2 (the molecular weight) and B (the index of solution non-ideality), to be calculated directly from the intercept and slope, respectively, from a plot of π / C_2 *versus* C_2.

11.4.2 The Donnan effect

When solute molecules, such as proteins, have charge and exist in solution as polyelectrolytes, there will be an additional Donnan effect in which the concentration differences in ionic species across the membrane contribute to the osmotic pressure by a factor that varies as the square of the charge/mass ratio. This effect will cause the solution to become non-ideal. However, for studies on the osmotic pressure of a protein measured at a pH near its iso-electric point and that is dissolved in a high salt solution, the Donnan effect becomes negligible compared to the colloidal effect. This is because the counterions that remain with the protein to maintain electrical neutrality are insignificant in comparison to the excess salt that equilibrates across the membrane (Tanford 1961).

11.4.3 Physical properties of protein solutions: colloid osmotic pressure

Proteins are macromolecules that take on specific conformations in solution based on their intramolecular interactions and their interactions with solvent. Native, mammalian hemoglobins fold into a dense structure due to their strong side-chain interactions that give them a spherical, globular conformation with a low radius of gyration (R_G). R_G provides an estimate of the volume occupied by the extended macromolecule in solution. Since folded proteins are compact, this number is close to the actual molecular size of the protein. But as a globular protein denatures, it takes on more of a random-coiled structure as intramolecular interactions are lost, the protein unfolds, and R_G increases. Other random-coil structures that are of interest to HBOC design are synthetic polymers such as polyoxyethylene (polyethylene glycol) with repeating units $-CH_2-CH_2-O-$, some forms which have been conjugated to the surface of hemoglobin (see below). Molecules with large radii of gyration normally increase the non-ideality of the solution, because in general, a solution becomes more non-ideal as the molecular size of the solute increases.

The effective volume occupied by a solute can be calculated based on virial coefficients. For example, for a compact spherical molecule in dilute solution, the center of mass of the macromolecule of radius R can approach another solute macromolecule only to within a distance of 2R. This gives a value called the excluded volume of the solute molecule (Λ). Λ can be calculated as a function of solute molecular weight and specific volume ($\upsilon_2 = 1/\rho$, reciprocal density) (Tanford 1961),

$$(13)\quad \Lambda = \frac{8M_2\upsilon_2}{N}$$

where N is Avogadro's number. The specific volume, υ_2, is a composite that includes both the actual volume occupied per gram of the dry molecule and the volume occupied by the solvent associated with each gram of dry molecule. Furthermore, the specific volume is related to B (Tanford 1961),

$$(14)\quad \upsilon_2 = \frac{BM_2}{4}$$

which allows Λ to be calculated as a function of M_2 and B,

$$(15)\quad \Lambda = 2M_2^2 \frac{B}{N}$$

Since the volume of a sphere is equal to $(4/3)\pi R^3$, and a solute macromolecule can approach to within a distance of 2R of any other solute molecule, the excluded volume can be used to calculate R_G for a sphere,

$$(16)\quad \Lambda = (\tfrac{32}{3})\, \pi\, R_G^3$$

11.5 Experiments

11.5.1 Evaluations of colloid osmotic properties of HBOCs

The colloid osmotic pressure of several proteins were measured as a function of their concentration. The proteins included: human serum albumin (HSA) (Baxter Healthcare Corp.), purified human hemoglobin A_0 (HbA_0) (preparation described in Baines *et al.* 1995) (a gift from Hemosol Inc.), human hemoglobin cross-linked between αLys99 residues (αα–Hb) (preparation described in Winslow and Chapman 1994) (a gift from the U.S. Army), trimesoyl tris(methyl phosphate) cross-linked human hemoglobin (Tm-Hb) (Schumacher *et al.* 1995) (a gift from Hemosol Inc.), human hemoglobin polymerized with *o*-raffinose (*o*-R-poly-Hb) (preparation described in Baines *et al.* 1995) (a gift from Hemosol Inc.), and hemoglobins conjugated at surface amino residues to a synthetic polymer of polyoxyethylene (POE): one to human hemoglobin reacted with pyridoxal 5′-phosphate (Benesch and Benesch 1981) and then conjugated to POE (Yabuki *et al.* 1990, Iwashita 1995), which is now manufactured by Apex BioScience, Inc. in which the conjugation is Hb-$(OCH_2CH_2)_n$-COO^- (n ≈ 70 with an approximate molecular weight for each POE unit of 3,000 Daltons [T. Talarico, personal communication]) (PHP) (a gift from Apex BioScience, Inc.); the second conjugation reaction is to unmodified bovine hemoglobin (Bradley *et al.* 1994) in which the conjugation is Hb-$(OCH_2CH_2)_n$-O-CH_3 (n ≈ 110 with an approximate molecular weight for each POE unit of 5,000 Daltons [R. Shorr, personal communication]) (PEG-Hb) (a gift from Enzon, Inc.).

COP as a function of concentration for each of these proteins is shown in Figure 11.1. The HbA_0 data in Figure 11.1 agree well with data previously reported for sheep hemoglobin (Adair 1925, 1928). Adair (1925) showed that the osmotic pressures of purified hemoglobin were the same in distilled water as in the presence of 0.1 N salt, so that these results reflect the colloidal properties of the hemoglobin molecule rather than a Donnan effect. This is consistent with the linear fits to the HSA, HbA_0, cross-linked tetrameric and polymeric hemoglobin data (Figure 11.1), implying that these globular proteins behave in a nearly ideal manner in the range of protein concentrations reported here and that the volume of

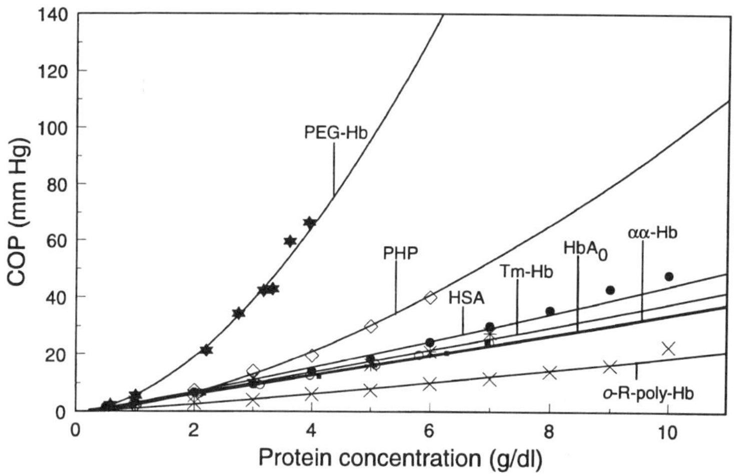

Figure 11.1. Colloid osmotic pressure as a function of protein concentration. Abbreviations for the proteins are given in the text. The symbols are measured data points: HSA, (closed circles), HbA_0 (open circles), αα–Hb (filled squares), Tm-Hb (asterisks), *o*-R-poly-Hb (crosses), PHP (open diamonds), PEG-Hb (filled stars). The solid lines going through the HSA, HbA_0, αα–Hb, Tm-Hb, and *o*-R-poly-Hb data are fitted linear regression lines; the solid lines going through the PHP and PEG-Hb data are fitted power series regression curves.

osmotically-inactive solvent water associated with the surface of these proteins is insufficient to increase the osmotic pressure. Deviation from ideal solution behavior for hemoglobin has been seen only at much higher concentrations than what were used here (*i.e.*, 29 g/dl) (Cameron and Fullerton 1990). In contrast, the non-linear fits required for the polyconjugated hemoglobins, PHP and PEG-Hb shown in Figure 11.1, reveal non-ideal solution behavior, suggesting that within this range of protein concentration, these surface-modified hemoglobins have a much greater stationary phase of solvent water molecules associated with them.

Linear plots of the same data using Equation 12 are shown in Figure 11.2. Slopes and intercepts were calculated by linear regression (see Table 11.1). Using the gas constant R = 62.364 mm Hg M^{-1} K^{-1} and temperature ranging from 293-295 K, RT is in units of mm Hg/M. The molecular weight (*i.e.*, the first virial coefficient) of each protein was calculated from the intercept in Figure 11.2 as (RT)/0.1*(intercept) in units of g/mol. The second virial coefficient, B, was calculated as the slope/(RT), and the units have been converted to cm^3mol/g^2. S_i was calculated from Equation 7, using a protein concentration of 5 mg/ml for C_2

(this concentration was chosen as one that would be close to that used physiologically). Exclusion volumes were calculated from Equation 15, and R_G was calculated from Equation 16 using the calculated values for Λ. All of these values are presented in Table 11.1.

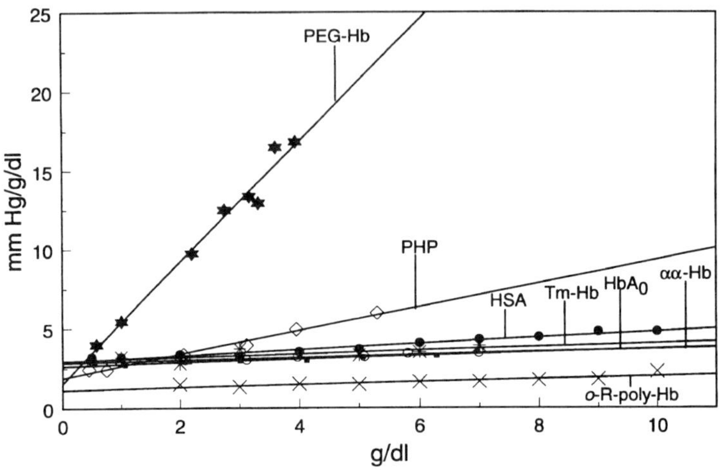

Figure 11.2. Colloid osmotic pressure data plotted as π/C_2 *versus* C_2, where π is colloid osmotic pressure in mm Hg and C_2 is protein concentration in g/dl. The symbols are measured data points and are designated in the legend to Figure 11.1. The solid lines are fitted regression lines to the data points.

Table 11.1

Sample	slope	intercept (mm Hg/ g/L)	M_2 (g/mol)	B (cm^{3}mol)/g^2 x 10^5	S_i*	Λ (nm^3)	R_G (nm)
HSA	0.1895	2.908	63,000	10.3	1.03	1,370	3.4
HbA_0	0.0881	2.828	65,000	4.8	1.02	660	2.7
αα–Hb	0.1087	2.640	69,000	5.9	1.02	950	3.1
Tm-Hb	0.1107	2.957	61,800	5.5	1.01	860	3.0
o-R-poly-Hb	0.0862	1.144	159,690	4.7	1.38	4,000	4.9
PHP	0.7446	1.899	97,000	40.5	1.20	13,000	7.2
PEG-Hb	3.8227	1.564	117,000	207.0	2.21	94,000	14.1

*Assuming C_2 = 5 g/dl.

11.5.1.1 Calculations of molecular weights

A comparison of these measured values for M_2 (Table 11.1) with reported values is shown in Figure 11.3, where reported values are (in units of g/mol = Daltons): HSA = 66,000 (Haeberli 1992); tetrameric hemoglobins = 65,000 (Dickerson and Geis 1983); *o*-R-poly-Hb = 128,000 (average) (G.

Adamson, personal communication); PHP= 90,000 (average) (T. Talarico, personal communication), and PEG-Hb = 125,000 ± 15,000 (Nucci, Shorr and Abuchowski 1996). The high correlation coefficient (R^2 = 0.94) provides confidence that these measurements are accurate within reasonable experimental error.

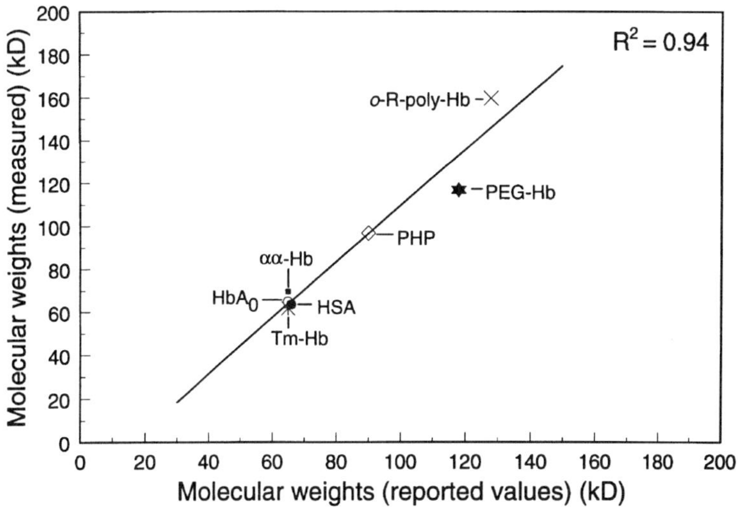

Figure 11.3. Molecular weights (kDaltons, kD) of proteins measured by osmotic pressure (given in Table 11.1) compared to reported values. The symbols are data points and are designated in the legend to Figure 11.1. The solid line is a fitted line with a regression coefficient of R^2 = 0.94.

For most HBOCs, the protein solutions are not homogeneous due to chemical modification reactions. For heterogeneous solutes, osmotic pressure measurements yield an average of molecular weights and thus determine the mean molecular weight of the solute; the same average would be obtained from measurements of any colligative property (van Holde 1985).

Our measurements demonstrate that PHP and PEG-Hb have similar molecular weights (97 *versus* 117 kD). However, the estimated number of POE units (OCH_2CH_2) in the polymers conjugated to PHP is less than that for PEG-Hb (n ≈ 70 *versus* ≈ 110). Assuming that both conjugation reactions are to tetrameric hemoglobins (which cannot be strictly correct since neither PHP nor PEG-Hb is intramolecularly cross-linked), the number of polymer-conjugations to the hemoglobins can be estimated as follows: for PHP, the average number of POE strands is equal to (97,000-65,000)/3,000 ≈11. This number is nearly double that reported for an earlier PHP product (~6 POE units per tetramer) (Yabuki *et al.* 1990, Iwashita 1995). For PEG-Hb, the average number of POE strands is equal to (117,000-65,000)/5,000 ≈ 10. It has been reported that the preferred PEG-Hb solutions are conjugates with an average degree of substitution of at least 11 POE units/hemoglobin molecules (Shorr, Cho and Nho 1995). These calculations suggest that these surface-modified hemoglobins have a similar number of surface conjugation sites. Either the length of the polyoxyethylene unit (5,000 *versus* 3,000 Daltons for PEG-Hb and PHP, respectively) or the termination group for the synthetic polymers (PHP terminates with carboxyl groups, whose charge may reduce the osmotic pressure, while PEG-Hb terminates with methoxy groups) is the important determinant in the final COP of the protein solution, or both.

11.5.1.2 Calculations of second virial coefficients

The idealities of the hemoglobin solutions were estimated from the value of the second virial coefficient (*B* in Table 11.1, all units for *B* given below are cm^3mol/g^2). The values for human serum albumin and native human hemoglobin determined here (10.3×10^{-5} and 4.8×10^{-5}, respectively) are slightly higher than published values for bovine serum albumin and bovine methemoglobin of 2.9×10^{-5} and 1.3×10^{-5} , respectively (Castellino and Barker 1968). The human hemoglobin number agrees well with the standard value of 4×10^{-5} for a spherical protein with a molecular weight of $\sim 10^5$ Daltons (Tanford 1961). The average *B* value for the cross-linked hemoglobin tetramers is 5.5×10^{-5}, and the value for the polymerized hemoglobin is 4.7×10^{-5}. All of these tetrameric and polymerized HBOC solutions exhibit nearly ideal solution behavior, giving S_i values near 1 (calculated at 5 g/dl).

In marked contrast, the polyconjugated hemoglobins show very different solution behavior. The second virial coefficient (*B*) for PHP-conjugated hemoglobin is an order of magnitude larger than for the non-conjugated hemoglobins at 41×10^{-5} , and the value of *B* for PEG-conjugated hemoglobin is two-orders of magnitude higher than for non-conjugated hemoglobins at 207×10^{-5}. At 5 g/dl, these correspond to S_i values for PHP and PEG-Hb of 1.2 and 2.2, respectively, indicating that these solutions are non-ideal, as reflected by the nonzero slopes of their regression lines in Figure 11.2.

All of the data in Figure 11.2 were fit well by linear regression. This justifies disregarding higher order terms in Equation 12, so that higher order virial coefficients are not necessary to describe these data. This leads to the following considerations: (1) the near-zero slopes for the albumin, tetrameric, and polymeric hemoglobins show that over the range of protein concentrations studied here, these solutions are nearly ideal, suggesting a fixed number of solvent interactions with these proteins. (2) The positive slopes for the polyconjugated hemoglobins demonstrate that within this same range of protein concentration these solutions are non-ideal, indicating an increased fixed, solvent-accessible surface area for these proteins. POE polymers are highly hydrophilic: three molecules of water associate with each POE unit (Liu and Parsons 1969, Maxfield and Shepard 1975). (3) The absence of significant higher order virial coefficients implies that there is no protein aggregation at these protein concentrations.

11.5.1.3 Calculations of specific volumes and densities

An advantage of osmotic pressure data analysis is that specific volumes are not required to evaluate the proteins' molecular weights. This is particularly important in the case of modified hemoglobins, because the modification may change the macromolecule's specific volume and density ($\upsilon_2 = 1/\rho$) (see Equation 13). In addition, the COP data allow an estimation of υ_2 from the calculation shown in Equation 14 by using experimentally determined values for M_2 and B. Our calculation for native hemoglobin (0.77 ml/g) is close to the reported value of 0.75 ml/g (Ross and Minton 1977). We have used these numbers to estimate relative densities of HBOC solutions. The numbers for native and tetrameric hemoglobins have densities that are close to that of water (i.e., ~1 g/ml), while the polymeric hemoglobin, *o*-R-poly-Hb, has a calculated density about half that of water, and the polyconjugated hemoglobins have calculated densities that are 10 to 60-fold less than water. The marked decreases in density for PHP and PEG-Hb is consistent with the known physical properties of synthetic polymer solutions in that density decreases with increasing chain length (Tanford 1961).

11.5.1.4 Calculations of excluded volumes and radii of gyration

Calculation of values for the radii of gyration and for the excluded volumes for these proteins are given in Table 11.1 and are represented graphically in Figures 11.4 and 11.5, respectively. Of all of the physical parameters determined here, these numbers probably best illustrate the differences between solution properties of these HBOCs.

The molecular radius of a native human hemoglobin tetramer is approximately 3.2 nm (Dickerson and Geis 1983). This number, based on x-ray structural data, agrees well with the values of R_G determined here for HbA_0, ααHb, and Tm-Hb (average value = 2.8 nm) (Figure 11.4). The R_G value for *o*-R-poly-Hb is slightly higher at 4.9 nm, as would be expected for a branched, polymerized hemoglobin. Even though the PHP and PEG-Hb are tetrameric, their R_G values are significantly higher: 8.4 and 14.1 nm, respectively.

In terms of effective volume in solution, compared to the average value for the tetramers (~800 nm^3), the polymerized hemoglobin, with a 2.5-fold higher molecular weight, has only a 5-fold higher excluded volume.

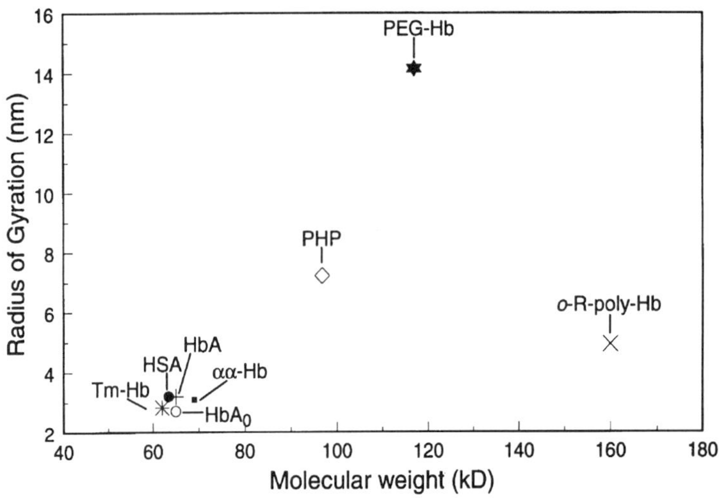

Figure 11.4. Radius of gyration (RG) as a function of protein molecular weight. RG was calculated from Equation 16 using the excluded volumes given in Table 11.1. RG is in units of nm. Molecular weights are in kDaltons (kD). The symbols are data points and are designated in the legend to Figure 11.1. The known radius of native HbA based on its x-ray crystallographic structure (Dickerson and Geis 1983) is shown by the symbol (+).

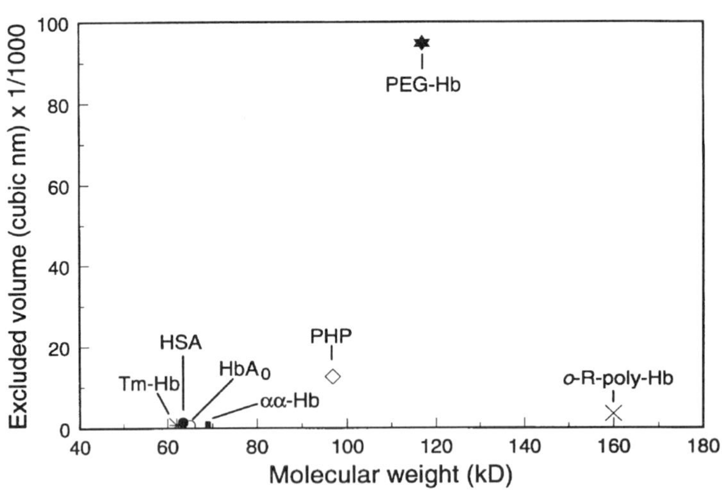

Figure 11.5. Excluded volumes as a function of protein molecular weight. Excluded volume was calculated from Equation 15 using the values for M_2 and B given in Table 11.1. The symbols are data points and are designated in the legend to Figure 11.1. Excluded volumes are in units of $nm^3 \times 10^{-3}$. Molecular weights are in kDaltons (kD).

In contrast, the molecular weights of PHP and PEG-Hb are less than that of the polymeric hemoglobin, but their excluded volumes are much larger. Compared to the hemoglobin tetramers, PHP and PEG-Hb have 16-fold and 120-fold greater excluded volumes, respectively (Figure 11.5). A schematic illustration of the differences between excluded volumes for these macromolecules is represented in Figure 11.6.

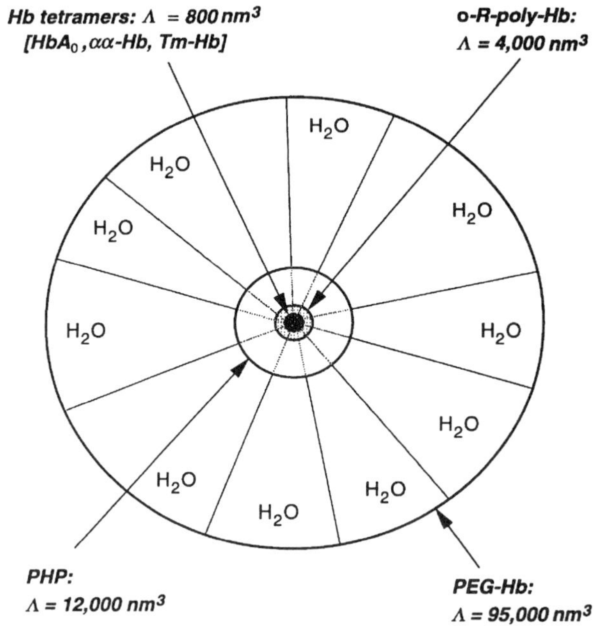

Figure 11.6. Schematic diagram representing the excluded volumes of hemoglobin tetramers (HbA_0, αα-Hb, and Tm-Hb), *o*-poly-R-Hb, PHP, and PEG-Hb.

In conclusion, these surface-polymer modification reactions increase the molecular radius of the hemoglobin molecule in solution by 3-4 times. The hydration of the conjugated POE units thus essentially forms larger macromolecules by trapping solvent and greatly increasing the volume of the macromolecule in solution. The result is a greater reduction in the chemical potential of the solvent and an increase in the colloid osmotic pressure exerted by these proteins.

11.5.2 Blood volume measurements

In a previously reported series of experiments, plasma volumes were measured in rats using Evan's blue dye after 50% exchange transfusions with either Ringer's lactate (RL), αα–Hb (7.9 g/dl), or PEG-Hb (5.5 g/dl) (Migita *et al.* 1997). Total blood volume was calculated by multiplying the plasma volume by 100/(100 - hematocrit). These volumes are given in Table 11.2 as a function of time after completion of the exchange transfusion. The control represents the blood volume of rats that were not exchange transfused.

Table 11.2

Time Post-exchange (minutes)	*Blood Volume (ml/kg) Samples*			
	Control	**RL**	**αα-Hb**	**PEG-Hb**
0	58 ± 1.9	48 ± 1.2	49 ± 1.2	74 ± 3.5
30		47 ± 2.6	48 ± 3.5	66 ± 11.5
60		42 ± 0.2	45 ± 2.9	62 ± 3.9
120		42 ± 5.8	42 ± 2.8	61 ± 3.8

Adapted from Migita *et al.* 1997.

The 5.5 g/dl solution of PEG-Hb (COP ≈ 100 mm Hg) significantly increased the blood volume in rats immediately after the 50% exchange transfusion which then returned to near control blood volume after two hours. In contrast, the 7.9 g/dl solution of αα–Hb, which is iso-oncotic (COP ≈ 24 Torr), showed a persistent decrease in total blood volume that became significantly lower than control 60 and 120 minutes post-exchange. The Ringer's lactate-exchanged animals also showed a persistent and more rapid decrease in blood volume, because crystalloid clears rapidly from the intravascular space. The increase in blood volume exhibited in the PEG-Hb-transfused animals is translated to an increase in cardiac output, presumably due to increased cardiac filling.

11.5.3 Total blood exchange with hyperoncotic HBOC

As discussed earlier, blood volume is tightly regulated. Plasma and tissue fluids shift in order to keep blood volume constant, and lymph flow adjusts as a result. However, the ability of the body to adjust to large infusions of hyperoncotic HBOC solutions have not been documented. To study this effect, preliminary experiments were carried out using a 100% exchange-transfusion protocol in rats with PEG-Hb (5.5 g/dl). Blood gases, acid-base status, and COP were monitored during the exchange. COP continued to rise during the exchange and did not reach equilibrium during the time period of the experiment; COP rose rapidly during the first 50% of the exchange and then more slowly during the last half of the exchange. By the end of the exchange, all of the circulating hemoglobin was plasma-derived, and the hematocrit was reduced to zero with a total hemoglobin concentration of ~3 g/dl. During this procedure, blood gases did not change substantially: arterial pO_2 increased slightly, arterial pCO_2 decreased slightly, base excess decreased slightly, and blood lactate and pH remained constant during the experiment.

Thus, 100% exchange transfusion was achieved with a large increase in blood COP and near normal acid-base status. Further experimentation in this area is necessary to understand the physiological responses to this procedure.

11.6 Conclusions

Blood replacement with cell-free, hemoglobin-based oxygen carriers is being considered as a substitute for blood transfusions. These hemoglobin solutions, being acellular solutions rather than particulate, do not have the same properties as blood, both in terms of oxygen delivery and solution properties. While oxygen delivery is a primary concern, blood volume restitution is an equally essential factor. In this regard, intravascular oncotic pressures that arise from administration of HBOCs may play a major role in their eventual clinical success. The impact of these solutions on recovery from blood loss may not be predicted *a priori* based on blood transfusions: hemostatic compensatory mechanisms might not respond in a typical manner following infusions of large amounts of cell-free proteins, leaving the system in an abnormal state of fluid balance. Specific treatment protocols and optimal formulations of HBOCs should be evaluated further before these products are used routinely in transfusion medicine with confidence in patient outcome.

11.7 Acknowledgment

We thank A. Gonzales, M.L. Gonzales, M.D. Magde, Jr., and M. McCarthy for technical assistance. This work was supported in part by USPHS/NHLBI Program Project No. HL48018.

11.8 References

Adair, G.S. The osmotic pressure of haemoglobin in the absence of salts. *Proc. R. Soc. Lond. A* 109: 292-300, 1925.

Adair, G.S. A theory of partial osmotic pressures and membrane equilibria, with special reference to the application of Dalton's law to hemoglobin solution in the presence of salts. *Proc. R. Soc. Lond. A* 120: 573-603, 1928.

Baines, A.D., B. Christoff, D. Wicks, D. Wiffen, and D. Pliura. Cross-linked hemoglobin increases fractional reabsorption and GFR in hypoxic isolated perfused rat kidneys. *Am. J. Physiol.* 269: F628-F636, 1995.

Benesch, R., and R.E. Benesch. Preparation and properties of hemoglobin modified with derivatives of pyridoxal. *Meth. Enzymol.* 76: 147-159, 1981.

Bradley, R., S. Sloshberg, K. Nho, B. Czuba, D. Szesko, and R. Shorr. Production of PEG-modified bovine hemoglobin: economics and feasibility. *Artif. Cells, Blood Substitutes, Immobil. Biotech.* 22: 657-667, 1994.

Cameron, I.L., and G.D. Fullerton. A model to explain the osmotic pressure behavior of hemoglobin and serum albumin. *Biochem. Cell Biol.* 68: 894-898, 1990.

Castellino, F.J., and R. Barker. Examination of the dissociation of multichain proteins in guanidine hydrochloride by membrane osmometry. *Biochemistry* 7: 2207-2217, 1968.

Dickerson, R.E., and I. Geis. *Hemoglobin: Structure, Function, Evolution, and Pathology*. Menlo Park: Benjamin/Cummings Publishing Co., 1983.

Ganong, W.F. *Review of Medical Physiology.* Los Altos: Lange Medical Publications, 1983, pp. 462-476.

Guyton, A.C. *Textbook of Medical Physiology (7th edition).* Philadelphia: Saunders, 1986.

Guyton, A.C., A.E. Taylor, and H.J. Granger. *Circulatory Physiology. II. Dynamics and Control of Body Fluids.* Philadelphia: WB Saunders, 1975, pp. 149-193.

Haeberli, A. (Editor). *Human Protein Data.* Meinheim: VCH, 1992.

Hess, J.R., C.E. Wade, and R.M. Winslow. Filtration-assisted exchange transfusion using ααHb, an erythrocyte substitute. *J. Appl. Physiol.* 70: 1639-1644, 1991.

Iwashita, Y. Hemoglobin conjugated with polyoxyethylene. In *Artificial Red Cells* (Tsuchida, E., ed.) New York: John Wiley & Sons, 1995, pp. 151-176.

Landis, E.M. Micro-injection studies of capillary permeability. II. The relation between capillary pressure and the rate at which fluid passes through the walls of single capillaries. *Am. J. Physiol.* 82: 217-238, 1927.

Liu, K.J., and J.L. Parsons. *Macromolecules* 2: 529-533, 1969.

Maxfield, J., and I.W. Shepard. Conformation of poly(oxyethylene oxide) in solid state, melt and solution measured by Raman scattering. *Polymer* 16: 505-509, 1975.

Migita, R., A. Gonzales, M.L. Gonzales, K.D. Vandegriff, and R.M. Winslow. Blood volume and cardiac index in rats after 50% exchange transfusion with hemoglobin-based oxygen carriers. *J. Appl. Physiol.* (In press) 1997.

Nucci, M.L., R.G.L. Shorr, and A. Abuchowski. PEG-hemoglobin. Oxygen carrying blood substitute. *Drugs of the Future* 21: 29-32, 1996.

Reed, R.K., Woie, K., and K. Rubin. Integrins and control of interstitial fluid pressure. *News Physiol. Sci.* 12: 42-48, 1997.

Ross, P.D., and A.P. Minton. Analysis of non-ideal behavior in concentrated hemoglobin solutions. *J. Mol. Biol.* 112: 437-452, 1977.

Schumacher, M.A., M.M. Dixon, R. Kluger, R.T. Jones, and R.G. Brennan. Allosteric transition intermediates by cross-linked haemoglobins. *Nature* 375: 84-87, 1995.

Shorr, R.G.L., M.-O.P. Cho, and K. Nho. Fractionation of polyalkylene oxide-conjugated hemoglobin solutions. *U.S. Patent No.* 5,478,805, 1995.

Starling, E.H. On the absorption of fluids from connective tissue spaces. *J. Physiol. Lond.* 19: 312-326, 1896.

Tanford, C. *Physical Chemistry of Macromolecules.* New York: John Wiley & Sons, Inc., 1961, pp. 180-274.

Tsai, A.G., H. Kerger, and M. Intaglietta. Microvascular oxygen distribution: effects due to free hemoglobin in plasma. In *Blood Substitutes: New Challenges* (R.M. Winslow, K.D. Vandegriff, and M. Intaglietta, eds.) Boston: Birkhäuser, 1996, pp. 124-131.

van Holde, K.E. *Physical Biochemistry (2nd Edition).* Englewood Cliffs: Prentice-Hall, Inc. 1985.

West, J.B. *Respiratory Physiology - the Essentials (3rd Edition).* Baltimore: Williams & Wilkins, 1985, pp. 44-46.

Winslow, R.M. *Hemoglobin-based Red Cell Substitutes.* Baltimore: The Johns Hopkins University Press, 1992.

Winslow, R.M., and K.W. Chapman. Pilot-scale preparation of hemoglobin solutions. *Meth. Enzymol.* 231: 3-16, 1994.

Yabuki, A., K. Yamaji, H. Ohki, and Y. Iwashita. Characterization of a pyridoxalated hemoglobin-polyoxyethylene conjugate as a physiologic oxygen carrier. *Transfusion* 30: 516-520, 1990.

11.9 Discussion

Woodson: In terms of measuring volumes of these animals using Evan's blue dye, does the Evan's blue find its way into the water of hydration of these large molecules, how large is that volume of water in relation to the total, and does that, if corrected for, change the blood volume of the animal in a range which would be clinically important?

Vandegriff: I can tell you a little bit about how much water we think is involved. The numbers are about three molecules of water per polyoxyethylene unit. With the PHP product, we have calculated that there are approximately 70 units per polymer and about 10 polymers per molecule. The PEG-hemoglobin with a 5000 molecular weight polymer has approximately 110 units, and Rob Shorr has said that there may be up to 150 polyoxyethylene units per polymer and, again, 10 polymers per tetramer. So, it's a large amount of water. However, as Dr. Torchilin showed us, because of the flexibility of these polymer chains, it has a tendency to lower the density of the water in the macromolecule's fixed-water stationary phase so that the distribution of water is completely changed. The Evan's blue dye is a small enough molecule, from what I've learned at this meeting, that it could partition into that space.

Winslow: One more brief comment on that question. I don't think it's introducing a large area if there is one because if you calculate the hematocrits based on mass balance, that is red cells out and the final measured hematocrit, it comes out to be about what you expect, so I don't think it's a very big effect if there is one.

Hess: Several years ago in *The New England Journal of Medicine* there was a case report about a surgical resident who, left to his own devices, managed to get a patient's albumin concentration up to about 12 grams per deciliter. The obvious result of this was that he shut down glomerular filtration. Have you looked at what happens to the urine output in these animals when you give them the PEG-hemoglobin?

Vandegriff: We have not done that quantitatively. This molecule has not been in Roland Blantz's kidney model. I think it needs to be done.

Meiselman: You mentioned the difficulty, or at least a technical difficulty, involved in measuring colloid osmotic pressure, and that you had used a 30,000 molecular weight membrane cut-off and were looking for a 10,000. I wonder if you've used other physical chemical techniques. There's a variety of molecular weights that you can calculate; you get them by viscometry or by light scattering. Particularly, do you have any feeling for molecular weight distribution? Are we talking number average, weight average, viscosity average, molecular weight?

Vandegriff: We're talking about molecular weight average. COP is a colligative property, so the number that is calculated from these measurements is the average molecular weight.

Meiselman: And if you did intrinsic viscosity determinations, do you think you'd be picking up some new information, or would it be the same sort of information?

Vandegriff: I think I should ask you that question.

Meiselman: It might.

Vandegriff: Okay. We're measuring viscosity as well as COP.

Meiselman: I think for the hemoglobins you're probably okay because you expect a monodispersed molecular weight distribution where the weight number average would be very close to 1. I don't know anything on the molecular weight distribution for the polyhemoglobins. Is the weight-to-number average close to 1, or is it much more polydisbursed?

Vandegriff: For the polymerized hemoglobin (*o*-R-poly-Hb) used here there is a range in molecular size so that there is a distribution of species from dimer, 32 kD, up to 526 kD, but those two extremes are a small fraction, and the majority fraction is basically a di- or tri-tetramer. I believe the surface-conjugated hemoglobins have less distribution because there is less intermolecular interaction.

Bonaventura: Starling's work is analogous, I think, to what Tanford said about the laws of thermodynamics. He said he could understand thermodynamics with absolute clarity every time he learned it. And so that's what I do with Starling. However, I'm still in the dark about Tanford's 1961 paper. Would you please repeat what you said about that?

Vandegriff: It's a book written by Tanford called Physical Chemistry of Macromolecules, and it is referenced in the chapter for this book.

Wong: It's fascinating to see the range of oncotic pressure that you can achieve with different kinds of blood substitutes, and of course, in the design of blood substitutes, one wants to pack more heme for oxygen capacity, but then what would end up is the varying end point of the oncotic pressure. Now, what is the ideal clinical target? So, let's say now that we have a whole range of blood substitutes achieving all kinds of oncotic pressure, should we be targeting at 20 or up to 70? Where is the ideal?

Vandegriff: I think what we have is the capability to target whatever the clinicians feel that they need depending on the indication. If you need blood volume restitution, I would go with something with high oncotic pressure. If you want a pharmacologic effect for a pressor effect, you may not need to worry about that as much. So, I think that the range of products and molecules that we're studying can address different clinical indications. I think it's a field that we need to address a bit more.

As far as your comment about trying to have more oxygen-carrying capacity, I would refer to Bob Winslow's talks yesterday and today to restate that we're not sure what's absolutely necessary. We must have appropriate oxygen delivery, but we also must have appropriate perfusion, or the oxygen delivery becomes insignificant in relation to the pharmacologic effects. Bob Przybelski showed very clearly that they are going after a therapeutic pressor effect right now. So, I think if we're talking in terms of oxygen delivery, we need to balance a lot of things, and solution properties are one of those to ensure that all organ systems are perfused.

Sakai: Hemoglobin concentration of PEG-hemoglobin is very low, and P50 is also very low, and so the A-V difference is very low, and you stressed the importance of oncotic pressure. It seems that oncotic pressure is much more important than the oxygen transport by the hemoglobin itself.

Vandegriff: I think the data that you presented yesterday showed some of that effect. I think you're absolutely correct that if we're not perfusing tissues, it doesn't matter what the P50 is.

Sakai: PEG-modified albumin doesn't have a heme. Do you think it will work very well?

Vandegriff: As a control for oncotic pressure and viscosity in the animal studies, we've been using Pentastarch, which has similar oncotic and viscosity properties at PEG-hemoglobin but doesn't carry oxygen. Yesterday, Bob Winslow showed data that the oxygen carrier showed a much greater survival rate than a solution that had identical solution properties but no oxygen-carrying capacity; but, as far as the starting concentration, the PEG-Hb is 5%, so we're really beginning to question how much oxygen-carrying capacity we need in tandem with red blood cells on board to have adequate delivery to tissue.

Baldwin: When you were talking about different colloid osmotic pressures when you add different hemoglobins to the blood, you were talking about the colloid osmotic pressure of the samples, but, as you know, when we're talking about fluid exchanges, it's the colloid osmotic pressure difference across the vessel wall that's important. Do you have any idea about how the colloid osmotic pressure in the tissue fluid changes as you add different hemoglobins?

Vandegriff: That's a very interesting question. Of course, the physical measurements that we made were all diluted in a Ringer's lactate, and so the only blood sample measurements that we have were in the 100% exchange transfused animals where it continued to climb. I think that initially there has to be a shift of water from the interstitium during that initial rapid rise in blood COP; however, as you've shown, there appears to be extravasation through the endothelial junctions or whatever, possibly of the intact protein, so I don't know the answer to that, and it's left for future research.

Woodson: As I think about the problems of measuring blood volume under these circumstances, I continue to realize how complex it really might be. If you do an exchange transfusion with a molecule that has a very high colloid osmotic pressure, and you try to measure the blood volume at time points during the exchange, you may actually be looking at a blood volume which is in evolution, so that maybe if one did a stepped exchange and left the animal alone after, let's say, a 20% exchange or a 50% exchange for an interval of time like an hour or two, the blood volume would be completely different at the end of that time than it was before, particularly if the animal had continuing access to water and didn't lose water during a procedure, as small animals are infamous for doing.

So, I have a concern about that. Even if you think that it doesn't contribute very much, one usually injects Evan's blue and then takes two or three samples at maybe 5, 10 or 15 minutes to get a curve and then extrapolate back to what would have been at time zero at pre-mixing. So, a further question is whether that kind of equilibration would be complete, or whether the major perturbation in fluid exchange, which is diluting the Evan's blue dye, does not reach completion very fast, but it's a different kinetic curve.

This leads me to answer the question. One would need to make a much more involved and difficult-to-do series of measurements in a small furry animal, such as a simultaneous radioactive hemoglobin measurement of the blood substitute you're putting in, in order to keep track of the total number of counts and where the counts wind up and the same thing for plasma, relate that to measured hemoglobin concentration and hematocrit and turn this into a two-year research project, because I'm really not sure that we can make very good inferences about whether those volume-change curves are right.

Winslow: Let me make a comment on the technical aspect because we haven't gone into detail about these volume measurements. This will be in the Migita *et al.* paper which is in press in the *Journal of Applied Physiology*. The first point is that we don't do serial volume measurements in a single animal. Because of the presence of Evan's blue, it's very difficult to make a second injection and a second measurement. So, each time point represents a different animal; that's the first point.

The second point is that when we inject Evan's blue, we then sample every five minutes for at least five samples, get a regression disappearance curve, and then extrapolate to time zero and, indeed, you do see a disappearance slope for Evan's blue dye after injection. It's a very shallow slope, but one of the things that we observed--and it's in the paper--is that the slope of that disappearance curve is dependent to some degree on the type of hemoglobin that you have used. And, we speculate that that may have to do with vascular leakiness, particularly the movement of albumin, and I think that, in fact, may be a very interesting observation that could be followed up on. We are aware of the technical problems you mentioned, and we have been very careful to do regression analysis on every single point.

Vandegriff: In addition, I'd like to say that the cardiac output measurements were measured independently. Perhaps there's a mechanism to increase cardiac output without increasing volume that I am unaware of, but the blood volumes and cardiac outputs are consistent.

Phillips: I think it's interesting that the colloidal osmotic pressure continues to rise during the whole course of the 100% exchange transfusions, and does that mean that the intercellular volume and the interstitial fluid just can't give up any more water?

Vandegriff: Keep in mind that this was a continuous exchange, so as blood was coming out more of the oncotically active material was going in, and those two were parallel. I would assume at some point, if we followed it longer, it would reach equilibrium.

Winslow: There's another interesting point that I mentioned yesterday, and that is if you do this exchange in an animal with the high oncotic pressure material and then you hemorrhage, the hematocrit doesn't change during the hemorrhage, which, I think means that you have very little shift of fluid back into the vascular space as you hemorrhage in these animals who have high oncotic pressure.

Vandegriff: There is some evidence that high molecular weight polymers somehow may plug capillary leakiness. Of course, Ann Baldwin is not seeing this. I don't know if that's happening in this case or not.

Chapter 12

Dextran-Hemoglobin

Sheung-Pun Tsai, Ph.D. and J. Tze-Fei Wong, Ph.D.

12.1 Introduction

In recent years the quest for a safe blood substitute has accelerated rapidly, propelled both by the hazardous nature of the whole blood supply in many parts of the world and by the increasingly satisfactory replacement of various plasma components by their recombinant counterparts. To replace the functions of erythrocytes and the bulk of plasma, a blood substitute needs to maintain effectively the oncotic pressure and volume of the circulation, and to carry oxygen from the lungs to support tissue respiration. Hemoglobin (Hb) is an attractive oxygen carrier in the development of a clinical blood substitute, given its attributes as a respiratory pigment of extensive solubility, uptake and release of oxygen at appropriate partial pressures, buffering power, and above all its capability of transporting a large quantity of oxygen (Odling-Smee and Wilson 1988). However, one fundamental disadvantage of free Hb itself as a blood substitute arises from its relatively small molecular size and consequent hemoglobinuria and rapid clearance from the circulation. Therefore, methods such as encapsulation, polymerization, interdimeric cross-linking and covalent conjugation have to be applied in order to prevent renal excretion and to prolong its plasma half-life (Chang 1992). The advantage of the conjugation method is based on the wide range of carrier polymers, with respect to chemical nature and size, that can be employed, as well as the type of linkage between Hb and carrier that can be constructed. Dextran-hemoglobin (Dx-Hb) was the first conjugate introduced as a blood substitute, but the approach of covalent conjugation has since been extended to the use of other carriers including hydroxyethylstarch, polyvinylpyrrolidone and polyethylene glycol (Table 12.1).

The dextran employed is a poly 1$\rightarrow$6-α-D-glucose containing randomly distributed 1$\rightarrow$3-α-glucopyranosyl branch residues (Yalpani 1988). Since dextran has been used for decades as a clinical plasma volume expander, its biocompatibility is well established. Its selection as carrier polymer in a Hb-based blood substitute is further suggested by its beneficial actions on blood flow. The permeability from plasma to lymph of dextrans of MW 8,000-500,000 daltons decreases with molecular weight (Muranishi 1991), and dextrans of less than MW 51,300 are not immunogenic in man (Kabat and Bezer 1958). Dextran is completely metabolized or excreted from the body after brief storage in the cells of the reticuloendothelial system, and it can be chemically modified by a variety of methods to form defined and stable compounds. Indeed, the combination of water solubility, availability in a wide range of molecular sizes, and lack of significant toxicity or tissue tropism, renders dextran an excellent drug carrier among biodegradable polymers. Dextran conjugation has been employed to prolong the plasma half-lives of asparaginase (Wileman, Foster and Elliott 1986), carboxypeptidase (Melton *et al.* 1987), adenosine deaminase (Rosemeyer, Körnig and Seela 1982) and arginase (Sherwood *et al.* 1977). The coupling of proteins to dextran is therefore an important means to enhance their therapeutic efficacies.

Table 12.1 Polymers conjugated covalently to hemoglobin in potential blood substitutes.

Polymer	Reference
Natural biopolymers	
Dextran	Tam, Blumenstein and Wong 1976
Inulin	Iwasaki, Ajisaka and Iwashita 1983
Biopolymer derivatives	
Hydroxyethylstarch	Cerny *et al.* 1984
Dextran Sulfate	Barberousse, Sacco and Dellacherie 1986
Dextran phosphate	Sacco *et al.* 1990
Dextran benzene hexacarboxylate	Prouchayret *et al.* 1992
Synthetic polymers	
Polyethylene glycol	Ajisaka and Iwashita 1980
Monomethoxypolyoxyethylene	Leonard and Dellacherie 1984
Polyvinylpyrrolidone	Schmidt 1979

12.2 Preparation and characteristics of Dx-Hb

12.2.1 Synthesis of Dx-Hb

Covalent conjugation of dextran to hemoglobin increases the effective size of the molecule, prevents its renal excretion and slows down its disappearance from the circulation. For this purpose, dextran is activated with cyanogen bromide at alkaline pH for 5 minutes, and diaminoethane is added to introduce free amino groups. The resultant aminoethylamino-dextran is acylated with bromo-acetylbromide at neutral pH prior to dialysis against water and lyophilization (Tam, Blumenstein and Wong 1976). This bromodextran is stable for 2-3 years upon storage at -20°C, and its bromine content, determined on the basis of bromide analysis after incubating the bromodextran in 0.1 N NaOH for 30 minutes at 100°C to hydrolyze the bromo function, is indicated to be in the range of 8-10 glucose residues per bromine atom.

The conjugation reaction (Figure 12.1) between the bromodextran and Hb is carried out in bicarbonate buffer of pH 9.5. That the linkage be-

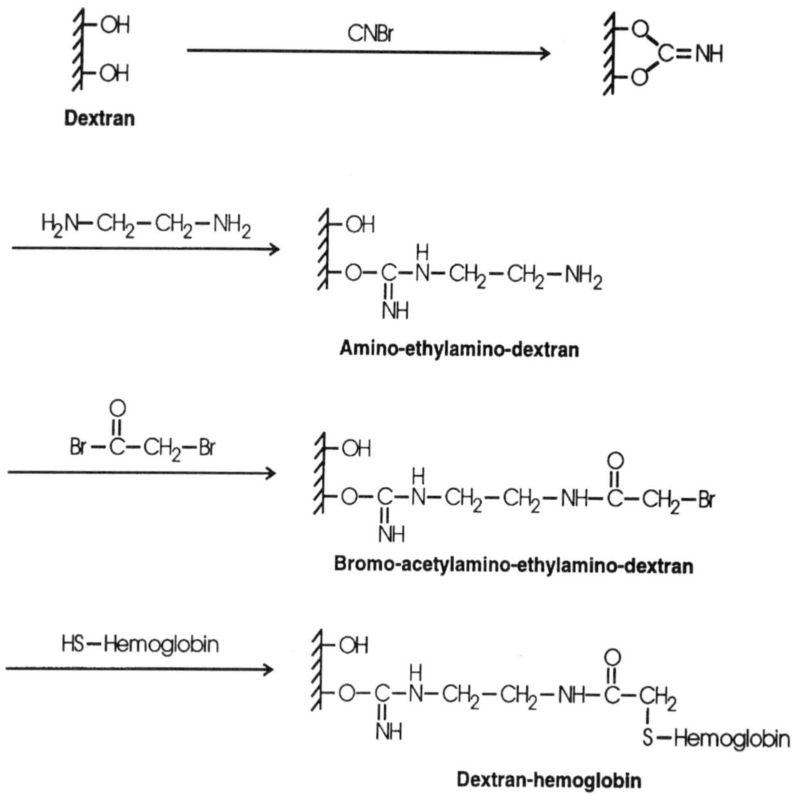

Figure 12.1. Activation of dextran and subsequent conjugation with hemoglobin in the alkylation method.

tween bromodextran and Hb is through the reactive sulfhydryl group of β-93 cysteine is evidenced by the close correlation between the loss of sulfhydryls and the formation of Dx-Hb (Chang and Wong 1977). The conjugate, therefore, has the chemical form of hemoglobin-S-acetylamino-ethylamino-dextran. This synthetic condition yields, in the case of dextran MW 20,000, a complete conjugation of Hb with a dextran-to-hemoglobin molar ratio close to unity. The high yield of the

Dx-Hb conjugate effectively renders unnecessary its cumbersome fractionation from any residual free Hb before use in transfusions.

12.2.2 Stability of Dx-Hb

In addition to a high conjugation yield, a long shelf life of Dx-Hb is essential to its practical use. Sterile solutions of Dx-Hb routinely may be stored at 4°C for at least six months without the metHb content exceeding 5% of total Hb. Upon prolonged storage at 4°C, however, Dx-Hb solutions display an increase in viscosity on account of continued reaction between residual bromo groups on the bromodextran and hemoglobin. This rise in viscosity is prevented by treatment with sulfhydryl containing compounds such as L-cysteine or β-mercaptopropionic acid to remove excess bromo groups, resulting in a stable solution viscosity (Figure 12.2). Thus treatment with β-mercaptopropionic acid enables maintenance of Dx-Hb solution at a lower viscosity compared to that of whole blood.

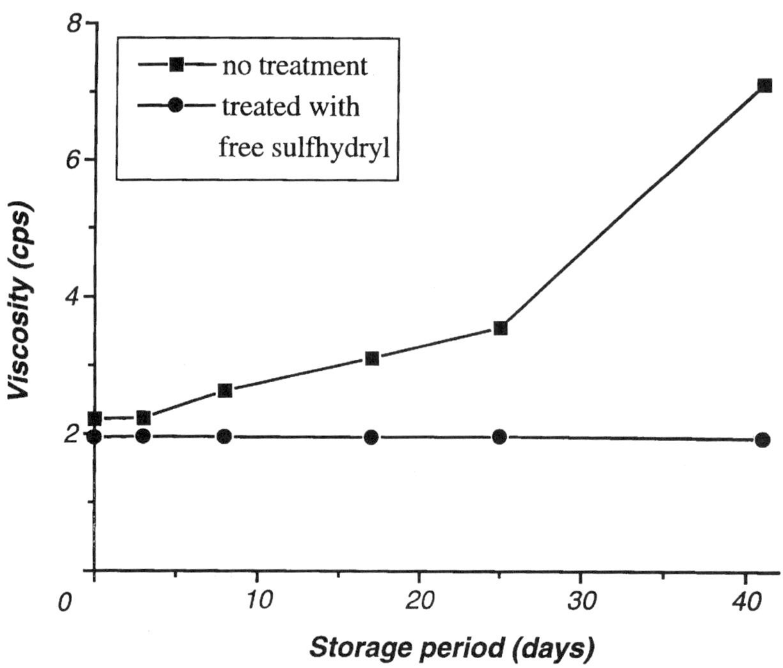

Figure 12.2. Viscosity stabilization of 6% Dx-Hb by treatment with 16 mM β-mercaptopropionic acid at pH 9.5.

12.2.3 Right-shifted Dx-Hb

Another property that can be controlled in the development of a blood substitute is its oxygen affinity. While the conjugation process does not bring about any damage to the heme that can be observed by spectral analysis, and Dx-Hb binds and releases oxygen reversibly, the conjugate binds oxygen 2.5-fold more tightly than does Hb itself, giving rise to a half-saturating oxygen partial pressure (P_{50}) of 7 mm Hg (Tam, Blumenstein and Wong 1976). The low P_{50} of Dx-Hb can be increased by the covalent attachment of the strong right-shifting agent, oxidized inositol tetrakisphosphate (oxyIP_4), without prior deoxygenation of the Dx-Hb, which is an important practical convenience in the large-scale production of right-shifted Dx-Hb. The oxyIP_4 is obtained by partial phytase digestion of inositol hexakisphosphate, namely phytate, followed by periodate oxidation to yield a dialdehyde function. Its covalent attachment to Dx-Hb is achieved through reductive alkylation with dimethylamine borane as reducing agent (Wong 1988). Since the attachment effectively abolishes further right-shifting response of the Hb molecule to phytate, oxyIP_4 evidently is attached to the same polyphosphate site as phytate (Xue, Wu and Wong 1992). The P_{50} of oxy-IP_4 right-shifted Dx-Hb, at 23 mm Hg (Figure 12.3), is three-fold that of Dx-Hb. Because of the re-

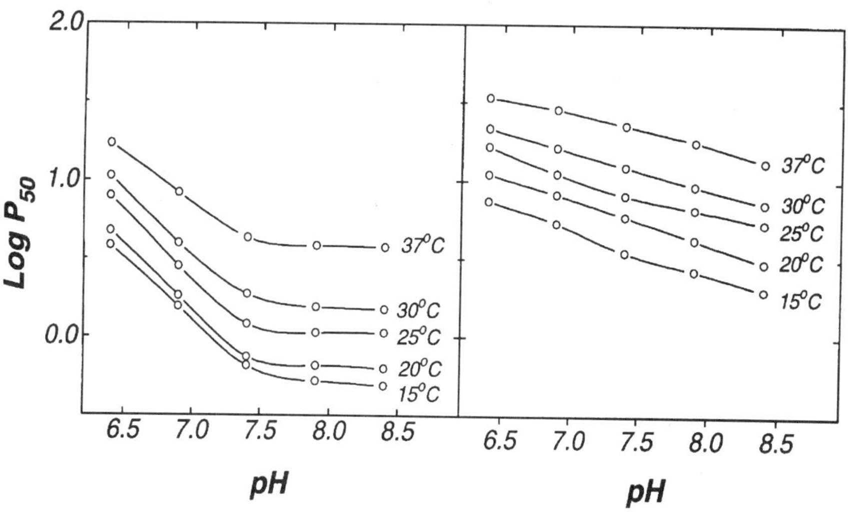

Figure 12.3. Variation of oxygen dissociation curves of Hb (left panel) and right-shifted Dx-Hb (right panel) with pH and temperature. After Xue, Wu and Wong (1992).

duced Hill coefficient of Dx-Hb relative to erythrocytes, during oxygen unloading from 100% down to 50% saturation, which is the normal operating range of unloading *in vivo*, the oxygen dissociation curve for right-shifted Dx-Hb will be slightly right-shifted relative to the erythrocyte curve over much of this range.

12.2.4 Other properties of Dx-Hb

In order to define further the behavior of Dx-Hb in circulation, it becomes important to examine its potential interactions with other components of blood. Haptoglobin is known to bind plasma Hb specifically and plays a role in its metabolic clearance. Covalent coupling of Hb to dextran increases steric hindrance and reduces its affinity for haptoglobin (Tam and Wong 1980). It also enhances its stability against acid denaturation. Since neither the presence of free dextran in solution nor alkylation of the Hb sulfhydryls by iodoacetamide alters the kinetics of acid denaturation of Hb, the enhanced stability of Dx-Hb must arise directly from the attachment of bulky dextran. This enhanced stability would usefully protect the Dx-Hb blood substitute against denaturation and precipitation even under conditions of extreme local or systemic acidosis.

The resistance of Dx-Hb to precipitation also holds in the presence of ethanol. Unlike Hb, which begins to precipitate when ethanol concentration exceeds 10%, Dx-Hb only begins to precipitate at 30% ethanol. This opens the way to possible sterilization of Dx-Hb solutions with organic solvents (Wong 1988).

Investigation of the immunological properties of Dx-Hb showed that, with dog, rabbit and sheep, administration of homologous Dx-Hb does not induce a significant antibody response towards either the protein or carbohydrate component as long as homologous Hb is employed for the synthesis of Dx-Hb. Since negative results were observed at both high and low doses of Dx-Hb, the lack of response could not be due to the induction of a state of tolerance by excess antigen. With heterologous Hb, the similarity between anti-Hb titers in animals immunized with Dx-Hb or uncoupled Hb suggests that conjugation to dextran makes little difference to the immunogenicity of heterologous Hb (Cunnington *et al.* 1981).

12.3 *In vivo* Behavior

12.3.1 Renal and non-renal clearance

The conjugation of Hb to dextran prevents both renal excretion of hemoglobin and kidney damage. When Dx-Hb synthesized from three different sizes of dextran (MW 20,000, 40,000 or 70,000) are infused into anesthetized rabbits, their clearance rates do not vary with the size of the dextran moiety (Blumenstein *et al.* 1978). Therefore MW 20,000 is sufficient to prevent renal excretion of Dx-Hb. The non-excretion also could not be the result of interference of renal function by Dx-Hb, because inulin excretion remains unimpaired in its presence (Tam, Blumenstein and Wong 1976).

Results from a rat model have shown that infusion of stroma-free Hb causes a marked decrease in glomerular filtration rate and an extensive elevation in urinary N-acetyl-β-D-glucosaminidase (NAG) activity (Figure 12.4), the latter being an indicator of the structural damage to renal tubular cells caused by the passage of hemoglobin into the tubules. In contrast, infusion of Dx-Hb, probably because of its larger molecular size, does not pass through the glomeruli into the tubules and leads to only a minor appearance in urinary NAG with no significant impairment in the glomerular filtration rate (Tam and Wong 1988).

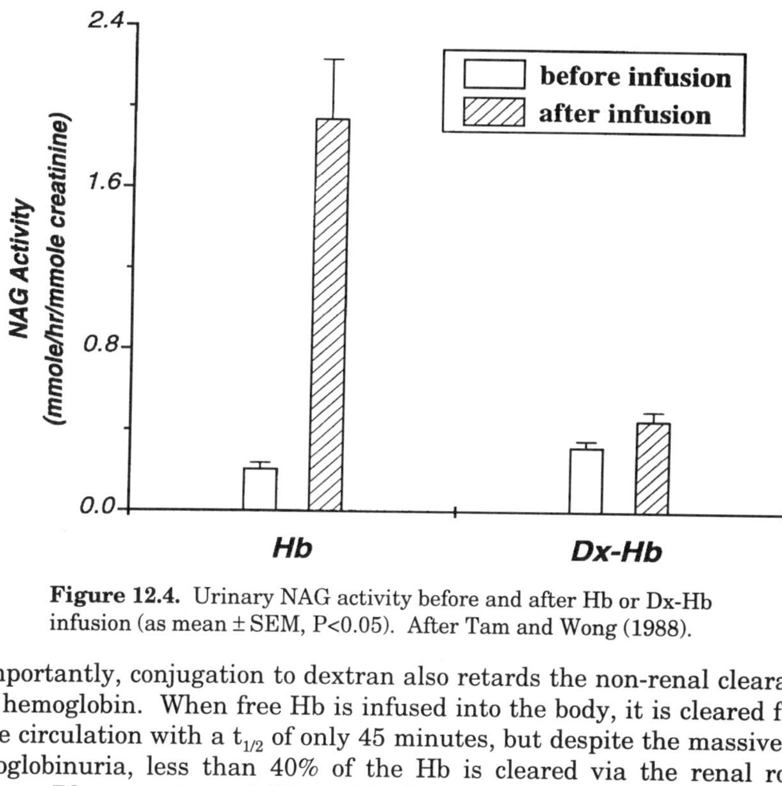

Figure 12.4. Urinary NAG activity before and after Hb or Dx-Hb infusion (as mean ± SEM, $P<0.05$). After Tam and Wong (1988).

Importantly, conjugation to dextran also retards the non-renal clearance of hemoglobin. When free Hb is infused into the body, it is cleared from the circulation with a $t_{1/2}$ of only 45 minutes, but despite the massive hemoglobinuria, less than 40% of the Hb is cleared via the renal route (Tam, Blumenstein and Wong 1976). Therefore, there occurs a rapid non-renal clearance of the molecule. Such non-renal escape of Hb into extravascular space is of utmost clinical significance for it may aggravate tissue edema. It is noteworthy in this regard that different Hb-based blood substitutes, albeit renally non-excretable, vary greatly with respect to their apparent circulatory $t_{1/2}$, evidently as a result of different rates of non-renal clearance. The $t_{1/2}$ of Dx-Hb in excess of two days, being one of the longest among Hb-based blood substitutes, offers important potential advantages. Extravasation-compounding tissue edema is decreased by its slow non-renal clearance, and frequent topping-up in order to maintain plasma Hb level is also rendered unnecessary.

One of the causes of the slow non-renal clearance of Dx-Hb is suggested by Figure 12.5, which shows that, when Dx-Hb or Hb was infused into sheep, Hb entered rapidly into the lymph, but Dx-Hb entered very slowly if at all.

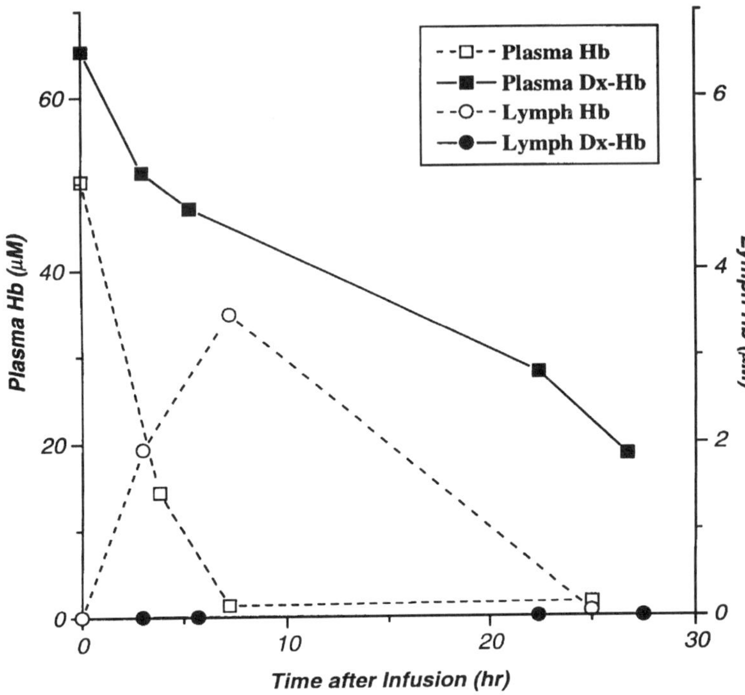

Figure 12.5. Significant entry of Hb but not Dx-Hb into sheep lymph from plasma. Blood samples were drawn from the jugular vein following infusion of Hb or Dx-Hb, and lymph samples were taken from the left efferent prefemoral lymphatic.

12.3.2 Exchange transfusion

When beagle dogs were exchange transfused with either 10% dextran or 6% Dx-Hb (with respect to Hb moiety) in kidney dialysis fluid, the animals exchange transfused with dextran could not survive when the hematocrit (Hct) was reduced to the 6-10% range, presumably because of lack of oxygen-delivering capacity (Figure 12.6). In contrast, the Hct could be lowered to 2% or less in the Dx-Hb exchange transfused dogs, whereby the animals depended on oxygen delivery by Dx-Hb for life support. The infused Dx-Hb exhibited a physical plasma $t_{1/2}$ of 2.4 days and a functional plasma $t_{1/2}$, after correcting for non-functional Dx-metHb, of 1.9 days. Because of the prolonged circulatory half-life of Dx-Hb and the vigorous erythropoiesis following the blood replacement, the animals went on to complete recovery under room air without any need for further transfusion (Figure 12.7). Hemoglobin was synthesized by these recovering animals at an average rate of 5% Hct/day, or ten-times the normal rate. Such a ten-fold rise in erythropoiesis is about the maximum that can be stimulated, and its vigor points to the excellent health of Dx-Hb oxygenated bone marrow, which is one of the most sensitive tissues in the body toward injury.

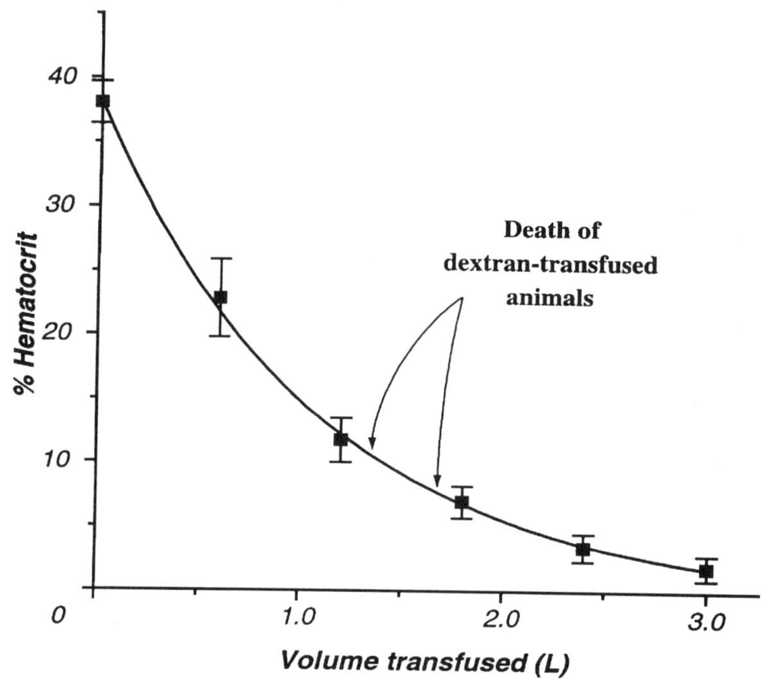

Figure 12.6. Lowering of hematocrit by exchange transfusion with a solution of either 10% dextran or 6% Dx-Hb. After Tam, Blumenstein and Wong (1978).

When cats were exchange transfused with 6% Dx-Hb in Tyrode solution, 8/9 survived after the Hct was lowered to 1% or below. When Hb in Tyrode was used, only 1/5 survived to 1% Hct, the mean lowest survivable Hct being 1.5 ± 0.5%. Cats exchange transfused with the following solutions all failed to survive to 1% Hct or below, the mean lowest survivable Hct being:

(a) 6% Dextran MW 20,000 in Tyrode: 2.4 ± 0.6% Hct

(b) 6% Dextran MW 20,000 in saline: 2.5 ± 0.5% Hct

(c) 6% Dextran MW 110,000 in 5% dextrose: 3.5 ± 0.5% Hct

(d) Isotonic saline: 7.0 ± 1.5% Hct

Therefore, Dx-Hb supported life more effectively than either Hb or any of the other solutions (Humphries *et al.* 1981).

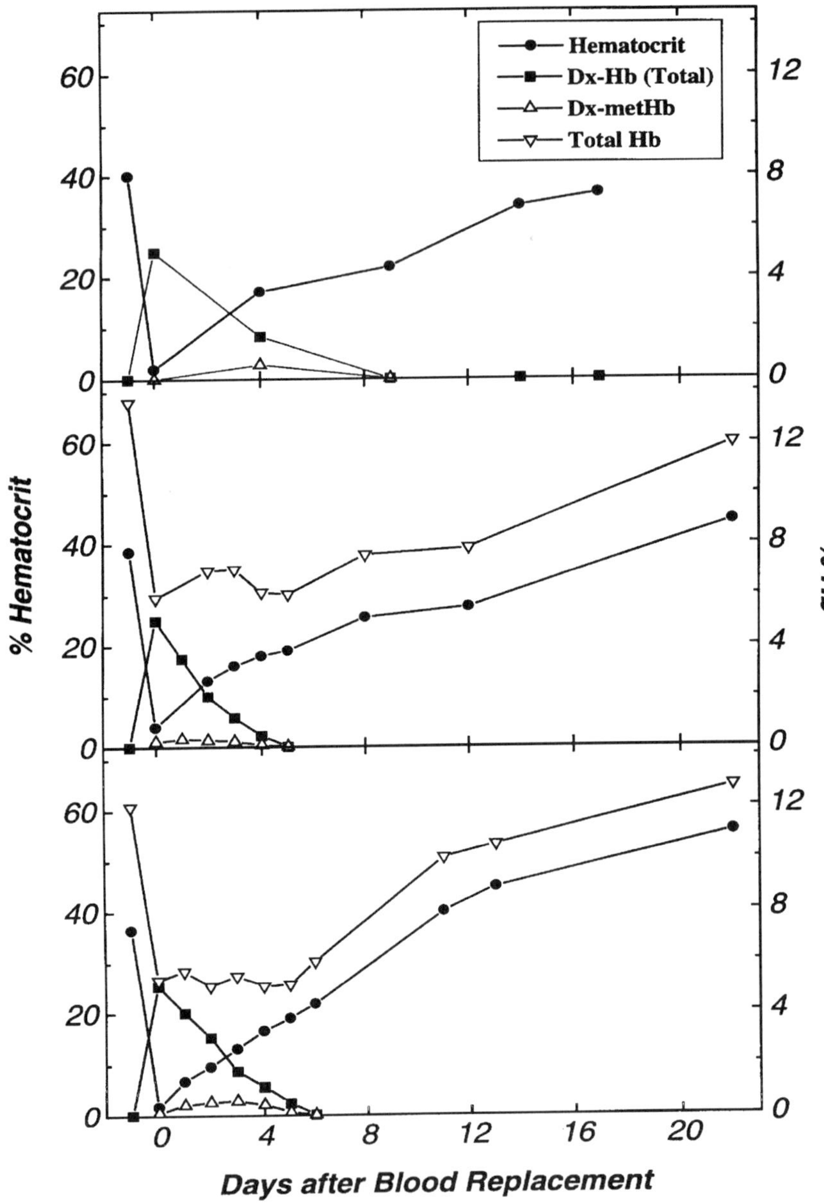

Figure 12.7. Course of recovery of three dogs exchange transfused with Dx-Hb containing 6% Hb moiety. The plasma half-life of Dx-Hb was 2.4 days. Subtracting the loss of oxygen-carrying function due to oxidation to Dx-metHb, the half-life for functional Dx-Hb was 1.9 days. The total blood hemoglobin was determined as the sum of Dx-Hb and erythrocytic hemoglobin. After Tam, Blumenstein and Wong (1978).

12.3.3 Tissue oxygenation

The myocardium is highly sensitive to hypoxia, and effects of hypoxia are readily detected. Macaques exchange transfused to 4% Hct with 6% right-shifted Dx-Hb not only recovered under room air without further transfusion, but also displayed no detectable myocardial hypoxia in their electrocardiogram at 4% Hct (Wong 1988).

In a canine myocardial ischemia model, following occlusion of the LAD branch of the coronary artery, infusion of Dx-Hb distal to the occlusion fully maintained work performance of downstream myocardium with no significant decrease in segmental shortening as measured by sonomicrometer crystals (C.W. Christensen, personal communications, Christensen *et al.* 1987).

Among all the organs of the body, the brain is one of the most demanding of oxygen. It can withstand total oxygen deprivation for only a few minutes, and it is estimated that the cerebral cortex could survive anoxia for only 1-5 minutes. When macaques had first been trained in reversal learning by means of the Wisconsin General Test Apparatus (which is sufficiently sensitive to reveal intelligence differences among different primates) prior to blood replacement to half the normal Hct with 6% Dx-Hb, and subsequently tested for reversal learning, no significant deficit in learning performance was detected. Thus oxygenation by an admixture of whole blood and Dx-Hb is compatible with maintenance of cerebral integrity (Handley *et al.* 1983).

12.3.4 Potential application to radiation therapy

Because anoxic cells are three-fold more resistant to radiation damage than oxygenated ones, cells in the anoxic centers of solid tumors are endowed with an inherent survival advantage over surrounding normal tissues in radiation therapy. To overcome this undesirable advantage, oxygen could either be delivered to the anoxic or hypoxic tumor cells or taken away from the surrounding normal tissues.

It is recognized that soluble Hb-based blood substitutes find potential application to the radiation therapy of cancers by improving the oxygenation of tumors through enhancement of flow penetration of the often poorly developed vascular beds of solid tumors. Although less commonly recognized, such blood substitutes may also contribute to radiation therapy by removing oxygen from the surrounding normal tissues. When deoxygenated Dx-Hb was infused as an oxygen-sequestering agent to induce hypoxia into a porcine internal thoracic artery during X-ray irradiation, the induced hypoxia effectively protected the irradiated pig skin by a factor of 2 against radiation damage monitored in terms of the area of resultant necrosis (Figure 12.8). This opens up the novel clinical application of Dx-Hb to radiotherapy, which is facilitated by the much more rapid deoxygenation of tissues by deoxy Dx-Hb compared to nitrogen breathing (Wong and Hill 1986).

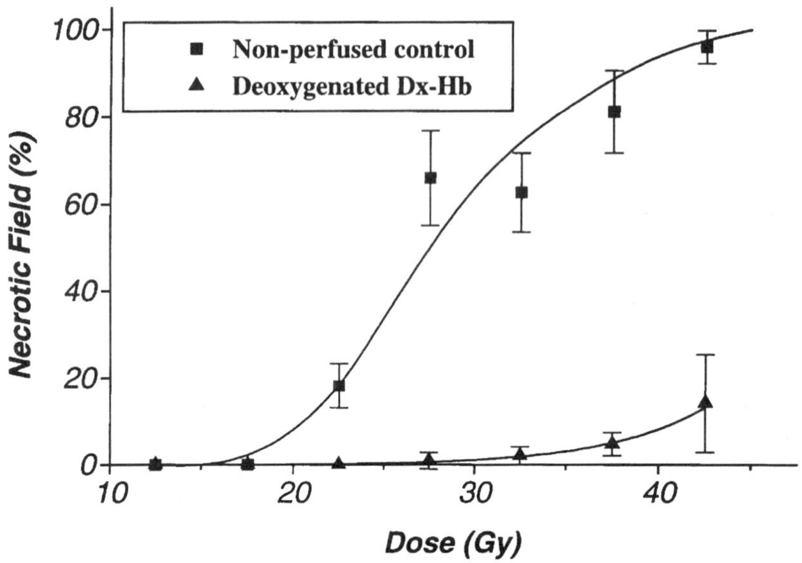

Figure 12.8. Radioprotection of pig skin. Sites were irradiated with 130kVp X-rays with 1-mm Al added filtration at a rate of 2.2 Gy/min. Damage was measured in terms of % area of irradiated field found to be necrotic. After Hill *et al.* (1984).

12.4 Conclusions

Dextran-hemoglobin is the first soluble blood substitute to sustain without any need for further transfusion complete recovery under room air of animals that have undergone essentially complete replacement of erythrocytes. This is made possible by its relatively long persistence time in plasma, such that its disappearance is adequately compensated for by the vigorous erythropoiesis it supports. The long persistence time is in turn the result of non-clearance through the renal route, thereby protecting the integrity of kidney function and structure, as well as slow clearance through non-renal routes, which include extravasation and cellular uptake processes. Slow extravasation would usefully limit tissue edema, and the long persistence time reduces the frequency of blood substitute infusion required to maintain an adequate hemoglobin level in the recipient. This reduction economizes the metabolic iron load imposed on the recipient, as well as the cost of blood substitute, which is expected to be a critical factor limiting the widespread application of hemoglobin-based blood substitutes.

While Dx-Hb adequately supports life and tissue function, recently it has been found that large blood substitute molecules could cause not only high viscosity but also significant rouleaux formation of erythrocytes (Tsai and Wong 1996). The detailed effects of all hemoglobin-based blood substitutes, including Dx-Hb, on viscosity and erythrocyte rouleaux formation, and consequently on the microcirculation, yet remain to be investigated.

12.5 References

Ajisaka, K., and Y. Iwashita. Modification of human hemoglobin with polyethylene glycol: a new candidate for blood substitute. *Biochem. Biophys. Res. Commun.* 97: 1076-1081, 1980.

Barberousse, V., D. Sacco, and E. Dellacherie. Chromatographic evaluation of the binding of haemoglobin to poly-anionic polymers. *J. Chromatogr.* 369: 244-247, 1986.

Blumenstein, J., S-C. Tam, J.E. Chang, and J.T. Wong. Experimental transfusion of dextran-hemoglobin. *Prog. Clin. Biol. Res.* 19: 205-212, 1978.

Cerny, L.C., E.L. Cerny, J. Roback, M. Reath, and L. Pontero. A blood substitute from hydroxyethyl starch and hemoglobin. *Appl. Biochem. Biotech.* 10: 151-153, 1984.

Chang, J.E., and J.T. Wong. Synthesis of soluble dextran-hemoglobin complexes of different molecular sizes. *Can. J. Biochem.* 55: 398-403, 1977.

Chang, T.M.S. Blood substitutes based on modified hemoglobin prepared by encapsulation or crosslinking: an overview. *Biomater. Artif. Cells Immobil. Biotech.* 20: 159-179, 1992.

Christensen, C.W., J.T. Wong, L.C. Daley, M.A. Rieder, and W.C. Reeves. Subendocardial steal induced by oxygenated Fluosol but not stroma free hemoglobin. A comparative study on regional blood flow in an acute myocardial ischemia model. *Circulation* 76: 211, 1987.

Cunnington, P.G., S.N. Jenkins, S-C. Tam, and J.T. Wong. Oxygen-binding and immunological properties of complexes between dextran and animal haemoglobins. *Biochem. J.* 193: 261-266, 1981.

Handley, C.S., G.E. Chaudron, L.S. Porter, and J.T. Wong. Use of a reverse-learning model to evaluate brain oxygenation by dextran-hemoglobin. *Prog. Clin. Biol. Res.* 122: 430, 1983.

Hill, R.P., L.S. Porter, S.A. Ives, and J.T. Wong. Initial studies of hypoxic radioprotection by deoxygenated dextran-hemoglobin. *Int. J. Radiation Oncology Biol. Phys.* 10: 369-373, 1984.

Humphries, R.G., P.G. Killingback, J. Mann, J. Sempik and J. Wilson. Exchange transfusion with dextran-haemoglobin, haemoglobin and dextran solutions in anaesthetized cats. *Brit. J. Pharmacol.* 74: 266, 1981.

Iwasaki, K., K. Ajisaka, and Y. Iwashita. Hemoglobin-inulin conjugate as an oxygen carrying blood substitute. *Biochem. Biophys. Res. Commun.* 113: 513-518, 1983.

Kabat, E.A., and A.E. Bezer. Effect of variation in molecular weight on the antigenicity of dextran in man. *Arch. Biochem. Biophys.* 78: 306-318, 1958.

Leonard, M., and E. Dellacherie. Acylation of human hemoglobin with polyoxyethylene derivatives. *Biochim. Biophys. Acta* 791: 219-225, 1984.

Melton, R.G., C.N. Wiblin, R.L. Foster, and R.F. Sherwood. Covalent linkage of carboxypeptidase G_2 to soluble dextrans - I. properties of conjugates and effects on plasma persistence in mice. *Biochem. Pharmacol.* 36: 105-112, 1987.

Muranishi, S. Drug targeting towards the lymphatics. *Adv. Drug Res.* 21: 1-38, 1991.

Odling-Smee, G.W., and B.G. Wilson. Haemoglobin as a blood substitute. In *Blood Substitutes* (K. C. Lowe, ed.) New York: VCH, 1988, pp.71-86.

Prouchayret, F., G. Fasan, M. Grandgeorge, C. Vigneron, P. Menu, and E. Dellacherie. A potential blood substitute from carboxylic dextran and oxyhemoglobin I. Preparation, purification and characterization. *Biomater. Artif. Cells Immobil. Biotech.* 20: 319-322, 1992.

Rosemeyer, H., E. Körnig, and F. Seela. Adenosine deaminase covalently linked to soluble dextran. The effect of immobilization on thermodynamic and kinetic parameters. *Eur. J. Biochem.* 122: 375-380, 1982.

Sacco, D., D. Klett-Zygmunt, C. Vigneron, and E. Dellacherie. Covalent fixation of hemoglobin to dextran phosphates decreases its oxygen affinity. *Biochim. Biophys. Acta* 1041: 279-284, 1990.

Schmidt, K. Polyvinylpyrolidone-fixed hemoglobin as an oxygen carrying blood substitute. *Klin. Wochenschr.* 57: 1169-1175, 1979.

Sherwood, R.F., J.K. Baird, T. Atkinson, C.N. Wiblin, D.A. Rutter, and D.C. Ellwood. Enhanced plasma persistence of therapeutic enzymes by coupling to soluble dextran. *Biochem. J.* 164: 461-464, 1977.

Tam, S-C., J. Blumenstein, and J.T. Wong. Soluble dextran-hemoglobin complex as a potential blood substitute. *Proc. Natl. Acad. Sci. USA.* 73: 2128-2131, 1976.

Tam, S-C., J. Blumenstein, and J.T. Wong. Blood replacement in dogs by dextran-hemoglobin. *Can. J. Biochem.* 56: 981-984, 1978.

Tam, S-C., and J.T. Wong. Modification of hemoglobin upon covalent coupling to dextran: enhanced stability against acid denaturation and reduced affinity for haptoglobin. *Can. J. Biochem.* 58: 732-736, 1980.

Tam, S-C., and J.T. Wong. Impairment of renal function by stroma-free hemoglobin in rats. *J. Lab. Clin. Med.* 111: 189-193, 1988.

Tsai, S.P., and J.T. Wong. Enhancement of erythrocyte sedimentation rate by polymerized hemoglobin. *Artif. Cells, Blood Subs. Immobil. Biotech.* 24: 513-523, 1996.

Wileman, T.E., R.L. Foster, and P.N.C. Elliott. Soluble asparaginase-dextran conjugates show increased circulatory persistence and lowered antigen reactivity. *J. Pharm. Pharmacol.* 38: 264-271, 1986.

Wong, J.T. Right-shifted dextran-hemoglobin as blood substitute. *Biomat. Art. Cells Art. Organs.* 16: 237-245, 1988.

Wong, J.T., and R.P. Hill. Biophysical basis of hypoxic radioprotection by deoxygenated dextran-hemoglobin. *Int. J. Radiation Oncology Biol. Phys.* 12: 1303-1306, 1986.

Xue, H., X-F. Wu, and J.T. Wong. Properties of hemoglobin and dextran-hemoglobin right-shifted by oxidized inositol tetrakisphosphate. *Artif. Organs.* 16: 427-431, 1992.

Yalpani, M. *Polysaccharides.* New York: Elsevier Science, 1988, pp. 8-49.

12.6 Discussion

Winslow: Jeffrey, I know that you did this work with dextran-hemoglobin quite some time ago, and the obvious question is why hasn't it been developed commercially? Is there a reason for that?

Wong: The answer is very simple. The biggest dextran manufacturers are Pharmacia and Fisons in England, and so Fisons became very interested and supported our work on dextran hemoglobin. But over the past 10 years, Fisons has been on a monotonic curve going downhill and finally sold to Rhône-Poulenc last year, so I think that is a very important reason why this has not been developed, but it does give us more time to understand more about the blood substitute and improve it even more.

Intaglietta: I was curious that you tried a range of molecular weights on dextran, and you decided on the 20,000 Dalton molecular weight, but did you observe any adverse effect or any peculiarities when you went up in molecular weight, and I think you went up as far as 200,000 did you say?

Wong: Yes, 200,000 Daltons.

Intaglietta: What were the observations when you had conjugates made of 200,000 Dalton molecular weight dextran with hemoglobin?

Wong: With the 200,000 Dalton dextran, we mainly were just looking at renal excretion in the rabbit using fairly small doses of dextran-hemoglobin. For example, we have never used very big dextran-hemoglobin and tried to perform a total blood replacement in the dog. So, basically, we were only looking at an excretion question, but I think it would be a very interesting experiment to do.

Baldwin: You showed that the dextran-hemoglobin did not extravasate significantly. I was wondering if it had any effect on blood-to-tissue transport of other materials because I worked with dextran, not dextran-hemoglobin, but I found that dextran altered the charge on the endothelial glycocalix.

Wong: I see. That would be very important to look at, but we haven't really looked at other solutes. What was your cut-off point with dextran to go into lymph? How big a dextran do you use?

Baldwin: I wasn't looking at the transport of dextran into the lymph. I was looking at the effect of dextran on the charge of the endothelial surface, and I would test that using differently charged ferritins.

Wong: I see.

Winslow: I wonder if we could induce Dr. Cokelet or Meiselman to comment on the utility of following the sedimentation rate as an indicator of flow properties *in vivo*. This seems to me a fairly complicated issue.

Cokelet: Of course, the sedimentation rate and the low shear-rate viscosity of red cell suspensions go hand in hand. However, there is not necessarily a 1:1 relationship. You can get different forms of aggregates and in a sense of almost like a density of the aggregate dependent on what you use to aggregate the cells and how much of it is present. In that case, the sedimentation rate will go up, but so will the yield stresses of blood or the low shear-rate viscosity but not necessarily proportionally, so you'd have to do some tests to get the details, but roughly, they go in parallel.

Wong: But let me ask—it's good to have the expertise here—we try to avoid high ESR, but at the same time, we understand that there are a lot of people walking around with very high ESR in their blood, presumably suffering from nothing very adverse. Is that correct?

Cokelet: Well, I think that the effect of increased low shear-rate viscosity is going to be mostly on the venous side unless the patient is bedridden for long periods of time or something like that in which the flow rate might go down in a more general way, but I think ordinarily you'd never expect to see much influence of low shear-rate viscosity except on the venous side.

Wong: So that sounds like something more chronic in its implication, so it's not particularly foremost for blood substitutes.

Cokelet: I would think so.

Meiselman: Let me disagree with Dr. Cokelet. I think there is a role for ESR-type measurements because what you are really looking at is red-cell aggregation. That's what you're seeing with erythrocyte sedimentation rate, and as long as it isn't terribly confounded by increasing the suspending phase viscosity, plasma viscosity, then you have some measure, although indirect, of red-cell aggregation and, therefore, a measure of low-shear viscosity, and I agree with Dr. Cokelet that it's primarily of importance on the venous side of the circulation, but it also can affect the distribution of red cells within a given microcirculatory bed; you may have more preferential movement of red cells through the larger vessels and a little bit more shunting of red cells away from the capillaries. So, I think there is an importance here for red-cell aggregation.

And, as a closing comment, I feel older than I look because all of these questions about where does dextran go and how much goes out and what the cut-off point, of course, is Pharmacia's strong point way back in the sixties, and a man named Dr. H.C. Hint who was, at that time, director of research at Pharmacia in Uppsala, did amazing studies in rabbit ears. He would inject dextran into rabbit ears and then macerate the tissue and then do a molecular weight distribution of the dextran that was then in the tissue. And it was surprising to me, and he claims that it's absolutely the truth, that if you inject into the ear and perfuse the ear with a wide range of molecular weight, that is an unfractionated dextran fraction having a wide distribution of molecular weights, and then macerate the tissue, you see the identical distribution in the tissue space indicating it has gone across the capillary walls, so I don't know the answer to the distribution, the cut-off point. I suspect it has to do with how long you're willing to wait.

Hess: Yes, last year I presented that data here as an abstract on the diffusion of various size molecules across the endothelial barrier, and because the dextran is getting into the interstitial space, when you didn't see it in the lymphatics, where is it going?

Wong: Well, it's going very slowly. The half-life is about two days, but...

Hess: And yet it's moving across, it's not being recirculated. Then it's simply moving back and forth across the endothelium.

Wong: So, I think there's really very little that we know of in terms of systematic knowledge about why the different blood substitutes have such vastly different half lives, and where are they going? Who is going where? I think there are a lot of interesting questions ahead.

Winslow: There is likely some breakdown simply in plasma, is there not? There must be some protease activity.

Wong: But dextran is known to undergo very slow metabolism in the body.

Winslow: You mentioned in the end the need for blood substitutes in a country like China, and I was wondering if you have any thoughts on the supply of outdated blood, let's say, to be used in blood substitutes? Are there any special problems, or do you see that as a viable thing to collect a sufficient amount of blood to process into blood substitutes?

Wong: Well, of course, there is some outdated blood in China, but it is probably a lot less. Often, each company pledges to donate so much blood every year. So, when the blood bank runs low, it will call in, for example, Shanghai auto factory, and all the workers go in and donate blood. So, the intake is a lot more programmed. Of course, this evens out the fluctuations you have in donation rates. As a result, the outdated blood supply is much lower.

Chapter 13

Modification of Molecules and Particles With Polyethylene Glycol (PEG): Long-circulating Pharmaceuticals

Vladimir P. Torchilin, Ph.D.

13.1 INTRODUCTION: Rationale for Long-circulating Pharmaceuticals

Currently, long-circulating pharmaceuticals and pharmaceutical carriers represent a huge and still fast growing area of biomedical research. The critical evaluation of the state-of-the art, long-circulating drugs and drug carriers, reviews and discussions on the current approaches and strategies in the design and practical application of these systems, as well as a theoretical background of their biological behavior, can be found in many important publications (Müller 1991, Rolland 1993, Lasic and Martin 1995, Cohen and Bernstein 1996, Torchilin and Trubetskoy 1995, Torchilin 1996).

We can name several reasons why the search for long-circulating drugs and drug carriers is so extensive. ***First***, in some cases we need to keep certain substances in the blood compartment long enough. Thus, long-circulating, slow-release systems may be used to create desirable levels of a drug or diagnostic (imaging) agent in the blood ("depot" effect) for extended time intervals for better drug availability (Langer 1985), *i.e.* better treatment and diagnosis. In case of therapeutical intervention, a drug can be attached to a long-circulating carriers via stable or biodegradable bonds, as well as a carrier itself may be made to degrade into smaller and easier to clear fragments (Ringsdorf 1975). Long-circulating diagnostic agents are of primary importance for the visualization of the blood pool. Blood pool imaging is of special interest for the evaluation of the current state of blood flow and for the discovery of its irregularities caused by atherosclerotic lesions, thrombi or tumors. Interestingly, some authors (Phillips and Goins 1995) consider blood pool imaging as an "antitargeting" application, though it might be also considered as a targeting into the blood compartment. Based on the longevity of imaging agent in blood, blood perfusion and various cardiac parameters (ventricular ejection fraction, cardiac output, and wall motion being among them) can be evaluated (Unger *et al.* 1993, Woodle 1993b) applying different imaging modalities, such as gamma-scintigraphy, computed tomography, magnetic resonance imaging, and sonography. Many long-circulating carriers (including liposomes) loaded with ^{111}In, ^{67}Ga, Gd, heavily iodinated organic compounds, and gas bubbles are already described as promising contrast agents for this purpose. It seems that certain of these agents may serve as a good alternative for those currently used for the same purposes, such as ^{99}Tc-labeled red blood cells, which do not allow acquisition of desirable quality images because of the fast accumulation of the latter in the liver and insufficient stability of label association with the cells. Blood substitutes represent another important area for the use of long-circulating pharmaceuticals, when artificial oxygen carriers or plasma expanders should present in the circulation long enough to provide sufficient time for the restoration of the normal physiological mechanisms for blood cell production (Winslow, Vandegriff and Intaglietta 1996).

Second, long-circulating drug-containing microparticulates or large macromolecular aggregates can slowly accumulate ("passive" accumulation via an impaired filtration mechanism) in pathological sites with affected vasculature (such as tumors, inflammations, and infarcted areas) and improve or enhance drug delivery in those areas, as it was shown in numerous experimental studies (Caride and Zaret 1977, Palmer *et al.* 1984, Gabizon 1995). This approach led to a clear success in cancer treatment, when doxorubicin-loaded long-circulating liposomes demonstrated enhanced efficacy and sharply decreased toxicity compared to a free drug both in animal experiments and in preliminary clinical trials (Gabizon 1995 and references therein).

Third, prolonged circulation can help to achieve a better targeting effect for those targeted (antibody-modified) drugs and drug carriers which are supposed to reach pathological areas with diminished blood flow or with a low concentration of a target antigen. The idea of using certain vectors (mainly, immunoglobulins or their fragments) to facilitate and enhance drug delivery into a prerequested area has been developed experimentally within the last 20 years (Gregoriadis 1977, Goldberg 1983, Torchilin 1985). Numerous attempts have been made to make drugs and drug carriers target-specific by attaching organ- or tissue-specific monoclonal antibodies (mAb) to their surface. Despite evident success in the development of mAb-to-carrier coupling technique and improvements in the targeting efficacy, the majority of mAb-modified microparticulate carriers or drug aggregates still ends in the liver, which is usually a consequence of insufficient time for the interaction between the target and targeted pharmaceuticals. This is especially true in cases when a target of choice has diminished blood supply (ischemic or necrotic areas). Even good drug/carrier affinity towards the target could not provide its high accumulation because of the small quantity of targeted drug passing through the target with the blood during the time period when the drug/carrier is still present in the circulation. The same lack of targeted accumulation can happen if the concentration of the target antigen is very low, and even sufficient blood flow (and consequently, targeted drug/carrier passage) through the target still does not result in good accumulation effect due to the small number of productive collisions between antigens and mAb-modified drugs. It is quite evident that in both cases much better accumulation can be achieved if drugs/carriers can stay in the circulation long enough. This will increase the total quantity of targeted drug/carrier passing through the target in the first case and the number of productive collisions between targeted drugs and target antigens in the second (Torchilin 1996).

These are some principal considerations which make a basis for the development of long-circulating drugs and drug carriers.

13.2 Steric Protection: Which Polymers Can Provide it and How?

13.2.1 Polymers for steric stabilization

Usually, certain chemical modification is applied to provide the *in vivo* longevity to low-molecular- or high-molecular-weight drugs and drug carriers. Recent trends involve the increasing use of different polymers for such modification. Synthetic or natural polymers have been shown to protect individual molecules and solid particulates from interaction with different solutes. The phenomenon is closely connected with the stability of various aqueous dispersions and has a tremendous practical significance (Molyneux 1977), especially within the pharmaceutical field where the polymers might protect drugs and drug carriers from undesirable interactions with biological milieu components. As we will see further, there exist two principal ways to couple the protective polymer with the substance to be protected. The first one involves the covalent attachment of the polymer chain with a drug molecule or "grafting" this chain onto the surface of a particulate substance. The other way (especially applicable to particulate systems) employs so called amphipathic (or amphiphilic) polymers composed of at least two different parts in their molecule with pronounced hydrophobic and hydrophilic properties. Such polymers demonstrate the ability to be easily adsorbed (or incorporated) onto the surface of a particulate carrier via hydrophobic interactions, while their hydrophilic portions are exposed into the solution and effectively protect those particulates from interactions with plasma proteins in the blood upon intravenous administration (Blunk *et al.* 1993). The term "steric stabilization" has been introduced to describe this polymer-mediated protection (Naper 1983).

We will consider here, what are the peculiar properties of certain polymers which provide them with the ability to serve as effective steric stabilizer or steric protectors? At this point we will temporarily concentrate our attention on artificial phospholipid vesicles called liposomes (Lasic 1993 and references therein). Being a member of a large family of microparticular carriers, liposomes may serve as a good model for the understanding of grafted polymer influence on carrier properties, and many regularities found for liposomes might be successfully applied to many microparticulate drug carriers and even individual drug molecules (with some limitations in the latter case). One of the most popular and successful methods to obtain long-circulating biologically stable liposomes is by coating them with certain hydrophilic and flexible polymers, first of all, with poly(ethylene glycol), or PEG (Klibanov *et al.* 1990, Mori *et al.* 1991, Torchilin *et al.* 1992).

13.2.2 Mechanism of PEG-mediated protection

Starting from the first description of such liposomes (Klibanov *et al.* 1990), the mechanism of PEG protective action has been under continuous investigation (Senior *et al.* 1991, Gabizon and Papahadjopoulos 1992, Needham, McIntosh and Lasic 1992, Woodle *et al.* 1992, Blume and Cevc 1993). The general opinion expressed in several reviews on properties of PEG-liposomes, see for example (Allen 1994, Woodle 1993a), is that on the biological level, coating liposomes with PEG sterically hinders interactions of blood components with the liposome surface. This prevents liposome interaction with opsonins which would result in fast capture of liposomes by the reticuloendothelial system (RES). To confirm this, the reduced binding of plasma proteins with PEG-liposomes has been demonstrated (Senior *et al.* 1991, Allen 1994, Chonn, Semple and Cullis 1991, 1992). The role of the inhibition of opsonization of PEG-liposomes in the prolongation of their circulation time also seems evident (Senior 1987).

The mechanisms by which PEG (or similar polymers) prevent opsonization and interaction of liposomes with proteins are also in the literature. Thus, from the properties of colloids it is known that repulsive interactions between colloidal particles can be enhanced by coating these particles with soluble, well-hydrated, and chemically inert polymers (Naper 1983). Such modification might decrease surface hydrophobicity and interaction of particles with RES. Coating of different nanoparticles with amphiphilic polymers, when hydrophobic block serves as an anchor to fix the polymer on the surface and hydrophilic block forms the protective layer around the particle, was shown to drastically decrease particle capture by RES and strongly influence particle biodistribution; many experiments were performed with particles coated with poloxamers (Illum, Hunneyball and Davis 1986, Moghimi *et al.* 1993, 1994). Special importance was also prescribed to the role of surface charge and hydrophilicity of PEG-coated liposomes (Gabizon and Papahadjopoulos 1992).

13.2.3 The role of polymer flexibility

In our studies, we demonstrated that the important feature of protective polymers is their flexibility (free rotation of individual polymer units around inter-unit linkages). This means that the molecular mechanism of polymer protective action is determined by the properties of a flexible polymer in solution and includes the formation of the polymeric layer over the liposome (particle, molecule) surface which is impermeable for other solutes, even at relatively low polymer concentrations (Torchilin *et al.* 1993, 1994a, 1994b, 1994c, Torchilin and Papisov 1994). Evidently, the protective layer of a polymer over the particle surface has to combine abilities to escape recognition by cells (the best way to be invisible is to look like a water) and to prevent the penetration of opsonizing proteins to the surface (which requires the polymer coat to be dense enough).

Considering the diffusional movement of a macromolecule from a solution towards the liposome (particle) surface as the initial step of its interaction with liposome, we can express the degree of liposome protection as the probability (***P***) for the protein to collide with a polymer instead of liposome (Torchilin and Papisov 1994). The higher ***P*** value, the better protection, and when ***P*** equals ***1***, no interaction between protein and liposome surface is possible. To analyze the probability values, we described the behavior of a surface-grafted polymer in terms of a simplified statistical model of polymer solution (des Cloizeaux and Jannik 1990). Within this model, the solution is considered as a three-dimensional network, where each unit cell is occupied either with a polymer unit or with a solvent (water) molecule. The more flexible the polymer, *i.e.*. the more independent the motion of any polymeric unit relative to the neighboring one, the larger the total number of its possible conformations and the higher the transition rate from one conformation to another. As a result, water-soluble, flexible polymer statistically exists as a distribution ("cloud") of probable conformations (Figure 13.1). The polymer flexibility correlates with its ability to occupy, with high frequency, many cells in solution, temporarily squeezing water molecules out of them and making them impermeable for other solutes which require free water for diffusion. Thus, a relatively small number of water-soluble and very flexible polymer molecules can create sufficient density of conformational "clouds" over the liposome surface and protect the latter from destruction or opsonization. Kinetic aspects of this model were discussed in (Torchilin and Papisov 1994).

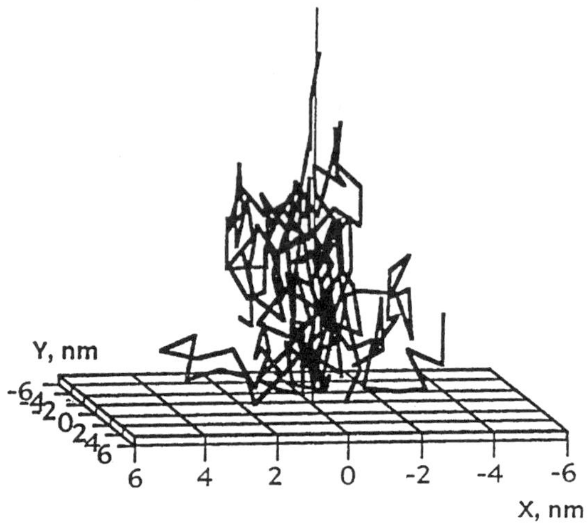

Figure 13.1. Computer simulation of a conformational "cloud" formation by a surface-attached polymer. Polymer molecule is conditionally assumed to consist of 20 segments, 1 nm each. This simulation was produced by random flight simulation. Unrestricted segment motion was assumed. Space restriction: Z > 0. Superposition of 11 random conformations. Adapted from Torchilin and Papisov (1994).

In a rigid-chain polymer unit, motion is hindered, and even good water-solubility and hydrophilicity may not provide sufficient protection for the liposome surface, such as has been noticed for liposome-grafted dextran (Blume and Cevc 1993, Torchilin *et al.* 1994a). The number of possible conformations for such polymers is lower, and conformational transitions proceed at a slower rate than for flexible polymers. The density of the conformational "cloud" for a rigid polymer should be much smaller. Enough free water remains within the "cloud" permitting the diffusion of plasma proteins toward the liposome surface. So, to be an effective steric protector, the polymer has to combine hydrophilicity (solubility) and flexibility (which is characteristic of, for example, PEG).

13.2.4 Some practical consequences

The size of the area on the liposome surface protected with a single polymer molecule of a given molecular weight and the number of polymer molecules required for the effective protection of the liposome of a given size were calculated by us using the parameter, $R_{0,sol}$ (Torchilin and Papisov 1994), which is the average end-to-end distance of a polymer random coil in solution. Using $R_{0,sol}$ values for PEG of different molecular weights published (Kurata and Tsunashima 1989), we estimated the area of the liposome surface which can be protected by a single PEG molecule and the molar ratio PEG-to-lipid required for complete protection of the liposome surface, which match well with published experimental data (Torchilin *et al.* 1992, Allen and Hansen 1991), see Figure 13.2.

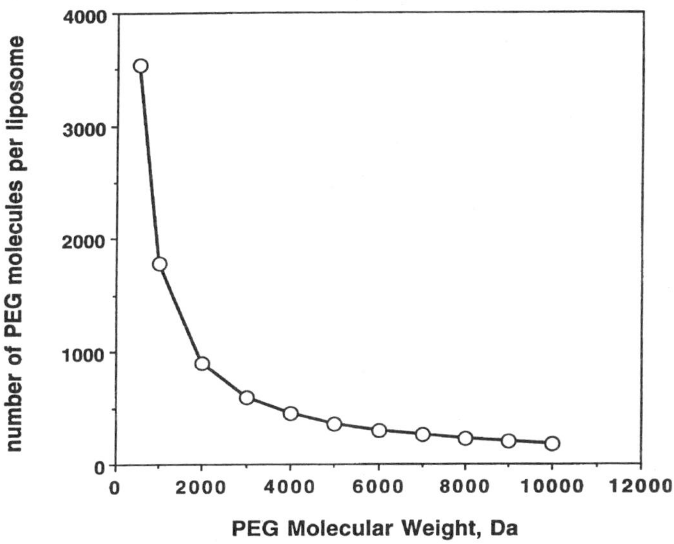

Figure 13.2. The dependence of the number of PEG molecules required for complete protection of a 100-nm liposome on PEG molecular weight.

By applying computer simulation, we were able to "visualize" flexible polymer behavior on the particle surface (Torchilin *et al.* 1994a). Spatial distribution of liposome surface-grafted polymers was simulated using a 3-dimensional random flight model, where polymer was assumed to consist of absolutely rigid segments with free-segment rotation around inter-segmental conjunction (the segment length 1 nm was taken for a flexible polymer and 5 nm for a rigid one). From the computer analysis it follows (the cross-section of the calculated protective "cloud" is presented in Figure 13.3A) that the flexible polymer forms the high density conformational cloud. A rigid polymer of the same length forms a broad but loose and permeable cloud.

An important (especially, from the pharmacological point of view) consequence of the model is that if there exist any reactive centers on the surface of protected particle or macromolecule (*e.g.*, binding sites for certain molecules, antibodies, antigens, or other ligands), the presence of PEG in concentrations below saturating leads to the appearance of two populations of those centers. The first population will consist of reactive moieties excluded from the PEG-occupied volume. Such reactive centers should possess the same properties and reactivity as on non-modified surfaces. However, centers remaining within the polymer cloud form the second population with sharply decreased ability to participate in "normal" interactions (Torchilin and Papisov 1994, Torchilin *et al.* 1994a), Figure 13.3B.

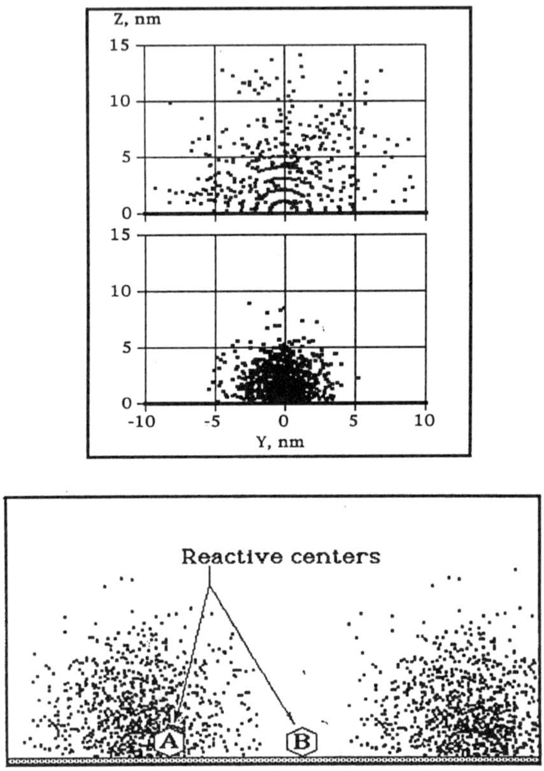

Figure 13.3. A - Distribution of polymer conformations (density of the conformational "cloud") in space; slice X = 0 ± 0.25 nm. The solution was produced by random flight simulation (Z > 0, polymer length 20 nm, 440 conformations). Upper panel - segment length is 5 nm (rigid polymer); lower panel - segment length is 1 nm (flexible polymer). Calculations for the rigid polymer have been done under the assumption that only every fifth 1-nm segment may change the direction. The "rings" on the upper panel are the result of the assumption that the net mass is concentrated at the remote termini of "frozen" shorter segments. **B** - The scheme of reactive site location on the liposome surface at low PEG concentration. The site can be either sterically hindered by a polymer "cloud" (A) or exposed and readily available for a variety of interactions (B). Kinetic parameters of chemically identical but differently located sites may differ. From Torchilin *et al.* (1994a).

13.2.5 Important theoretical considerations

More detailed analysis within the suggested model permits the answer to several important questions (Torchilin and Hoop, unpublished). For example, how are the PEG coils distributed in the space above the surface of the particle (molecule, liposome)? The thickness t of the PEG protective surface (the extent to which the PEG chain sticks up above the particle surface) can be represented with a class of probability distributions $c(t)$ (chi-squared distributions):

$$c(t) = \frac{c_0 \rho}{\Gamma(\rho)} \frac{\rho t}{\tau}^{(\rho-1)} e^{\frac{\rho t}{\tau}}$$

where c_0 is a normalizing factor, τ is a mean length of the PEG coil above the particle (liposome) surface, and ρ is a "shape" factor which determines the width of the distribution. The width of distribution is given by ρ^{-1}, and $\Gamma(\rho)$ is the corresponding Gamma function. For a value of $\rho = 0.01$, the distribution peaks at the surface, whereas for large ρ $(=20)$, the distribution approaches a Gaussian shape centered about a normalized mean length $t/\tau=1$. That is, as ρ goes from near zero to very large, the probability distribution goes from hyperbolic ($\rho=0.01$; the PEG molecule is most likely lying on the surface) to approximately Gaussian ($\rho=20$; the PEG molecule is most likely stretched out to its full length perpendicular to the surface). The effective volume (bare liposome plus PEG-coated sheath) would then be just $V=4/3\pi(R+\langle r\rangle)^3$, where R is the bare liposome (particle, protein globule) radius and $\langle r\rangle$ is the mean sheath thickness [mean length τ weighted by $c(t)$].

The other important question is what is the thickness of the spherical volume around a protected particle which can be entirely filled with PEG molecules? To answer this question, we may consider anchoring of some PEG molecules, each of length N monomers, onto the surface of the bare particle (liposome). Hydrophobic tails have to be placed as closely as possible. If λ is the distance between them, the total number of anchored PEG molecules will be $4\pi R_0^2\lambda/\lambda^3 = 4\pi R_0^2/\lambda^2$. Assuming that each monomer element of PEG molecule can occupy a volume λ^3, we will need $N4\pi R_0^2/\lambda^2$ cells above the surface to accommodate the PEG molecules. Within a radial distance r above the bare surface we will have

$$(4\pi/3)[(R_0 + r)^3 - R_0^3/\lambda^3$$

empty cells. Setting this equal to $4\pi R_0^2N/\lambda^2$ gives a cubic equation in r, of which a positive real root is the minimum radial distance away from the bare surface within which all N monomers of all $4\pi R_0^2/\lambda^2$ PEG molecules can, in principle, be accommodated. The two extreme volumes in this model will be: (a) the minimum volume $V_{min}=4\pi/3(R_0+r)^3$ (compared with the bare liposome volume V_0) and (b) the maximum volume

V_n or V_{max}=$4\pi/3(R_0+\lambda N)^3$, which is the volume defined by all of the PEG molecules sticking radially straight out of the surface. Taking the real values for the parameters used (such as liposome or particle size, distance between surface-grafted PEG molecules, and the number of monomeric units in PEG molecule) we can easily estimate V_{min}/V_{max} and the volume providing optimal protection. These are just two examples of possible application of the approach. There are a few other important questions which can be analyzed within the suggested model. The answers for these questions might contribute to further understanding of the mechanism of polymer-mediated liposome (particle) protection and development of optimized long-circulating microparticular drug carriers.

13.2.6 Experimental confirmation of the model

The theoretical model discussed above was confirmed experimentally by studying the efficacy of liposome-incorporated, fluorescent-marker quenching by macromolecular quencher from the solution, depending on the polymer presence on the liposomal membrane (Torchilin *et al.* 1994a). Two different systems were investigated: (a) the quenching of liposome-incorporated N-[7-nitrobenz-2-oxa-1,3-diazol-4-yl]-dioleoyl-phosphatidyl ethanolamine (NBD-PE) with soluble rhodamine-modified ovalbumin (Rh-OVA) and (b) the quenching of liposome-incorporated phospholipid derivative of fluorescein with anti-fluorescein antibody. In both cases, the presence of even small quantities of flexible PEG (as low as 0.2 mol %) on the liposome sharply decreased the quenching compared with that for plain or rigid dextran-modified liposomes (Figure 13.4). Since the whole quenching process is limited only by macromo-

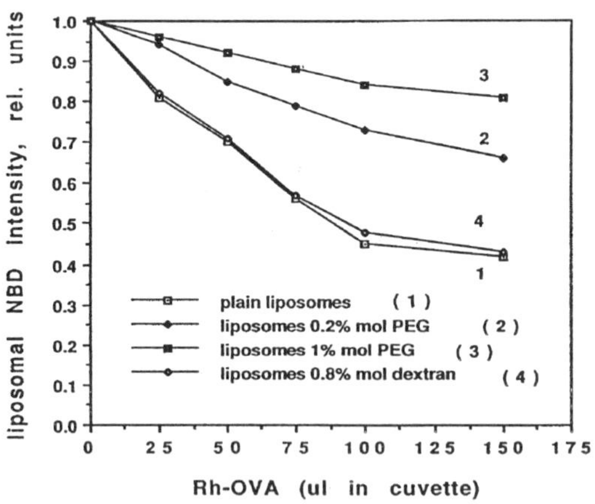

Figure 13.4. Quenching of liposome-incorporated NBD fluorescence with Rh-OVA from the solution at different Rh-OVA concentrations. 1 - plain liposomes; 2 - liposomes with 0.2 % mol PEG-PE; 3 - liposomes with 1 % mol PEG-PE; 4 - liposomes with 0.8 % mol dextran-stearylamine. Flexible PEG provides much better protection against quenching than more rigid dextran. Adapted from Torchilin *et al.* (1994a).

lecular quencher diffusion from the solution to the liposome surface, it is evident that the presence of PEG on the surface creates pronounced diffusional hindrances for this process (Torchilin *et al.* 1994a). Besides, the existence of two different fluorescein pools on the liposome surface was revealed at low PEG concentration. One of them was quenched with the same rate as fluorescein on plain liposomes, whereas the quenching kinetics for another was close to that for fluorescein on PEG-liposomes with higher PEG content. This reflects different location of fluorescein molecules on the liposome surface - between and inside PEG "clouds", as was predicted by theoretical analysis (see Figure 13.3B).

13.3 Chemistry of Polyethylene Glycol (PEG) and PEG-like Polymers

13.3.1 Attractive features of polyethylene glycol

The fact that the absolute majority of research on long-circulating drugs and drug carriers was performed with the use of PEG as a sterically protecting polymer can be explained by the very attractive combination of properties of PEG. The biological behavior of sterically-protected drugs and drug carriers is, to a great extent, determined by the properties of the protecting polymer. From this point of view, excellent solubility of PEG in aqueous solutions and its ability to bind a lot of water molecules, high flexibility of its polymer chain, very low toxicity, immunogenicity, and antigenicity, lack of accumulation in the RES cells, minimum influence on specific biological properties of modified pharmaceuticals make PEG highly pharmacologically acceptable (Zalipsky 1995a, Pang 1993, Powell 1980, Yamaoka, Tabata and Ikada 1994). It is also important that PEG is not biodegradable and subsequently does not form any toxic metabolites. On the other hand, PEG molecules with the molecular weight below 50 kDa are readily excretable from the body via kidneys.

13.3.2 Reactive derivatives of PEG and their coupling to other molecules

From the practical point of view, PEG is easily commercially available in a variety of molecular weights. PEGs which are normally used for the modification of drug and drug carriers have a molecular weight from 1,000 to 20,000 Da and represent quite homogeneous polymers of the general structure $HO\text{-}(CH_2CH_2O)_n\text{-}CH_2CH_2\text{-}OH$. Monomethyl derivatives of PEG (mPEGs) are often used for modification of pharmacologically important substances. The advantage of using such single-terminus reactive (semi-telehelic) polymers is the absence of cross-linked aggregates in the product and higher homogeneity of PEG conjugates with biomacromolecules or drug carriers. Currently, there exists many chemical approaches to synthesize activated derivatives of PEG and to couple these derivatives with a variety of drugs and drug carriers. The extensive review of these methods and their applicability towards different situations was recently done by Zalipsky (Zalipsky 1995a). To illustrate this variety, commonly used methods for preparation of activated PEGs and chemically couple them to proteins (and drug carriers) are presented on Figure 13.5.

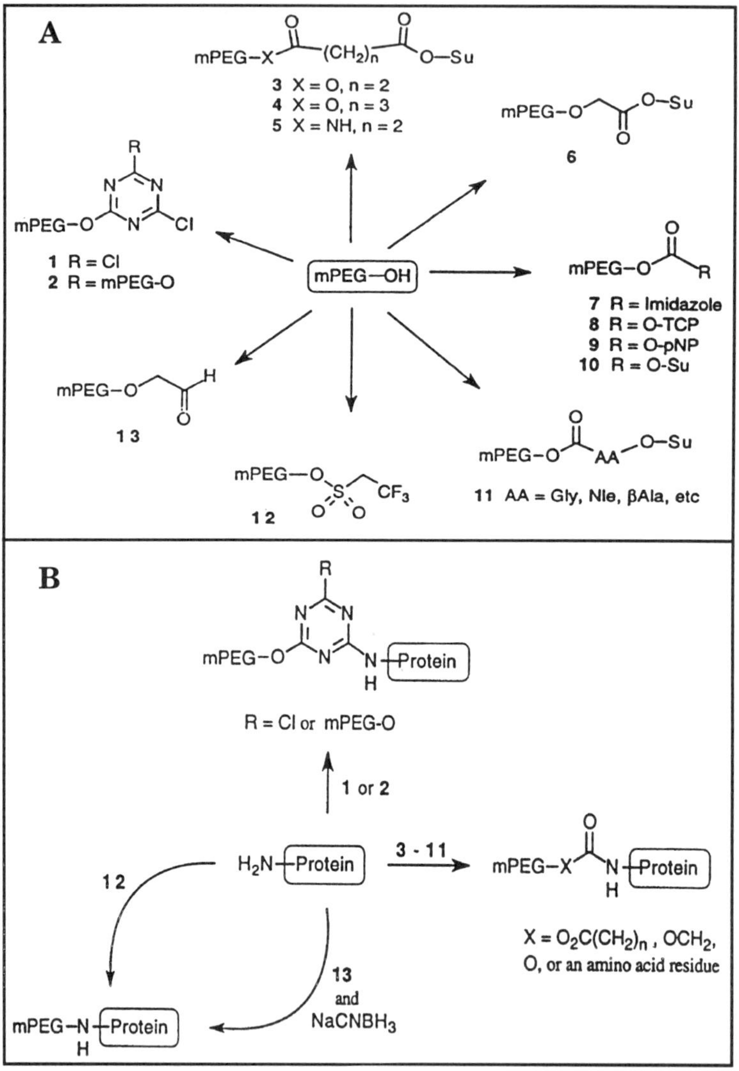

Figure 13.5. **A** - Commonly used methods for preparation of mPEG-based modifying reagents. **B** - Use of mPEG-based reagents 1-13 for preparation of conjugates. mPEG represents $CH_3(OCH_2CH_2)_n$-. Su, succiinmidyl; TCP, trichlorophenyl; pNP, *p*-nitrophenyl; AA, amino acid. From Zalipsky (1995a).

As noted by Zalipsky (Zalipsky 1995a, 1995b), since many of the beneficial properties of PEG-modified drugs and drug carriers, such as extended blood circulation time, reduced toxicity and immunogenicity, depend on the PEG content of corresponding conjugates, two-armed reagents (such as reagent **2** on Figure 13.5) have an advantage over single mPEG chain reagents, because at the same number of attachment sites, they can double the quantity of grafted polymer.

13.3.3 New polymers for steric protection of drugs and drug carriers

Despite well developed chemistry of PEG coupling to pharmaceuticals, the search for alternative sterically protecting polymers is quite active. This might be explained by both the patent situation around PEG and its derivatives and the hope to get even better control over the properties of modified drugs and drug carriers. The suggested theoretical model for the protecting protein behavior and available experimental data (partially discussed above) permitted us to formulate some general requirements towards polymers for steric protection of drugs and drug carriers. These polymers should be soluble and hydrophilic and have a highly flexible main chain. Polymer biocompatibility has to be added to the list if polymer-liposomes are intended for medical use. Synthetic polymers of vinyl series, such as poly(acryl amide) (PAA), poly(vinyl pyrrolidone) (PVP), and some others, may serve as the most evident examples of other potentially protective polymers (Torchilin, Milstein and Shtilman 1993, Torchilin *et al.* 1994a, 1994b, 1995). We reported recently the first experimental data on the synthesis and possible use of synthetic polymer other than PEG for steric protection of liposomes *in vivo* (Torchilin, Milstein and Shtilman 1994, Torchilin *et al.* 1994b, 1995). It was shown that amphiphilic derivatives of PAA and PVP can be synthesized by radical polymerization of the corresponding monomers in the presence of hydrophobic growing chain terminator, and the products obtained provide effective protection to liposomes *in vivo* (in mice experiments) similar to PEG-PE (Klibanov *et al.* 1990, Torchilin *et al.* 1994a, 1994b). Other amphiphilic polymers with well-soluble and a flexible hydrophilic moiety, such as amphiphilic poly(acryloyl morpholine) (PAcM), branched PEG in which two PEG chains are attached to a single hydrophobic phospholipid group (PEG2) and phospholipid-attached PVP, have been also successfully used as liposome steric protectors *in vivo* (Torchilin *et al.* 1995). Amphiphilic PEG2, PAcM, and PVP were prepared by synthesizing carboxyl-terminated polymers (PAcM-COOH, PEG2-COOH, PVP-COOH) (Monfardini *et al.* 1995, Ranucci *et al.* 1994, Sartore *et al.* 1994), which were then modified with PE according to the scheme presented in Figure 13.6.

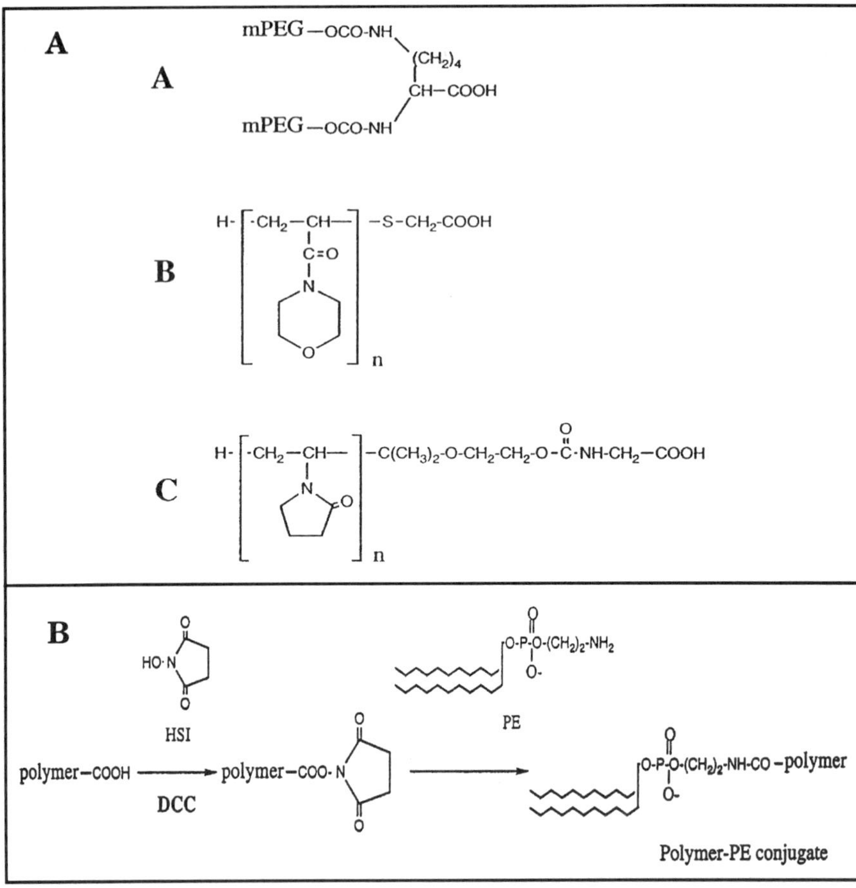

Figure 13.6. A - Chemical structures of carboxyl-terminated polymers used to prepare amphiphilic derivatives for steric protection of liposomes. A - branched poly(ethylene glycol)-COOH (Monfardini *et al.* 1995); B - poly(acryloyl morpholine)-COOH (Ranucci *et al.* 1994); C - poly(vinyl pyrrolidone)-COOH (Sartore *et al.* 1994). **B** - Reaction scheme of the modification of COOH-terminated polymers with PE. HSI, hydroxysuccinimide; DCC, dicyclohexylcarbodiimide.

13.4 PEG-modified Molecules

Historically, first attempts to modify drug properties by PEG were made with individual biologically active and therapeutically important molecules, such as various low-molecular-weight drugs, peptides, and proteins (enzymes). Therapeutical enzymes were grafted with reactive PEG derivatives in a hope to increase their conformational stability and to make them less sensitive towards proteolytic degradation under the action of natural enzymatic systems (Abuchowski and Davis 1979, 1981, Torchilin 1991). *E. coli* asparaginase, trypsin, catalase, uricase, arginase, urokinase, streptokinase, and phenylalanine ammonialyase were among the first enzymes chemically immobilized on soluble PEG, which resulted in their increased stability (in particular, resistance to proteases) without noticeable changes in normal catalytic activity (Holcenberg and Roberts 1981, Abuchowski and Davis 1981). Later, such enzymes as glucolactone oxidase, peroxidase, superoxide dismutase, alkaline phosphatase, ribonuclease, elastase, and tissue plasminogen activator were added to the list (Zalipsky 1995a and references therein).

Early modification protocols were non-specific, and modified enzymes contained PEG chains grafted to a variety of protein reactive groups. Later, however, methods of site-specific modification of proteins with PEG were developed. These methods involved specific attachment of amino-containing PEG molecules to periodate-oxidized oligosaccharide portions of glycoproteins (Urrutigoity and Souppe 1989) or even site-specific mutagenesis in order to obtain a protein containing a certain specially inserted group for further interaction with one of the active PEG derivatives (Goodson and Katre 1990, Kuan, Wang and Pastan 1994).

Among low-molecular-weight drugs attached to PEG, one can find hormones, such as dexamethasone and hydrocortisone (Khue and Galin 1985); atropin and quinidine (Zalipski, Gilon and Zilkha 1983); ibuprofen, penicillin V, aspirin and some others (Zalipsky 1995a and references therein). Numerous chemical approaches to prepare PEG conjugates with individual molecules, including polymerization of ethylene oxide onto a drug molecule (Geckeler and Mutter 1979, Khachadurian *et al.* 1981), are recently well reviewed by Zalipsky (Zalipsky 1995a, 1995b).

13.5 PEG-protected Liposomes

Liposomes (artificial phospholipid vesicles with varying size, charge and composition) since long ago have been widely considered as promising drug carriers (Gregoriadis 1988). Surface modification of liposomes with antibodies, chelating compounds, saccharides, and natural and synthetic polymers was often used to improve different physico-chemical properties of liposomes and, in particular, to make them more stable against destructive influence of the biological milieu and fast clearance from the body. To make PEG capable of incorporation into the liposomal membrane, the reactive derivative of hydrophilic PEG is single terminus-modified with a hydrophobic moiety (usually, the residue of phosphatidyl ethanolamine or a long chain fatty acid is attached to PEG-OSu) (Klibanov *et al.* 1990), see Figure 13.7.

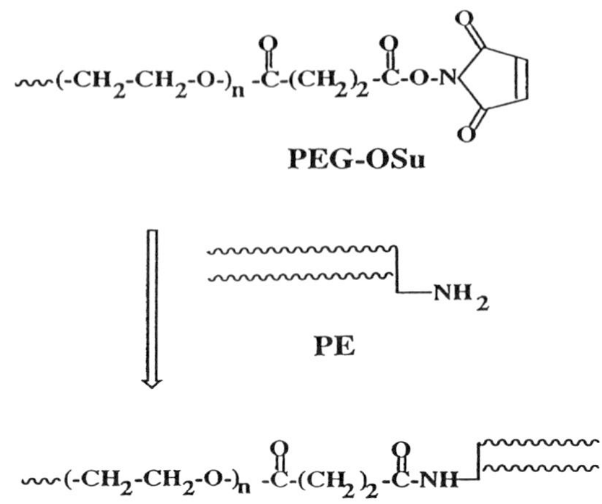

Poly(ethylene glycol)-phosphatidyl ethanolamine, PEG-PE

Figure 13.7. Synthesis of PEG-PE from PEG-hydroxysuccinimide ester (PEG-OSu) and phosphatidyl ethanolamine (PE). From Klibanov *et al.* (1990).

Currently, numerous studies on the preparation and properties of polymer-modified liposomes exist well reviewed in several important books (Gregoriadis 1993, Lasic and Martin 1995, Lasic and Barenholz 1996). Moreover, the understanding of the mechanism underlying the stabilizing effect of PEG onto liposomes, permitted suggestion that the whole number of other polymers which, together with PEG, can be used as effective steric protectors for liposomes (see above) (Torchilin and Trubetskoy 1995, Torchilin 1996). The structures of various polymers used so far for the steric protection of liposomes are presented on Figure 13.8.

Another interesting question is if it is possible to combine the unique properties of long-circulating (PEG-coated) nanocarriers (liposomes and others) and targeted antibody-modified carriers in one preparation? The concern about using PEG for immunocarrier protection is that the grafted polymer can create steric hindrances for normal antibody-target interaction. However, in certain cases this problem can be avoided. To understand it, one has to consider different cases for the co-immobilization of antibody and water-soluble flexible polymer on the same carrier (Torchilin and Papisov 1994). In the first case, the polymer does not cover the carrier surface completely. Antibody molecules are excluded from the volume occupied with PEG, and two separate zones appear on the surface - "clouds" of PEG and antibodies in between. Such immunocarriers should easily interact with target antigens, but their circulation time will be short because there still exists sufficient PEG-free surface area available for opsonization.

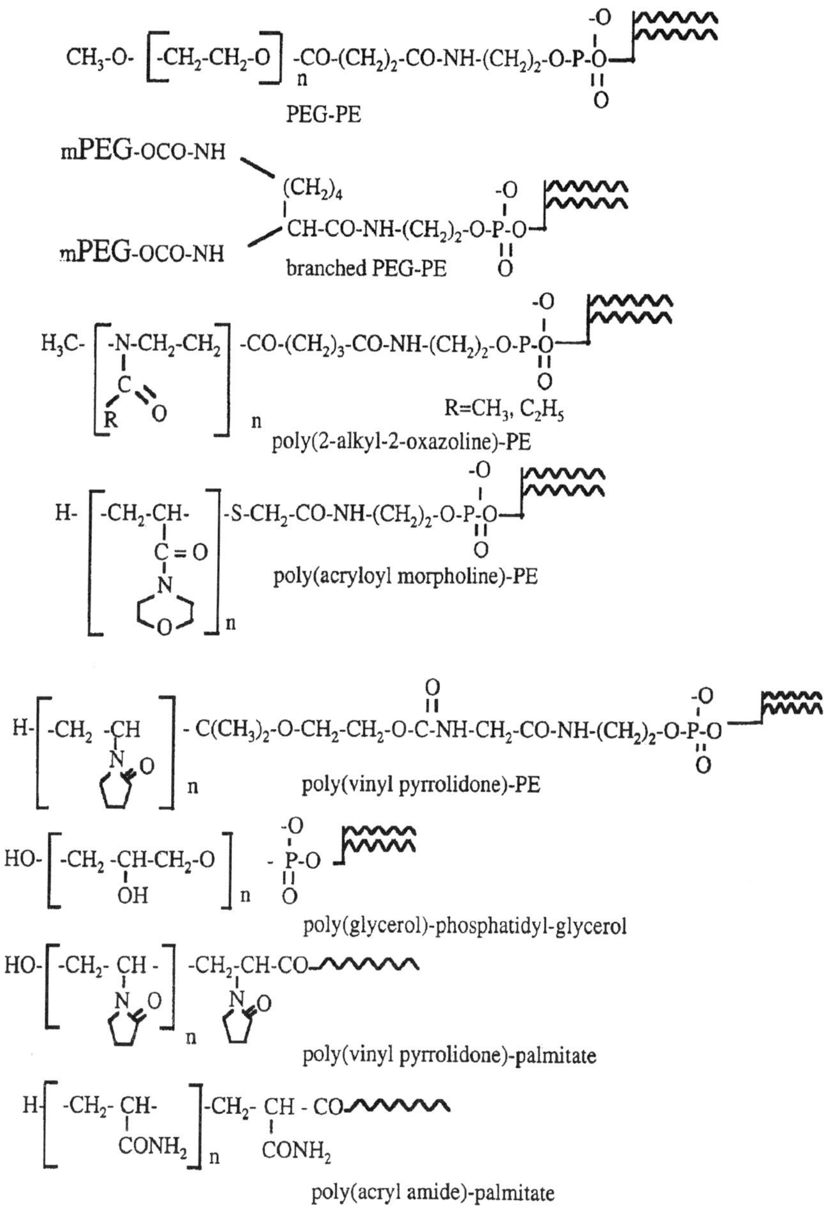

Figure 13.8. Amphiphilic synthetic polymers used for steric protection of liposomes. Synthetic scheme for amphiphilic PEG2, PVP, and PAcM see on Figure 13.6. Poly(2-alkyl-2-oxazoline)-PE is described by Woodle, Engbers and Zalipsky (1994); poly(glycerol)-phosphatidyl-glycerol is described by Maruyama *et al.* (1994).

In the second case, the carrier surface might be completely coated with overlapping "clouds" of PEG, but still some areas of more "loose" conformational density exist, into which free antibodies (capable of the lateral diffusion) can be squeezed from more dense PEG areas. In this case, opsonins have very limited opportunity for the interaction with the liposome, while antibodies are still able to recognize and to bind the target. This is the way in which we can get long-circulating, targeted drug carriers. At a very high degree of surface modification (the third case), PEG is forming conformationally stretched "brushes" (Milner 1991) on the surface. In this case, surface-immobilized antibody is trapped between polymer molecules, and can not overcome steric hindrances and bind to the target, though the carrier itself is well protected against opsonins and can circulate very long. However, brushes of this type can also be used to prepare the long-circulating immuno-carrier preparation if antibodies are immobilized on the surface via the long spacer group or even directly on termini of some PEG molecules (Blume *et al.* 1993, Allen *et al.* 1994).

13.6 PEG-protected Nanoparticles

Synthetic amphiphilic polymers have been used for steric stabilization of various nanoparticulate drug carriers in order to prolong their circulation in the blood and to alter their biodistribution. The detailed description of polymer-modified nanoparticulates was recently given in several good reviews (Moghimi 1995, Stolnik, Illum and Davis 1995). So we have no need to discuss all the related information. I would like, however, to present some data demonstrating the principal similarities underlying the behavior of sterically-protecting polymers on different surfaces.

There are several principal types of amphipathic polymers used so far for the coating of injectable nanoparticulate carriers. All of them consist of a hydrophobic moiety which easily adsorbs on the surface and performs anchoring function, and a hydrophilic moiety which protrudes into the solution and protects particulates from interactions with plasma proteins in the blood upon intravenous administration in accordance with the mechanism discussed by us earlier.

Polystyrene latex particles, commercially available in a number of sizes in the range of 0.05-1 mm, are the carriers of choice for the surface modification studies. Polystyrene latex particles have narrow size distribution, and, hence, might be a convenient model to study the phenomena connected with polymer modification of surfaces. The mechanism of protection is essentially the same as for PEG-coated liposomes - formation of a conformational "cloud" of polymer flexible chains which protects the particle hydrophobic core from the contact with opsonizing proteins (Torchilin *et al.* 1994a, Torchilin and Papisov 1994). Modification of the liposome surface with amphiphilic polymer usually requires the incorporation of the polymer's hydrophobic moiety into the liposomes phospholipid bilayer, which is impossible in the case of solid particle modification. In the latter case, surface modification can be performed by one of the following two methods: 1) physical adsorption of a polymer on a particle surface or 2) chemical grafting of polymer chains onto a particle.

One of the most commonly used is the series of linear or branched copolymers of polyethylene oxide and polypropylene oxide (Pluronic/Tetronic™ or Poloxamer/Poloxamine™). There are numerous studies on the coating of different surfaces with these polymers, including their use for protection of latex particles from the uptake by the reticulo-endothelial system upon i.v. injection (Moghimi *et al.* 1991, Moghimi 1995, Stolnik, Illum and Davis 1995). Hydrophilic linear polymers with terminal lipid or fatty acyl group can also be used for the same purpose. PEG-phosphatidyl ethanolamine (PEG-PE) is a typical representative of such polymers; see Figures 13.7 and 13.8 and reference (Klibanov *et al.* 1990). The third important type of amphipathic polymers are amphiphilic copolymers in which in the water media the hydrophobic block itself is able to form a solid phase (particle), while the hydrophilic part remains as a surface-exposed "protective cloud". The example of such structure is block-copolymer of PEG and polylactide-glycolide (PEG-PLAGA) (Krause, Schwartz and Rohdewald 1985, Gref *et al.* 1994, 1995). Using PLAGA-PEG copolymer, one can prepare long-circulating particles with an insoluble (solid) PLAGA core and a water-soluble PEG shell covalently linked to the core (Gref *et al.* 1994, 1995). The adsorption of Pluronic/Tetronic™ or Poloxamer/Poloxamine™ surfactants on the surface of polystyrene latex particles proceeds via the hydrophobic interaction with polypropylene oxide fragment. Interestingly, the adsorption of Poloxamer-type copolymers takes place only on the solid particles with clearly hydrophobic surface: no interaction is detected, for example, between such copolymers and the liposome surface (Moghimi *et al.* 1991, Jamshaid *et al.* 1988).

Hydrophilic linear polymers with terminal lipid or fatty acyl groups, such as PEG-PE or PAA-P (Klibanov *et al.* 1990, Torchilin *et al.* 1994b) have been also tried as potential steric protectors for nanoparticular carriers. To investigate the behavior of such polymers on the surface of nanoparticulates, Polybeads™ polystyrene latex particles with a diameter of 100 nm were used. PAA-P (MW 12,000) and PEG-PE (MW 5,000) have been used to coat the surface of latex particles. The particle diameter increase upon polymer adsorption was found to be approximately 5 nm for PEG-PE and approximately 20 nm for PAA-P, which proves the formation of a protective polymer layer over the surface of latex particle.

13.7 PEG-containing Micelles

Amphiphilic copolymers in aqueous environment spontaneously form polymeric micelles, particles with hydrophobic blocks forming a core protected with hydrophilic chains of the copolymer. Normally, the size of such particles vary from 5 to 50 nm. They are sufficiently stable in aqueous solutions and can entrap numerous hydrophobic substances, including drugs, into their hydrophobic core. So, micelles prepared from amphiphilic-block copolymers might be considered as another important example of particulate drug carriers, surface-modified with polymers (Kwon and Kataoka 1995, Trubetskoy and Torchilin 1995, 1996). These types of micelles exhibit relatively low critical micelle concentrations in solutions, a thermodynamic property which assures their existence as a particle. Eventually, upon indefinite dilution, micellar nanoparticulates dissociate into individual polymeric chains, a property which might be extremely useful *in vivo* (drug-carrying micelles can slowly dissociate in the body releasing the drug).

Several chemical designs for drug-carrying, long-circulating polymeric micelles have been proposed. Ringsdorf (1975) described the synthesis of a copolymer of PEG and polylysine partially modified with hydrophobic palmitoyl chains which, in a form of a micelle, interacts with rat peritoneal macrophages (Pratten *et al.* 1985). The micellar carrier of similar structure with the anti-cancer agent cyclophosphamide attached to the remaining non-palmitoylated amino groups of the polylysine exhibited prolonged release of the active drug (Bader, Ringsdorf and Schmidt 1984).

Another popular approach involves the use of micelle-forming block-copolymers consisting of a hydrophilic PEG block and a hydrophobic block of poly(L-aminoacid) (Kwon and Kataoka 1995). Copolymers may be of A-B or A-B-A type, and blocks made of benzyl-aspartate, benzyl-glutamate, lysine, and aspartic acid have been utilized to form the micelle's core. Drugs (such as cyclophosphamide, doxorubicine, and cisplatin) have been covalently coupled to hydrophobic blocks or non-covalently incorporated in the hydrophobic core during the process of micelle formation. Evident advantage of PEG-based micelles over traditional surfactant micelles is a very low value of critical micellization concentration (CMC) of the former. CMC for PEG-based micelles may be as low as 10^{-7} M, whereas traditional surfactant micells have CMC values in the range of 10^{-3} - 10^{-4} M. This makes PEG-based micelles much more stable in diluted solution (for example, after dilution of drug-containing micelle preparation in the blood).

Recently, we have proposed new polymeric micellar particles as a carrier for iodinated organic compounds to be used use as a contrast agent in x-ray imaging (Trubetskoy *et al.* 1994, 1996). The copolymer, ε,N-(triiodobenzoyl)polylysine-monomethoxy PEG, can form particles with hydrophobic iodine-containing nucleus which is sterically protected from the aqueous environment with flexible PEG chains (Figure 13.9).

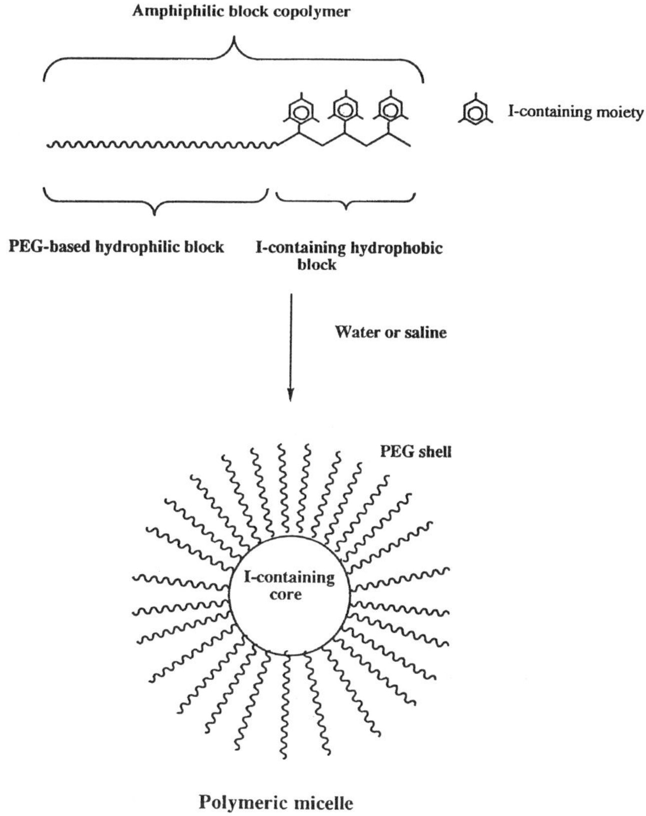

Figure 13.9. Schematic representation of micelle formation from amphiphilic iodine-containing block-copolymer.

13.8 Biological Consequences of PEG Modification

13.8.1 Molecules

The first and the most general result of the modification of individual molecules (primarily enzymes and proteins) is the increase in their stability towards various inactivating influences of the biological milieu (temperature, pH, proteolytic enzymes, *etc.*) (Holcenberg and Roberts 1981, Abuchowski and Davis 1981, Torchilin 1991). Thus, animal experiments demonstrated that many enzymes that normally inactivate in the blood within minutes retain their activity in the blood for 24 to 48 hours and even longer after modification with PEG and some other water-soluble polymers. This was explained by the stabilizing effect of such polymers on active conformations of these proteins and the polymer shielding effect against proteolytic enzymes. Such clinically significant enzyme as superoxide dismutase, after modification with PEG, was able to retain its activity in the blood for more than 9 hours compared with approximately 3 minutes for the native enzyme (Pyatak, Abuchowski and Davis 1980, Beauchamp *et al.* 1983, Morpurgo *et al.* 1996).

Another important consequence of PEG modification is the frequent decrease in immunogenicity of modified proteins, which was found for polymer-modified catalase, streptokinase, and bovine serum albumin (Abuchowski and Davis 1981, Torchilin 1991). However, in many other cases, immunogenicity and antigenicity of proteins (enzymes) conjugated with PEG was retained (Hadley and Sato 1989).

The preservation of a functional activity of PEG-conjugated biomolecules is, clearly, an important requirement towards such conjugates. Numerous studies on this subject have demonstrated that the preservation of specific properties in conjugates depends on modification degree and the type of expected biological activity (Abuchowski and Davis 1981, Torchilin 1991, Zalipsky 1995a). Naturally, the higher the modification the less initial activity preserved. On the other hand, it turned out that enzymatic activity towards low-molecular-weight substrates is less sensitive to modification than similar activity towards high-molecular-weight substrates. This was explained by steric hindrances created by polymer molecules for normal enzyme-high-molecular-weight substrate interaction. Thus, for example, PEG-modified elastase retained approximately 35% of initial activity towards its low-molecular-weight substrate and only approximately 17% of activity towards casein (Koide and Kobayashi 1983). Trypsin might be completely inactivated towards proteins but still preserve good activity towards specific small substrates (Abuchowski and Davis 1979). This problem is much less important in the case of PEG-modified, small, biologically active molecules, especially if they are able to detach from the polymer.

13.8.2 Liposomes

The most important consequence of liposome modification with protecting polymers is sharp increase in their circulation time and decrease in their RES (liver) accumulation (Klibanov *et al.* 1990, Torchilin *et al.* 1994a, 1995, Lasic and Martin 1995). Though PEG is still considered to be the most popular and clinically acceptable sterically protecting polymer for liposome modification, other polymers mentioned before can also provide similar control over the biological behavior of liposomes. Biodistribution and blood clearance experiments with polymer-modified ^{111}In-labeled liposomes in CD-1 mice clearly demonstrated that amphiphilic palmitoyl- or PE-containing derivatives of PAcM, PEG2, PAA, and PVP can also provide effective protection to liposomes *in vivo* similar to PEG-PE, which agrees well with our theoretical considerations and previous experiments (Torchilin *et al.* 1993, 1994a, 1994b, 1994c, Torchilin and

Papisov 1994); see also Figure 13.8 for the list of polymers used so far for the liposome surface modification.

The extent of protective activity for different polymers towards liposomes *in vivo* depends on the length of hydrophobic anchor, polymer molecular weight (*i.e.*, chain length and the energy of molecular motion), and the structure and quantity of protecting polymer on the liposome surface (Torchilin *et al.* 1994a, 1995), see Figure 13.10. When modified

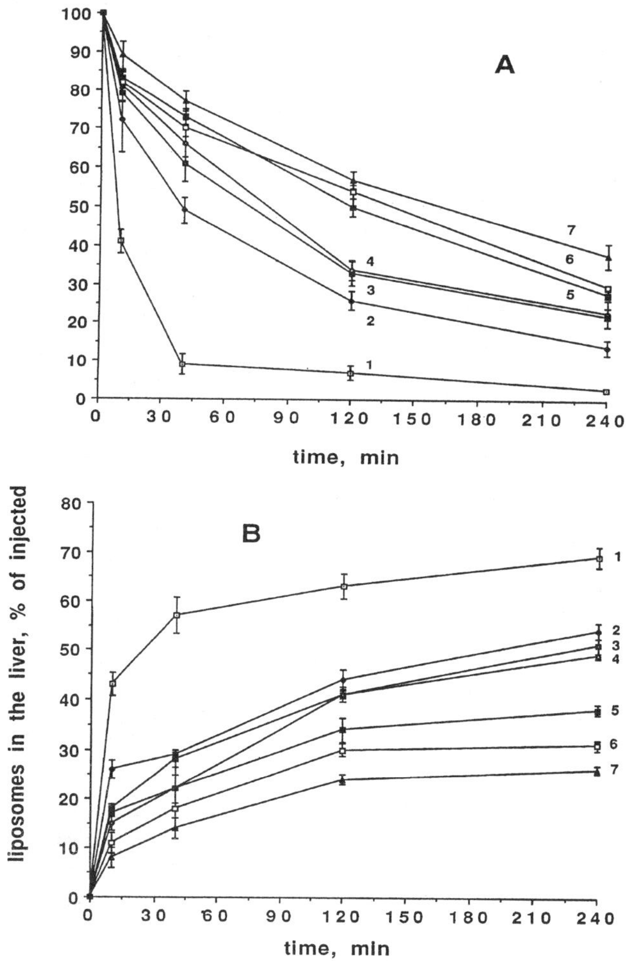

Figure 13.10. **A** - liposome clearance from the blood of experimental mice; **B** - liposome accumulation in the liver. **1** - "plain" liposomes; **2** - PVP-liposomes (2.5 % mol PVP); **3** - PAA-liposomes (2.5 % mol PAA); **4** - PEG-liposomes (2.5 % mol PEG); **5** - PVP-liposomes (6.5 % mol PVP); **6** - PAA-liposomes (6.5 % mol PAA); **7** - PEG-liposomes (6.5 % mol PEG). One can notice both, polymer content and polymer-type influence on liposome circulation time. Still, polymer content seems to be a more important factor. From Torchilin *et al.* (1994b).

with the same residue (such as PE or palmitoyl), PAA, PVP, and PEG of similar molecular weight (6,000 - 8,000) being used in similar concentration, all provide efficient steric protection for liposomes and noticeably increase the residence time of liposomes in the blood. Half-clearance times for PVP-, PAA-, and PEG-liposomes with 2.5% mol content of protective polymer are approximately 45, 80, and 80 minutes, and for PVP-, PAA-, and PEG-liposomes with 6.5% mol content of protective polymer, approximately 120, 140 and 170 minutes, respectively, whereas half-clearance time for "plain" liposomes of the same size is only about 10 - 15 minutes.

The protective activity of polymers with a shorter hydrophobic moiety (dodecyl) or with higher MW (12,000 - 15,000) is, however, much lower (corresponding half-clearance times do not exceed 40 minutes). This can be easily understood taking into account the supposed energy of interaction between the fatty acyl anchoring the polymer onto the liposome surface and the hydrophobic part of the liposomal membrane. From the thermodynamic point of view, a relatively short dodecyl group is unable to keep 6 - 8 kDa polymer molecule on the liposome surface: the energy of the polymeric chain motion in the solution might be higher than the energy of dodecyl group interaction with phospholipid surroundings within the liposomal membrane. As a result, dodecyl-terminated polymers might be relatively easily removed from the liposomal membrane, and demonstrate only slight and transient protective effect. The longer palmitoyl anchor provides much more firm polymer binding with liposome (higher energy of interaction with hydrophobic membrane core due to the larger number of membrane-embedded CH_2-groups) and thus much better liposome steric protection. On the other hand, even the length of palmitoyl anchor is insufficient to fix firmly 12 - 15 kDa polymer on the liposome surface because of much higher energy of polymer chain motion in solution compared with that for the shorter polymers (des Cloizeaux and Jannik 1990). So again, the liposome surface gradually looses the protective polymer coat; as a result, the liposomes are opsonized and captured by the liver and spleen.

Still, PEG-PE and PEG2-PE both most sharply increase the residence time of liposomes in the circulation. However, PEG2-PE seems to be noticeably more efficient than PEG-PE at low content of polymer in liposome, whereas at high molar content their effect on liposomes blood clearance is practically identical. Thus, half-clearance times for PEG- and PEG2-liposomes with 3% mol content of protective polymer are approximately 80 and 140 minutes, respectively, and for PEG- and PEG2-liposomes with 7% mol content of protective polymer - approximately 230 minutes for both preparations. The results obtained can be easily interpreted taking into account the structure of both polymers. In PEG2-PE, the single PE residue carries two PEG-5000 chains, whereas in PEG-PE, each PE residue is conjugated with single PEG-5000 chain. As a result, when 3% mol of PEG2 is used, the actual amount of protective PEG chains over the liposome surface is twice as high as for PEG-PE, which results in better protection. Similar phenomenon was described in Monfardini *et al.* (1995) where PEG2 was shown to be a better steric protector for proteins than PEG. When 7% mol of protected polymer is used, even single-chained PEG-PE can provide complete coating of the liposome surface and maximum protection, so there is no room for additional effect of extra PEG chains of PEG2-PE.

Liposomes containing 5 mol % of distearoyl-PE covalently linked to poly(2-methyl-2-oxazoline) or poly(2-ethyl-2-oxazoline), (see Figure 13.8) also exhibit extended blood circulation time and decreased uptake by the liver and spleen (Woodle, Engbers and Zalipsky 1994). A similar observation was made by Maruyama *et al.* (1994) where phosphatidyl polyglycerols (see structure in Figure 13.8) were shown to prolong liposome circulation time *in vivo*.

From the clinical point of view, it is extremely important that various long-circulating liposomes of a relatively small size (100-200 nm) were shown to effectively accumulate in many tumors via the "impaired filtration" mechanism (Gabizon 1995, Gabizon and Papahadjopoulos 1988). As a result, PEG-coated and other long-circulating liposomes were prepared containing a variety of anti-cancer agents, such as doxorubicine, arabinofuranosylcytosine, adriamycin, and vincristin (Huang *et al.* 1994, Gabizon *et al.* 1994, Boman *et al.* 1994, Allen *et al.* 1992). The biggest success was achieved with PEG-liposome-incorporated doxorubicine, which has already demonstrated very encouraging results in clinical trials (Gabizon 1995 and references therein).

13.8.3 Immunoliposomes

To confirm that under certain circumstances long-circulating PEG-coated liposomes (or other nanoparticulate drug carriers) can be made targeted by co-incorporation of an antibody onto their surface, *in vivo* studies have been performed with PEG-liposomes additionally containing anti-cardiac myosin antibody (Torchilin *et al.* 1992). This antibody effectively binds myosin inside ischemic or/and necrotic cardio-myocytes with affected or destroyed cellular membranes but does not interact with normal cells, being unable to penetrate the intact plasmic membrane (Khaw *et al.* 1984, 1987). This formed the basis for the targeted delivery of radiolabeled PEG-coated long-circulating liposomes in the region of ischemically compromised myocardium in rabbits and dogs with experimental myocardial infarction. Infarcts in rabbits and dogs were generated as described (Khaw *et al.* 1991, Torchilin *et al.* 1992). Different radiolabeled liposome preparations were injected intravenously after 30 to 60 minutes of reperfusion, and 5 to 6 hours after liposome injection, animals were killed by an overdose of pentobarbital. The hearts were excised, and tissue samples of normal and infarcted myocardium were weighed and counted in a gamma-counter. The data on the liposome accumulation in the heart were expressed as infarct-to-normal myocardium radioactivity ratio. It was demonstrated clearly that the increasing quantity of PEG increasingly protected liposomes from the clearance, and co-immobilization of an antibody and PEG decreased the half-life of liposomes only at the lower PEG concentration, while at intermediate PEG concentration (approximately 4% mol) liposomes demonstrated both longevity and targetability (Torchilin *et al.* 1992, 1996). The highest uptake ratio was achieved for PEG-immunoliposomes and reached 20:1. As soon as the target accumulation in this case can proceed, both via specific recognition and non-specifically via decreased filtration rate (liposomes can enter necrotic area via permeabilized capillaries but cannot leave it because of worsened drainage), in the case of PEG-antibody-liposomes, both mechanisms work in an additive fashion, so these liposomes demonstrated also the maximum "absolute" accumulation in the target.

Current methods are being developed permitting coupling of targeted devices (antibodies) to the distal ends of the grafted PEG molecules (Blume *et al.* 1993, Allen 1994). The preparations described advantageously combine longevity and targetability even at high concentrations of the surface-grafted PEG.

13.8.4 Nanoparticles

Numerous studies have been performed on blood clearance and biodistribution of various nanoparticles upon their coating with surfactants, including the use of surfactants for particle protection from the uptake by the reticulo-endothelial system upon intravenous injection (Illum and Davis 1983, 1984). Upon i.v. administration, hydrophobic particles of sub-micron size are believed to be opsonized with macrophage-recognizable but not yet identified serum proteins (Patel 1992). Protection of the particle surface with hydrophilic flexible polymeric chains results in substantial decline in phagocytosis by liver macrophages and subsequent prolongation of circulation time. The adsorption of the above copolymers leads not only to the decrease of particle uptake by resident macrophages in liver but, after coating with some specific copolymers, can redirect the injected nanoparticles to other organs (Porter *et al.* 1992). For example, the coating of 60-nm polystyrene latex with Poloxamer 407 results in increased particle accumulation in bone marrow. The same group has demonstrated that analogous procedure also helps substantially to alter the biodistribution of subcutaneously injected nanospheres. Coating of 60-nm diameter polystyrene nanospheres with certain Poloxamer/Poloxamine copolymers results in their increased accumulation in regional lymph nodes. The optimal length of the copolymer polyoxyethylene block for this particular purpose has been found to be 5-15 oxyethylene units. Non-coated particles normally stay at the injection site while particles coated with longer polyoxyethylene-containing copolymers are not retained in the nodes and eventually appear in systemic circulation (Moghimi *et al.* 1994).

There exist certain differences in the biological behavior of hydrophobic nanoparticulates and liposomes coated with the same polymers. Thus, the results of biodistribution studies in mice demonstrated that PEG-PE-coated Polybeads particles, as one can expect, stayed in the circulation for a long time ($t_{1/2}$=4 hours). However, unlike PAA-coated liposomes (Torchilin, Milstein and Shtilman 1994), PAA-coated nanospheres cleared from the blood as fast as non-coated particles with a similar pattern of liver accumulation. At the same time, spleen accumulation of PAA-coated particles was substantially reduced comparing to non-coated ones (Figure 13.11). Different biological effects of the same amphiphilic polymer coating on the behavior of different particulates *in vivo* has also been reported previously. It was shown that Poloxamer 407 can protect from RES uptake of latex nanospheres but not the liposomes of similar size (Moghimi *et al.* 1991). This difference in the *in vivo* behavior has been explained by the different orientation of poly(acrylamide) chains on the particle surface compared with the surface of the liposome, which results in a different degree of carrier protection from adsorbing plasma proteins.

In the recent review on long-circulating liposomes (Allen 1994), the way of polymer attachment to the surface was pointed out as the major difference in liposomes with poloxamers or PEG-PE. With poloxamers, the hydrophobic region lies perpendicular to the acyl-chain region of the bilayer, whereas for PEG-PE the hydrophobic anchor is parallel to the acyl chains. As a result, the thickness of coating is considerably less for poloxamers on liposomes than for poloxamers on nanoparticles (Jamshaid *et al.* 1988, Woodle, Newman and Martin 1992). For liposomes, PEG-PE works better than poloxamer F-108 (Woodle, Newman and Martin 1992). Still, we are talking about the differences in anchoring various protecting polymers onto different surfaces, whereas the behavior of hydrophilic moiety in the surrounding water solution should remain pretty much the same.

I have already mentioned about amphipathic copolymers in which in the water media the hydrophobic block is able to form a solid phase (particle), while the hydrophilic part remains as a surface-exposed protective "cloud". To demonstrate *in vivo* protective effect of hydrophilic polymer in such systems, block copolymers PLAGA-PEG have been synthesized. Using the solvent evaporation method (Gref *et al.* 1994), submicron particles with insoluble (solid) PLAGA core and water-soluble PEG shell covalently linked to the core were prepared. Several polymer preparations have been synthesized where the molecular weight of PEG block was 20 kDa, and it was connected with the PLAGA block at 1:9, 1:5 and 1:4 PLAGA:PEG w/w ratios (Trubetskoy, Langer and Torchilin, unpublished results).

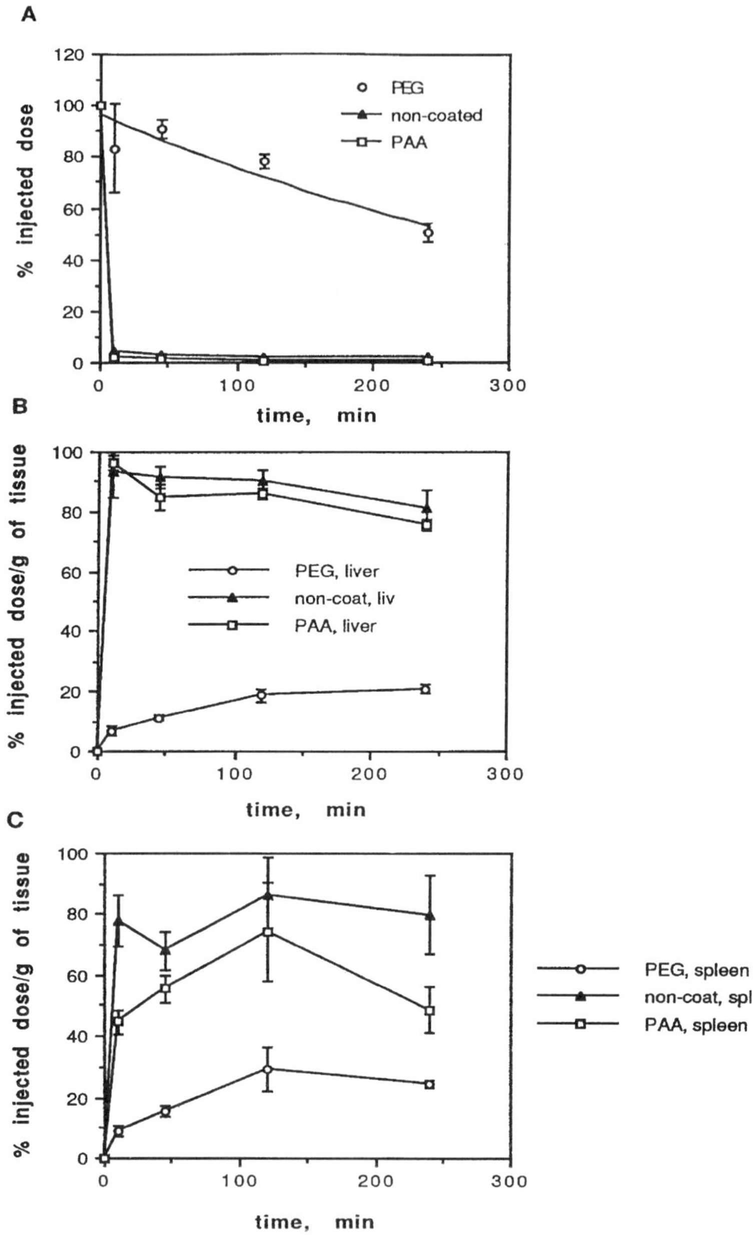

Figure 13.11. Blood clearance (A), liver (B) and spleen (C) accumulation of ^{111}In-labeled 100-nm polystyrene latex nanospheres with surface-adsorbed PEG and PAA in mice. Notice the different influence of PEG and PAA on nanoparticles, whereas in the case of liposomes, the effect of PEG and PAA did not differ much (see Figure 13.10).

To study the biological behavior of PEG-PLAGA nanospheres, they were labeled by incorporation of hydrophobic ^{111}In-diethylene teriamine pentaacetic acid stearylamine into the PLAGA core during the solvent evaporation procedure. Blood clearance and biodistribution experiments in BALB/c mice have demonstrated that protective effect of PEG in this system depends on the content of its block (Figure 13.12). Clearance and liver accumulation patterns reveal one basic feature of the preparations under discussion: the higher the content of PEG block, the slower the clearance and the better protection from the liver uptake. The splenic uptake reflects also the particle size-dependent filtering effect. As already demonstrated for liposomes, the vesicles with diameters exceeding 250 nm can be non-specifically detained in spleen (Klibanov *et al.* 1991). 1:5 and 1:4 PEG-PLAGA nanoparticles were 265 and 315 nm in size, respectively, so the elevated splenic uptake for these preparations can be explained by their passive retention in the spleen. Similar effects on longevity and biodistribution of microparticular drug carriers might be achieved by direct chemical attachment of protective polyethylene oxide chains onto the surface of preformed particles (Harper *et al.* 1991).

13.8.5 Micelles

Detailed studies of *in vivo* behavior and biodistribution of therapeutic polymeric micelles have been performed by Kataoka and coworkers, using the micelles formed by copolymer of polyethyleneoxide and poly(aspartic acid) with covalently bound adriamycin [PEO-p(Asp(ADR)] (Kwon and Kataoka 1995, Yokoyama *et al.* 1990). It has been found that upon intravenous injection, the circulation time and biodistribution of micelles depend on the relative size of the copolymer blocks. For example, it was found that [PEO-p(Asp(ADR)] micelles with a PEO block of 12 kDa in mice has a $t_{1/2}$ of approximately 7 hours, while micelles with 5 kDa PEO block have a $t_{1/2}$ of approximately 1.5 hours, and micelles with 1-kDa block have circulation half-time substantially lower than 1 hour. It seems that longer PEO blocks and shorter p(Asp) segments favor maintaining micellar structure in the blood and, consequently, longer circulation times and lower uptake by reticuloendothelial system (Kwon *et al.* 1994).

X-Ray computer tomography (CT) experiments with PEG-based iodine-containing micelles (Trubetskoy and Torchilin 1995, 1996, Trubetskoy *et al.* 1995, 1996) in rabbits demonstrated that such micelles are long-circulating and can be used for CT-imaging of the blood pool. Because of the protective action of PEG and the high stability (low CMC value) of such micelles even in diluted systems, the blood remained opacified for more than 24 hours after intravenous administration of the micellar agent.

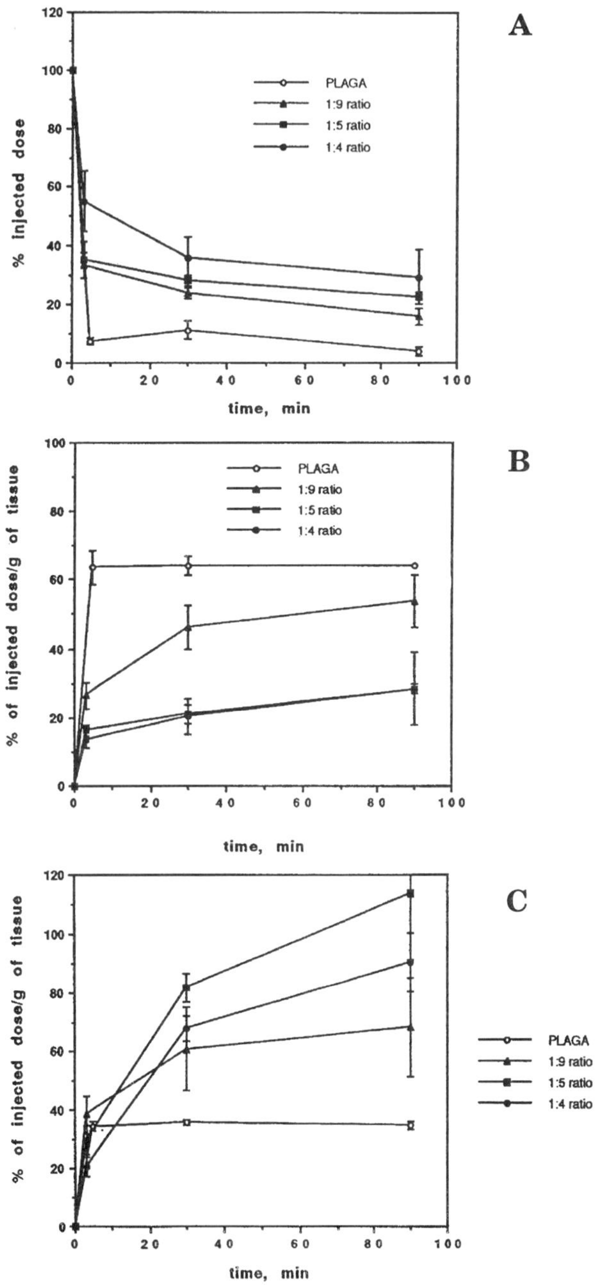

Figure 13.12. Blood clearance (A) liver (B), and spleen (C) accumulation of ^{111}In-labeled PEG-PLAGA nanospheres with different PEG:PLAGA w/w ratios in mice (Trubetskoy, Langer, and Torchilin, unpublished). Notice an important role of PEG-to-PLAGA molar ratio.

13.8.6 Pharmacokinetics and clearance

The most important pathways for the clearance of long-circulating drugs and drug carriers - extravasation, renal clearance, and uptake by cells from the blood - are independent processes. However, extravasation determines interstitial and lymphatic transport and interstitial and lymphatic uptake of long-circulating substances. With this in mind, it was suggested (Papisov 1995) to divide all long-circulating drugs/carriers into extravasating and non-extravasating ones. The main difference between these two groups is their size, with a border zone at approximately 5-10 nm. The non-extravasating group includes cells, cell ghosts, particles, and large liposomes, while the extravasating group includes small liposomes, proteins and their derivatives (including antibodies and PEG-modified enzymes) and various polymers which are large enough (more that 40,000 Da) to avoid fast renal clearance. Naturally, all said is true in the case of normal endothelium and in certain pathological areas with increased endothelial permeability, the pattern can change completely. However, such conditional division permitted two simple idealized models describing the biological behavior of different long-circulating substances to be built (Papisov 1995).

Interactions of non-extravasating or very slowly extravasating drugs/carriers are limited to blood components and cells exposed into the blood. Usually, such substances are removed from the circulation via opsonization-mediated phagocytosis. Opsonization (*i.e.*, binding of certain proteins facilitating the recognition and removal of foreign particles and macromolecules by phagocytic cells) might be enhanced by the presence of charged or chemically reactive groups on the surface of these particles, whereas surface coating with PEG or PEG-like polymers may prevent opsonization or, at least, significantly slow it down. Biological mechanisms and consequences of opsonization for long-circulating drugs and drug carriers are well discussed by Papisov (1995).

An important analysis of pharmacokinetics of long-circulating (PEG-coated) liposomes was recently performed by Allen (Allen, Hansen and de Menezes 1995). It clearly follows that association of drugs with carriers such as liposomes has pronounced effects of pharmacokinetic profiles of both the drug and the carrier. The most important consequences of such association for the drug are: delayed drug adsorption, restricted drug biodistribution, decreased volume of drug biodistribution, delayed drug clearance, and retarded drug metabolism (Hwang 1987). All these effects are determined by hindered interstitial penetration of a drug and lesser drug accessibility for the biological milieu because of entrapment into the liposome (or other drug carrier). The presence of a protective polymer on the carrier surface changes all of these parameters still further (Klibanov *et al.* 1990, Senior *et al.* 1991). Thus, while "plain" liposomes have non-linear, saturable kinetics, long-circulating liposomes demonstrate dose-independent, non-saturable, and log-linear kinetics

(Allen and Hansen 1991, Huang *et al.* 1992, Mayhew *et al.* 1992). The arrearance of log-linear kinetics for long-circulating liposomes (and, evidently, other sterically protected carriers) is explained by a significant decrease in the first phase of particulate carriers clearance into a high affinity and relatively low capacity system, such as the RES. All pharmacokinetic effects depend on the route of liposome administration and their size and composition and always are less expressed for sterically protected PEG-carriers (Allen, Hansen and Rutledge 1989, Maruyama *et al.* 1992, Liu, Mori and Huang 1991, 1992).

13.8.7 Diagnostic (imaging) applications

Diagnostic (medical imaging) represents a relatively new but fast growing area of biomedical application of long-circulating pharmaceuticals (Trubetskoy and Torchilin 1995, 1996, Trubetskoy *et al.* 1995, 1996, Weissleder *et al.* 1995, Bogdanov, Weissleder and Brady 1995). The ability of many drug carriers to stay in the circulation long enough after being sterically protected with PEG or PEG-like polymers naturally led to the idea of loading such carriers with diagnostic labels and subsequently using them for visualization of blood or lymphatic vessels. Polyoxyethylene-lipid conjugates were used to prepare micelles able to carry hydrophobic radiolabels, labels for magnetic resonance imaging, and for computed tomography, and these micelles were successfully used for visualization of lymph nodes and lymphatic flow in experimental animals (Trubetskoy and Torchilin 1995, 1996, Trubetskoy *et al.* 1995). Microparticles of iron oxide coated with certain polymers, including dextran and PEG, were used in experimental magnetic resonance imaging for visualization of the blood pool, RES, and neuronal transport (Weissleder *et al.* 1995). Long-circulating conjugates of chelating, agent-modified polylysine and PEG were loaded with Gd and also used for magnetic resonance imaging of the blood pool (Bogdanov, Weissleder and Brady 1995). Long-circulating iodinated polymers look to be promising agents for blood pool computed tomography (Revel *et al.* 1991). Those are just few examples from this rapidly developing field.

13.9 Conclusion

Thus, steric protection of various nanoparticulate drug carriers can be achieved by grafting their surface with many hydrophilic and flexible polymers including linear and branched poly(ethylene glycol), poly(acrylamide), poly(vinyl pyrrolidone), poly(acryloyl morpholine), and some others. The protective effect of these polymers on nanoparticulate carriers, including liposomes, may be interpreted in terms of statistical behavior of macromolecules in solution where polymer flexibility plays a key role. According to the mechanism proposed, surface-grafted chains of flexible and hydrophilic polymers form dense conformational "clouds" over the particle surface and prevent other macromolecules from the interaction with the surface even at low concentration of protecting polymer. The model permits the answer to various questions concerning spatial distribution and density of polymer molecules on the surface of nanoparticulate carriers. Principal behavior of protecting polymers on the surface of liposomes and particles is similar, though the architecture of polymer coats might differ. The scale of protective effect can be considered as the balance between the energy of hydrophobic anchor interaction with the surface and the energy of polymer chain free motion in solution. The whole approach opens wide opportunities for controlling the *in vivo* behavior of various microparticular drug carriers. Long-circulating pharmaceuticals have already been used successfully in various diagnostic modalities, in cancer therapy, and in experimental drug delivery into zones of ischemia and inflammation. Pharmacokinetic properties of such pharmaceuticals demonstrate their obvious advantages over many traditional drugs and drug carriers.

13.10 List of Abbreviations

PEG, poly(ethylene glycol); PEG2, branched PEG, containing two PEG chains attached to a single anchoring group; PAA, poly(acrylamide); PAA-P, PAA-palmitate; PAcM - polyacryloyl morpholine; PVP, polyvinyl pyrrolidone; PLAGA, polylactideglycolide; PEG-PLAGA, block-copolymer of PLAGA and PEG; PE, phosphatidyl ethanolamine; OSu - hydroxysuccinimide ester; NBD, N-(7-nitrobenz-2-oxa-1,3-diazol-4-yl); NBD-PE, NBD-dioleoyl phosphatidyl ethanolamine; Rh, sulforhodamine; Rh-OVA, Rh-ovalbumin conjugate; MW, molecular weight; CMC, critical micellization concentration; RES, reticulo-endothelial system; CT, computed tomography.

13.11 References

Abuchowski, A., and F.F. Davis. Preparation and properties of polyethylene glycol-trypsin adducts. *Biochim. Biophys. Acta* 578: 41-46, 1979.

Abuchowski, A., and F.F. Davis. Soluble polymer-enzime adducts. In *Enzymes as Drugs* (J.G. Holcenberg and G. Roberts, eds.). New York: John Wiley and Sons, 1981, Ch. 13.

Allen, T.M. The use of glycolipids and hydrophilic polymers in avoiding rapid uptake of liposomes by the mononuclear phagocyte system. *Adv. Drug Deliv. Rev.* 13: 285-309, 1994.

Allen, T.M., E. Brandies, C.B. Hansen, G.Y. Kao, and S. Zalipsky. Antibody-mediated targeting of long-circulating (Stealth) liposomes. *J. Liposome Res.* 4: 1-15, 1994.

Allen, T.M., and C. Hansen. Pharmacokinetics of stealth *versus* conventional liposomes: effect of dose. *Biochim. Biophys. Acta* **1068: 133-**141, 1991.

Allen, T.M., C.B. Hansen, and D.E.L. de Menenez. Pharmacokinetics of long-circulating liposomes. *Adv. Drug Delivery Rev.* 16: **267-284, 1995.**

Allen, T.M., C. Hansen, and J. Rutledge. Liposome with prolonged circulation times: factors affecting uptake by reticuloendothelial and other tissues. *Biochim. Biophys. Acta* 981: 27-35, 1989.

Allen, T.M., T. Mehra, C. Hansen, and Y.C. Chin. Stealth liposomes: an improved sustained release system for 1-β-D-arabinofuranosylcytosine. *Cancer Res.* 52: 2431-2439, 1992.

Bader, H., H. Ringsdorf, and B. Schmidt. Water soluble polymers in medicine. *Angew. Makromol. Chem.* 123/124: 457-462, 1984.

Beauchamp, C.O., S.L. Gonias, D.P. Menapace, and S.V. Pizo. A new procedure for the synthesis of polyethylene glycol-protein adducts: Effects on function, receptor recognition, and clearance of superoxide dismutase, lactoferrin and α2-macroglobulin. *Anal. Biochem.* 131: 25-33, 1983.

Blume, G., and G. Cevc. Molecular mechanism of the lipid vesicle longevity *in vivo*. *Biochim. Biophys. Acta* 1146: 157-168, 1993.

Blume, G., G. Cevc, M.D.J.A. Crommelin, I.A.J.M. Bakker-Woudenberg, C. Kluft, and G. Storm. Specific targeting with poly(ethylene glycol)-modified liposomes: coupling of homing devices to the end of the polymeric chains combines effective target binding with long circulation times. *Biochim. Biophys. Acta* 1149: 180-184, 1993.

Blunk, T., D.F. Hochstrasser, B.W. Müller, and R.H. Müller. Differential adsorption: effect of plasma protein adsorption patterns on organ distribution of colloidal drug carriers. In *Proc. 20th Int. Symp. Control. Release Bioact. Mater.* Washington: Controlled Release Society, Inc., **1993, pp. 256-257.**

Bogdanov, A.A., Jr., R. Weissleder, and T.J. Brady. Long-circulating blood pool imaging agents. *Adv. Drug Delivery Rev.* 16: 335-348, 1995.

Boman, N.L., D. Masin, L.D. Mayer, P.R. Cullis, and M.B. Bally. Liposomal vincristin which exhibits increased drug retention and increased circulation longevity cures mice bearing P388 tumors. *Cancer Res.* 54: 2830-2833, 1994.

Caride, V.J., and B.L. Zaret. Liposome accumulation in regions of ex**perimental myocardial infarction.** ***Science*** **198: 735-738, 1977.**

Chonn, A., S.C. Semple, and P.R. Cullis. Separation of large unilamellar liposomes from blood components by a spin column procedure: towards identifying plasma proteins which mediate liposome clearance *in vivo*. *Biochim. Biophys. Acta* 1070: 215-22, 1991.

Chonn, A., S.C. Semple, and P.R. Cullis. Association of blood proteins with large unilamellar liposomes *in vivo*: relation to circulation lifetimes. *J. Biol. Chem.* 267: 18759-18765, 1992.

Cohen, S., and H. Bernstein (eds.). *Microparticulate Systems for the Delivery of Proteins and Vaccines.* New York: Marcel Dekker, Inc., 1996.

des Cloizeaux, J., and G. Jannink. *Polymers in Solution. Their Modelling and Structure.* Oxford: Clarendon Press, 1990.

Gabizon, A. Liposome circulation time and targeting: implication for cancer chemotherapy. *Adv. Drug Delivery Rev.* 16: 285-294, 1995.

Gabizon, A., R. Catane, B. Uziely, B. Kauffman, T. Safra, R. Cohen, F. Martin, A. Huang, and Y. Barenholz. Prolonged circulation time and enhanced accumulation in malignant exudates of doxorubicin encapsulated in polyethylene-glycol coated liposomes. *Cancer Res.* 54: 987-992, 1994.

Gabizon, A., and D. Papahadjopoulos. Liposome formulations with prolonged circulation time in blood and enhanced uptake by tumors. *Proc. Natl. Acad. Sci. USA* 85: 6949-6953, 1988.

Gabizon, A., and D. Papahadjopoulos. The role of surface charge and hydrophilic groups on liposome clearance *in vivo*. *Biochim. Biophys. Acta* 1103: 94-100, 1992.

Geckeler, K., and Mutter, M. Soluble polymers for substitute of biopolymers in natural compounds. I. Replacement of the oligosaccharide chain in cinerubin A by polyoxyethylene. *Z. Naturforsch.* 34b: 1024-1025, 1979.

Goldberg, E.P. (ed.). Targeted Drugs. New York: John Wiley and Sons, 1983.

Goodson, R.J., and N.V. Katre. Site-directed glycosylation site. *Bio/Technology* 8: 343-346, 1990.

Gref, R., A. Domb, P. Quellec, T. Blunk, R.H. Muller, J.M. Verbavatz, and R. Langer. The controlled intravenous delivery of drugs using PEG-coated sterically stabilized nanospheres. *Adv. Drug Delivery Rev.* 16: 215-234, 1995.

Gref, R., Y. Minamitake, M.T. Peracchia, V.S. Trubetskoy, V.P. Torchilin, and R. Langer. Biodegradable long-circulating polymeric nanospheres. *Science* 263: 1600-1603, 1994.

Gregoriadis, G. Targeting of drugs. *Nature* 165: 407-411, 1977.

Gregoriadis, G. (ed.). *Liposomes as Drug Carriers.* Avon: John Wiley and Sons, 1988.

Gregoriadis, G. (ed.). *Liposome Technology*, Vol. 1-3, Boca Raton: CRC Press, 1993.

Hadley, K.B., and P.H. Sato. Catalytic activity of administered gulonolactone oxidase polyethylene glycol conjugates. *Enzyme* 42: 225-234, 1989.

Harper, G.R., M.C. Davies, S.S. Davis, T.F. Tadros, D.C. Taylor, M.P. Irving, and J.A. Waters. Steric stabilization of microspheres with grafted polyethylene oxide reduces phagocytosis by rat Kupffer cells *in vitro*. *Biomaterials* 12: 695-699, 1991.

Holcenberg, J.G., and G. Roberts (eds.). *Enzymes as Drugs*. New York: John Wiley and Sons, 1981.

Huang, S.K., E. Mayhew, S. Gilani, D.D. Lasic, F.J. Martin, and D. Papahadgopoulos. Pharmacokinetics and therapeutics of sterically stabilized liposomes in mice bearing C-26 colon carcinoma. *Cancer Res.* 52: 6774-6781, 1992.

Huang, S.K., P.R. Stauffer, K. Hong, J.W. Guo, T.L. Philips, A. Huang, and D. Papahadjopoulos. Liposomes and hyperthermia in mice: increased tumor uptake and therapeutical efficacy of doxorubicin in sterically stabilized liposomes. *Cancer Res.*54: 2186-2191, 1994.

Hwang, K.J. Liposome pharmacokinetics. In *Liposomes: from Biophysics to Therapeutics* (M. Ostro, ed.). New York: Marcel Dekker, Inc., 1987, pp.109-156.

Illum, L., and S.S. Davis. Effect of nonionic surfactant Poloxamer 338 on the fate and deposition of polystyrene microspheres following intravenous administration. *J. Pharm. Sci.* 72: 1086-1090, 1983.

Illum, L., and S.S. Davis. The organ uptake of intravenously administered colloidal particles can be altered using nonionic surfactant (poloxamer 338). *FEBS Lett.* 167: 79-82, 1984.

Illum, L., I.M. Hunneyball, and S.S. Davis. The effect of hydrophilic coatings on the uptake of colloidal particles by the liver and peritoneal macrophages. *Int. J. Pharm.* 29: 53-65, 1986.

Jamshaid, M., S.J Farr, P. Kearney, and I.W. Kellaway. Poloxamer sorption on liposomes: comparison with polystyrene latex and influence on solute efflux. *Int. J. Pharm.* 48: 125-131, 1988.

Khachadurian, A.K., C.H. Fung, T. Van Es, and F.F. Davis. Polyoxyethylated cholesterol derivatives: organic synthesis, cellular uptake and effect on lipid metabolism in cultures skin fibroblasts. *Biochim. Biophys. Acta* 665: 434-441, 1981.

Khaw, B.A., A. Klibanov, S.M. O'Donnell, T. Saito, N. Nossiff, M.A. Slinkin, J.B. Newell, H.W. Strauss, and V.P. Torchilin. Gamma imaging with negatively charge-modified monoclonal antibody: modification with synthetic polymers. *J. Nucl. Med.* 32: 1742-1751, 1991.

Khaw, B.A., J.A. Mattis, G. Melnicoff, H.W. Strauss, H.K. Gold, and E. Haber. Monoclonal antibody to cardiac myosin: imaging of experimental myocardial infarction. *Hybridoma* 3: 11-23, 1984.

Khaw, B.A., T. Yasuda, H.K. Gold, R.C. Leinbach, J.A. John, M. Kanke, M. Barlai-Kovach, H.W. Strauss, and E. Haber. Acute myocardial infarct imaging with indium-111-labeled monoclonal antimyosin Fab. *J. Nucl. Med.* 28:1671-1678, 1987.

Khue, N.V., and J.C. Galin. Antiinflammatory polymer-bound steroids for topical applications. I. Synthesis and characterization. *J. Appl. Polym. Sci.* 30: 2761-2778, 1985.

Klibanov, A.L., K. Maruyama, A.M. Beckerleg, V.P. Torchilin, and L. Huang. Activity of amphipathic poly(ethylene glycol) 5000 to prolong the circulation time of liposomes depends on the liposome size and is unfavorable for immunoliposome binding to target. *Biochim. Biophys. Acta* 1062: 142-148, 1991.

Klibanov, A.L., K. Maruyama, V.P. Torchilin, and L. Huang. Amphipathic polyethyleneglycols effectively prolong the circulation time of liposomes. *FEBS Lett.* 268: 235-237, 1990.

Koide, A., and S. Kobayashi. Modification of amino groups in porcine pancreatic elastase with polyethylene glycol in relation to binding activity towards anti-serum and to enzymatic activity. *Biochem. Biophys. Res. Commun.* 111: 659-667, 1983.

Krause, H.J., A. Schwartz, and P. Rohdewald. Polylactic acid nanoparticles, a colloidal drug delivery system for lipophilic drugs. *Int. J. Pharm.* 27: 145-155, 1985.

Kuan, C.-T., Q.-C. Wang, and I. Pastan. Replacement of surface exposed residues in domain II with cysteine residues that can be modified with polyethylene glycol in a site-specific manner. *J. Biol. Chem.* 269: 7610-7616, 1994.

Kurata, M., and Y. Tsunashima. Viscosity - molecular weight relationships and unperturbed dimensions of linear chain molecules. In *Polymer Handbook* (J. Brandup and E.H. Himmelgut, eds.) New York: John Wiley and Sons, 1989, pp. VII/1-VII/52.

Kwon, G.S., and K. Kataoka. Block copolymer micelles as long-circulating drug vehicles. *Adv. Drug Delivery Rev.* 16: 295-309.

Kwon, G.S., S. Suwa, M. Yokoyama, T. Okano, Y. Sakurai, and K. Kataoka. Enhanced tumor accumulation and prolonged circulation times of micelle-forming poly(ethylene oxide-aspartate) block copolymer-adriamycin conjugates. *J. Control. Release* 29: 17-23, 1994.

Langer, R. Bioavailability of macromolecular drugs and its control. In *Controlled Drug Bioavailability*, Vol. 3 (V.R. Smolen, ed.). New York: John Wiley and Sons, 1985.

Lasic, D.D. *Liposomes. From Physics to Applications.* Amsterdam: Elsevier, 1993.

Lasic, D.D., and Y. Barenholz (eds.). *Handbook of Nonmedical Applications of Liposomes.* Boca Raton: CRC Press, 1996.

Lasic, D.D., and F. Martin (eds.). *Stealth Liposomes.* Boca Raton: CRC Press 1995.

Liu, D., A. Mori, and L. Huang. Large liposomes containing ganglioside G_{M1} accumulate effectively in spleen. *Biochim. Biophys. Acta* 1066:159-165, 1991.

Liu, D., A. Mori, and L. Huang. Role of liposome size and RES blockade in controlling biodistribution and tumor uptake of G_{M1}-containing liposomes. *Biochim. Biophys. Acta* 1104: 95-101, 1992.

Maruyama, K., S. Okuizumi, O. Ishida, H. Yamauchi, H. Kikuchi, and M. Iwatsuru. Phosphatidyl polyglycerols prolong liposome circulation *in vivo*. *Int. J. Pharm.* 111: 103-107, 1994.

Maruyama, K., A.O. Yuda, S. Kojima, A. Suginaka, and M. Iwatsuru. Prolonged circulation time *in vivo* of large unilamellar liposomes composed of distearoylphosphatidylcholine and cholesterol containing amphiphatic poly(ethylene glycol). *Biochim. Biophys. Acta* 1128: 44-49, 1992.

Mayhew, E.G., D. Lasic, S. Babbar, and F.J. Martin. Pharmacokinetics and antitumor activity of epirubicin encapsulated in long-circulating liposomes incorporating a polyethyleneglycol-derivatized phospholipid. *Int. J. Cancer* 51: 302-309, 1992.

Milner, S.T. Polymer brushes. *Science* 251: 905-907, 1991.

Moghimi, S.M. Mechanisms regulating body distribution of nanospheres conditioned with pluronic and tetronic block co-polymers. *Adv. Drug Delivery Rev.* 16: 183-193, 1995.

Moghimi, S.M., A.E. Hawley, N.M. Christy, T. Gray, L. Illum, and S.S. Davis. Surface engineered nanospheres with enhanced drainage into lymphatics and uptake by macrophages of the regional lymph nodes. *FEBS Lett.* 344: 25-30, 1994.

Moghimi, S.M., H. Hedeman, N.M. Christy, L. Illum, and S.S. Davis. Enhanced hepatic clearance of intravenously administered sterically stabilized microspheres in zymosan-stimulated mice. *J. Leukoc. Biol.* 54: 513-517, 1993.

Moghimi, S.M., C.J.H. Porter, L. Illum, and S.S. Davis. The effect of poloxamer-407 on liposome stability and targeting to bone marrow: comparison with polystyrene microspheres. *Int. J. Pharm.* 68: 121-126, 1991.

Molyneux, P. *Water-Soluble Synthetic Polymers: Properties and Behavior*, Vol. 2. Boca Raton: CRC Press, 1977.

Monfardini, C., O. Schiavon, P. Caliceti, M. Morpurgo, J.M. Harris, and F.M. Veronese. A branched monomethoxypoly(ethylene glycol) for protein modification. *Bioconj. Chem.* 6: 62-69, 1995.

Mori, A., A.L. Klibanov, V.P. Torchilin, and L. Huang. Influence of steric barrier activity of amphipathic poly(ethyleneglycol) and ganglioside GM_1 on the circulation time of liposomes and on the target binding of immunoliposomes *in vivo*. *FEBS Lett.* 284: 263-266, 1991.

Morpurgo, E., R. Cardobbi, M. Morpurgo, P. Rigotti, F. Schavion, O. Schavion, P. Caliceti, E. Ancona, and F.M. Veronese. Protective effect of superoxide dismutase and polyethylene glycol-linked superoxide dismutase against warm ischemia/reperfusion injury. *Transplantation* 62: 1221-1223, 1996.

Müller, R.H. *Colloidal Carriers for Controlled Drug Delivery and Targeting.* Stuttgart: Wissenschaftliche Verlagsgesellschaft mbH, 1991.

Naper, D.H. *Polymeric Stabilization of Colloidal Dispersions.* New York: Academic Press, 1983.

Needham, D., T.J. McIntosh, and D.D. Lasic. Repulsive interactions and mechanical stability of polymer-grafted lipid membranes. *Biochim. Biophys. Acta* 1108: 40-48, 1992.

Palmer, T.N., V.J. Caride, M.A. Caldecourt, J. Twickler, and V. Abdullah. The mechanism of liposome accumulation in infarction. *Biochim. Biophys. Acta* 797: 363-368, 1984.

Pang, S.N.J. Final report of the safety assessment of polyethylene glycols (PEGs)-6, -8, -32, -75, -150, -14M, -20M. *J. Am. Coll. Toxicol.* 12: 429-456, 1993.

Papisov, I.M. Modeling in vivo transfer of long-circulating polymers (two classes of long-circulating polymers and factors affecting their transfer in vivo). *Adv. Drug Delivery Rev.* 16: 127-139, 1995.

Patel, H. Serum opsonins and liposomes: their interaction and opsonophagocytosis. *Crit. Rev. Ther. Drug Carriers Syst.* 9: 39-90, 1992.

Phillips, W.T., and B. Goins. Targeted delivery of imaging agents by liposomes. In *Handbook of Targeted Delivery of Imaging Agents* (V.P. Torchilin, ed.). Boca Raton: CRC Press, 1995, pp. 149-173.

Porter, C.J.H., S.M. Moghimi, L.L. Illum, and S.S. Davis. The polyethylene/polypropylene block copolymer Poloxamer-407 selectively redirects intravenously injected microspheres to sinusoidal endothelial cells of rabbit bone marrow, *FEBS Lett.* 305: 62-66, 1992.

Powell, G.M. Polyethylene glycol. In *Handbook of Water Soluble Gums and Resins* (R.L. Davidson, ed.). New York: McGraw-Hill, 1980, Ch. 18.

Pratten, M.K., J.B. Lloyd, G. Horpel, and H. Ringsdorf. Micelle-forming block copolymers: pinocytosis by macrophages and interaction with model membranes. *Makromol. Chem.* 186: 725-731, 1985.

Pyatak, P.S., A. Abuchowski, and F.F. Davis. Preparation of polyethylene glycol: superoxide dismutase adduct, and an examination of its blood circulating life and anti-inflammatory activity. *Res. Commun. Chem. Pathol. Pharmacol.* 29: 113-127, 1980.

Ranucci, E., G. Spagnoli, L. Sartore, and P. Ferruti. Synthesis and molecular weight characterization of low molecular weight end-functionalized poly(4-acryloylmorpholine). *Macromol. Chem. Phys.* 195: 3469-3479, 1994.

Revel, D., C. Chambon, P. Havard, G. Dandis, E. Canet, C. Corot, and M. Amiel. Iodinated polymer as blood-pool contrast agent. Computed tomography evaluation in rabbits. *Invest. Radiol.* 26: S57, 1991.

Ringsdorf, H. Structure and properties of pharmacologically active polymers. *J. Polym. Sci.* 51: 135-153, 1975.

Rolland, A. (ed.). *Pharmaceutical Particulate Carriers.* New York: Marcel Dekker, Inc., 1993.

Sartore, L., E. Ranucci, P. Ferruti, P. Caliceti, O. Schiavon, and F.M. Veronese. Low molecular weight end-functionalized poly(N-vinylpyrrolidone) for the modification of polypeptide aminogroups. *J. Bioact. Compat. Polym.* 9: 411-427, 1994.

Senior, J.H. Fate and behavior of liposomes *in vivo*: A review of controlling factors. *CRC Crit. Rev. Ther. Drug Carriers Syst.* 3: 123-193, 1987.

Senior, J., C. Delgado, D. Fisher, C. Tilcock, and G. Gregoriadis. Influence of surface hydrophilicity of liposomes on their interaction with plasma proteins and clearance from the circulation: studies with poly(ethylene glycol)-coated vesicles. *Biochim. Biophys. Acta* 1062: 77-82, 1991.

Stolnik, S., L. Illum, and S.S. Davis. Long circulating microparticulate drug carriers. *Adv. Drug Delivery Rev.* 16: 195-214, 1995.

Torchilin, V.P. Liposomes as targetable drug carriers. *CRC Crit. Rev. Ther. Drug Carrier Syst.* 2: 65-115, 1985.

Torchilin, V.P. *Immobilized Enzymes in Medicine.* Berlin: Springer-Verlag, 1991.

Torchilin, V.P. How do polymers prolong circulation time of liposomes. *J. Liposome Res.* 6: 99-116, 1996.

Torchilin, V.P., A.L. Klibanov, L. Huang, S. O'Donnell, N.D. Nossiff, and B.A. Khaw. Targeted accumulation of polyethylene glycol-coated immunoliposomes in infarcted rabbit myocardium. *FASEB J.* 6: 2716-2719, 1992.

Torchilin, V.P., A.M. Milstein, and M.I. Shtilman. Liposome protection in vivo with synthetic polymers other than poly(ethylene glycol). In *Proc. 21th Int. Symp. Control. Release Bioact. Mater.* Washington: Controlled Release Society, Inc., 1994, pp.604-605.

Torchilin, V.P., J. Narula, E. Halpern, and B.A. Khaw. Poly(ethylene glycol)-coated anti-cardiac myosin immunoliposomes: factors influencing targeted accumulation in the infarcted myocardium. *Biochim. Biophys. Acta* 1279: 75-83, 1996.

Torchilin, V.P., V.G. Omelyanenko, I.M. Papisov, A.A. Bogdanov, Jr., V.S. Trubetskoy, J.N. Herron, and C.A. Gentry. Poly(ethylene glycol) on the liposome surface: on the mechanism of polymer-coated liposome longevity. *Biochim. Biophys. Acta* 1195: 11-20, 1994a.

Torchilin, V.P., and M.I. Papisov. Why do polyethylene glycol-coated liposomes circulate so long? *J.Liposome Res.* 4: 725-739, 1994.

Torchilin, V.P., M.I. Shtilman, V.S. Trubetskoy, K. Whiteman, and A.M Milstein. Amphiphilic vinyl polymers effectively prolong liposome circulation time in vivo. *Biochim. Biophys. Acta* 1195: 181-184, 1994b.

Torchilin, V.P., and V.S. Trubetskoy. Which polymers can make nanoparticular drug carriers long-circulating? *Adv. Drug Delivery Rev.* 16: 141-155, 1995.

Torchilin, V.P., V.S. Trubetskoy, A.M. Milstein, J. Cannillo, G.L. Wolf, I.M. Papisov, A.A. Bogdanov, J. Narula, B.A. Khaw, and V.G. Omelyanenko. Targeted delivery of diagnostic agents by surface-modified liposomes. *J. Contr. Release* 28: 45-58, 1994c.

Torchilin, V.P., V.S. Trubetskoy, M.I. Papisov, A.A. Bogdanov, V.G. Omelyanenko, J. Narula, and B.A. Khaw. Polymer-coated immunoliposomes for delivery of pharmaceuticals: targeting and biological stability. In *Proc. 20th Int. Symp. Control. Release Bioact. Mater.* Washington: Controlled Release Society, Inc., 1993, pp. 194-195.

Torchilin, V.P., V.S. Trubetskoy, K.R. Whiteman, P. Caliceti, P. Ferruti, and F.M. Veronese. New synthetic amphiphilic polymers for steric protection of liposomes in vivo. *J. Pharm. Sci.* 84:1049-1053, 1995.

Trubetskoy, V.S., J.A. Cannillo, A. Milstein, G.L. Wolf, and V.P. Torchilin. Controlled delivery of Gd-containing liposomes to lymph nodes: surface modification may enhance MRI contrast properties. *Magn. Res. Imag.* 13: 31-37, 1995.

Trubetskoy, V.S., M.D. Frank-Kamenetsky, K.R. Whiteman, G.L. Wolf, and V.P. Torchilin. Stable polymeric micelles: lymphangiographic contrast media for gamma scintigraphy and magnetic resonance imaging. *Acad. Radiol.* 3: 232-238, 1996.

Trubetskoy, V.S., and V.P. Torchilin. Use of polyoxyethylene-lipid conjugates as long-circulating carriers for delivery of therapeutic and diagnostic agents. *Adv. Drug Delivery Rev.* 16: 311-320, 1995.

Trubetskoy, V.S., and V.P. Torchilin. Polyethyleneglycol-based micelles as carriers of therapeutic and diagnostic agents. *S.T.P. Pharma Sci.* 6: 79-86, 1996.

Trubetskoy, V.S., V.P. Torchilin, G.S. Gazelle, and G.L. Wolf. Amphiphilic radiopaque iodine-containing block-copolymer as micellar polymeric carrier with controlled in vivo performance. In *Proc. 21st Int. Symp. Control. Release Bioact. Mater.* Nice, France, 1994, pp. 676-677.

Unger, E., D.K. Shen, T. Fritz, P. Lund, G.L. Wu, B. Kulik, D. DeYoung, J. Standen, T. Ovott, and T. Matsunaga. Gas-filled liposomes as echocardiographic contrast agents in rabbits with miocardial infarction. *Invest. Radiol.* 28: 1155-1159, 1993.

Urrutigoity, M., and J. Souppe. Biocatalysis in organic solvents with a polymer-bound horseradish peroxidase. *Biocatalysis* 2: 145-149, 1989.

Weissleder, R., A.A. Bogdanov, Jr., E.A. Neuwelt, and M. Papisov. Long-circulating iron oxides for MR imaging. *Adv. Drug Delivery Rev.* 16: 321-334, 1995.

Winslow, R.M., K.D. Vandegriff, and M. Intaglietta (eds.). *Blood Substitutes. New Challenges.* Boston: Birkhauser, 1996.

Woodle, M.C. Surface-modified liposomes: assesssment and characterization for increased stability and prolonged blood circulation. *Chem. Phys. Lip.* 64: 249-262, 1993a.

Woodle, M.C. ^{67}Gallium-labeled liposomes with prolonged circulation: preparation and potential as nuclear imaging agents. *Nucl. Med. Biol.* 20: 149-155, 1993b.

Woodle, M.C., L.R. Collins, E. Sponsler, N. Kossovsky, and D. Papahadjopoulos. Sterically stabilized liposomes: reduction in electrophoretic mobility but not electrostatic surface potential. *Biophys. J.* 61: 902-910, 1992.

Woodle, M.C., C.M. Engbers, and S. Zalipsky. New amphipatic polymer-lipid conjugates forming long-circulating reticuloendothelial system-evading liposomes. *Bioconj. Chem.* 5: 493-496, 1994.

Woodle, M.C., M.S. Newman, and F.J. Martin. Liposome leakage and blood circulation: comparison of adsorbed block copolymers with covalent attachment of PEG. *Int. J. Pharm.* 88: 327-334, 1992.

Yamaoka, T., T. Tabata, and Y. Ikada. Distribution and tissue uptake of poly(ethylene glycol) with different molecular weights after intravenous administration in mice. *J. Pharm. Sci.* 83: 601-606, 1994.

Yokoyama, M., M. Miyauchi, N. Yamada, T. Okano, Y. Sakurai, K. Kataoka, and S. Ionue. Characterization and anticancer activity of the micelle-forming polymeric anticancer drug adriamycin-conjugated poly)ethylene glycol)-poly(aspartic acid) block copolymer. *Cancer Res.* 50: 1693-1700, 1990.

Zalipsky, S. Chemistry of polyethylene glycol conjugates with biologically active molecules. *Adv. Drug Delivery Rev.* 16: 157-182, 1995a.

Zalipsky, S. Functionalized poly(ethylene glycol) for preparation of biologically relevant conjugates. *Bioconj. Chem.* 6: 150-165, 1995b.

Zalipsky, S., C. Gilon, and A. Zilkha. Attachment of drugs to polyethylene glycols. *Eur. Polym. J.* 19: 1177-1183, 1983.

13.12 Discussion

Phillips: Do you think this polymeric cloud that is created by PEG could actually interfere with oxygen if it's on the outside of a liposome or else bound onto the hemoglobin protein as in PEG-hemoglobin?

Torchilin: It's a good question. It can be a little bit more generalized: what is the importance of this cloud for penetration of small molecules?

Phillips: That's a good question.

Torchilin: What is known from polymer chemistry is that the permeability of the polymeric gels, or so-called hydrogels, for small molecules is reasonably good. These gels are formed at a very low concentration of polymer in water, but because the polymer is very flexible, they form gel, and we know that now the polymeric chemistry can prepare real gels from the solution which carries concentration like around 1% of polymer only, and this is because of these particular properties of this polymer. According to the so-called cellular model of polymer solution, the polymer solution is considered as a three-dimensional network in which each cell is occupied by water molecule of a unit of a polymer chain. And because of the very fast motion of a polymer, water molecules might temporarily be squeezed from their cells, and those might be occupied not with actual polymer but with the probability of its occupation over there.

It was shown that at the concentration of which we are dealing with, on a level of one or two percent in solution, there is still quite good permeability for all low molecular weight substances. And even for relatively large molecules, there is a molecular weight up to, let's say 500. So, my guess would be (I never did this experiment, so I can only guess) that the presence of PEG in the quantities which can be described as diluted polymer gels, and were discussed in the audience during those days,, should not affect penetration of oxygen to hemoglobin much.

Intaglietta: It was my impression that the maximum half-life for clearance of most of the molecules that you showed us was in the range of about 4 hours. I didn't see anything that went like 12 hours, and I was curious as to what are the limitations for extending the half-life of these materials in the circulation where they are injected?

Torchilin: In one talk, it's impossible to present all the available data, but I can assure you that there exists the stuff which carries a circulation life-time up to like 48 hours. I just showed certain examples from what we did which might be built in a very logical construct. If I would talk about, for example, the influence of a polymer on the circulation time, I would show different pictures which will have half-lives of up to 12, 16 and 24, or even 48 hours.

Winslow: I wonder if you would mind commenting on these extraordinarily high oncotic pressures that we see with pegylated hemoglobin solutions. What is it about the PEG that raises oncotic pressures so much?

Torchilin: It's a very interesting question. I intentionally made one slide which carried some information about specific properties of PEG and its relationship towards water. PEG is known to destructure water sharply because it's so well solvated that it can carry water densely packed like single molecules along its chain while the normal water, as you know, exists as a tripod which occupies the must bigger volume that thin molecules put together.

So, from, let's say, a point of view of, for example, magnetic resonance imaging, if you put PEG on the surface of liposomes simultaneously with gadolinium, you get much better signals than without PEG because actually what you did was to create a higher concentration of water in water because you destructured it. The same property of PEG is used in the fusion of cells and liposomes to cells. If PEG is relatively short, let's say around 5000, it does not form very a firm globule; it's still partially unfolded, and this is why it can bind a lot of water and destructure water in the vicinity of surface which facilitates fusion. However, if you take, for example, PEG with a molecular weight like 20,000 and up, it doesn't work any more. It sounds strange, but this is because it's highly flexible, and from the thermodynamic point of view, being so flexible, it has a tendency to form as dense a globule as possible. And, this is how it squeezes water even out of its cell leaving it only on the outer surface.

My guess is that all these things with oncotic pressure are definitely connected with the property of relatively low molecular weight PEG, which is like around 5000 ± 3000, to destructure water and to change the density of different molecules in water. For example, it was shown by Dr. Lauffer that such replacement of water with something else can change magnetic resonance properties of many substances, and this is what you might expect in case of pegylated material.

Winslow: So it should be, in the case of pegylated hemoglobin, possible to produce molecules with different amounts of PEG not necessarily corresponding to the oncotic pressure?

Torchilin: Yes, sure.

Winslow: You may be able to select the properties that you like depending upon the nature of the PEG?

Torchilin: Yes. We played a little bit because of our own interests with certain pegylated molecules which turned out to behave pretty well like potential plasma expanders, and the properties of those expanders might depend a lot on the ratio between main polymer chain and grafted PEG, and even very small variations in this ratio. They can change properties, such as viscosity and pressure quite a lot.

Bonaventura: Your talk about these different polymers is extremely interesting, and it brings to mind some work done by Parsegian and Colombo of the NIH who are keenly interested in the role of water and structural water in conferring different activities in proteins, and they've used hemoglobin as their model, and by putting hemoglobin in various PEG solutions, but not the fancy ones, if you will, like you've described. They've been able to show that water activity around the protein is critically important to the functional properties, that is to say, water acts like an allosteric effector, like an effector molecule, and so forth, and so I think their work is really interesting, but coupled with what you're talking about, the work that you're doing and whether it has possibilities in terms of commercial development, but I think in terms of basic understanding of how proteins work. It might be very interesting to look at those things. Have you done anything like that?

Torchilin: Yes, we know about those studies, so we have independently confirmed the same idea from two different sides. So, why should we do what they have done already, and they did it very well, so we were glad to find very similar interpretation of our data. I believe that our data mutually confirm each other.

Bonaventura: But your polymers have the opportunity of probing structure-function relationships in membrane proteins, for example, that they could not do.

Torchilin: We did not try it. I would like to do it, but, you know, life is short, and this is what is unfortunately limited, so it's an excellent idea, but if somebody would find me a couple of more people and one million dollars, I will do it.

Winslow: I'd like to ask you one more question about the potential toxicities of PEG, because in the applications that we're talking about, we're talking about huge quantities being administered in opposition to some small-quantity drugs. Are there particular toxicities? It seemed to me that there is some literature on the effect of PEG itself on blood pressure, for instance.

Torchilin: No, I'm afraid I'm unfamiliar with this. Just recently, I mean two years ago, and I do have a reference, so I will be pleased to provide it to you, a big study was performed on the toxicity study of PEG of different molecular weights, from like 3000 to 200,000 molecular weight, and there were no toxicities even under circumstances when PEG was used in large quantities. This was one of the reasons, even before people understood what the mechanism of PEG action was, to use PEG as a pharmaceutical carrier, in many cases, because of complete lack of toxicity and antigenicity. In 1985, I was editing the special issue of *Advanced Drug Delivery Reviews*, which was completely devoted to long-circulating pharmaceuticals, drugs and drug carriers, and there were a couple of papers dealing with properties of PEG-modified molecules and the properties of PEG to be used as a pharmaceutical carrier. So I will be pleased to provide you with a reference for this, and you will find that all these papers usually start with a statement which is full of "no": why PEG is so good—because "no" toxic, "no" antigenic. The only thing they found is so-called physical toxicity. Physical toxicity is that in all polymers, like PEG or PEG-like polymers, which are usually cleared from the blood by the kidneys, and kidneys are able to filter well particles with a size of, roughly speaking, on a level of 40,000 Daltons. So, if you are dealing with PEG, which is below that, you'll find everything in urine reasonably fast, not fast, but reasonably fast. However, if something is above this value, it will not be filtered through. It will be deposited on the surface of kidney channels thus affecting the normal permeability of kidney channels, and this is called physical toxicity. As far as I know, this was the only negative side of PEG ever described in literature, at least in the literature that has been available for me.

Chapter 14

The Reaction of Nitric Oxide with Cell-free Hemoglobin Based Oxygen Carriers: Physiological Implications

Ronald J. Rohlfs, Ph.D., Kim D. Vandegriff, Ph.D. and Robert M. Winslow, M.D.

ABSTRACT

Changes in mean arterial pressure (MAP) were monitored in rats following 50% isovolemic exchange transfusion (ET) with a solution of either (1) human hemoglobin cross-linked with diaspirin between the α subunits at lysine 99 (αα–Hb), or (2) bovine hemoglobin surface modified by conjugation with methoxypolyethylene glycol (PEG-Hb). Within seconds of the start of ET with αα–Hb solution, MAP is observed to increase at least 25 mm Hg above the pre-exchange baseline value. This increase in MAP persists for at least two hours. In contrast, no significant increase in MAP is observed subsequent to 50% ET with a solution of PEG-Hb. In order to test the hypothesis that this difference in MAP response may be due to differences in reactivity between these hemoglobins and the endothelium-derived relaxing factor nitric oxide (NO), bimolecular association rate constants, dissociation rate constants, and overall equilibrium binding constants were determined for the reaction of these two hemoglobins with NO. Additionally, the bimolecular rate constants for the reaction of NO with the oxygen-bound form of these hemoglobins were also measured. No significant difference was observed between αα–Hb and PEG-Hb in either the bimolecular NO association rate or the rate of NO-induced oxidation *in vitro*. PEG-Hb binds NO a factor of two more tightly than αα–Hb at equilibrium. This suggests that some property of PEG-Hb either prevents reaction with NO *in vivo*, or prevents increases in MAP despite NO scavenging. These results also suggest that the increase in MAP observed upon ET with αα–Hb may not be the result of NO scavenging, but rather due to alternative physiologic mechanisms.

14.1 Introduction

14.1.1 Cell-free hemoglobin-based oxygen carriers and vasoconstriction

Hemoglobins from human, bovine and recombinant sources are being developed for use as a cell-free hemoglobin-based oxygen carrier (HBOC). These hemoglobins are highly purified and modified either chemically or through site-directed mutagenesis in order to make them suitable for clinical use. Chemical modifications currently under development include intramolecular cross-linking, polymerization, and surface modification. Recombinant techniques have also produced genetically engineered hemoglobin tetramers and polymers. These strategies have proven largely successful in eliminating toxicities due to impurities and hemoglobin dimer formation (Winslow 1992). There currently exists an impressive array of cell-free hemoglobin solutions that display a wide range of physical properties available for study. Intramolecularly cross-linked tetramers can display relatively strong or weak oxygen (O_2) binding affinities, depending upon the type of cross-linker used and conditions of the cross-linking reaction (Jones *et al.* 1993). The molecular mass of a polymerized hemoglobin can be controlled by reaction conditions (Wojciechowski 1996), and solution properties such as viscosity and colloid osmotic pressure can be altered by surface modification of the hemoglobin molecule (Vandegriff, Rohlfs, and Winslow 1997).

Several *in vivo* and *ex vivo* studies have shown that administration of a cell-free HBOC often results in vasoconstriction, hypertension and increased vascular resistance. This effect appears to be widespread and does not, in most cases, appear to be affected by hemoglobin source or the type of cell-free HBOC studied. Increases in systemic and pulmonary arterial pressure with concomitant increases in systemic and pulmonary vascular resistance have been demonstrated in sheep immediately following exchange transfusion (ET) with polymerized bovine hemoglobin (Lieberthal *et al.* 1987). Isolated rat kidney perfused with solutions of polymerized human hemoglobin have shown an increase in renal vascular resistance and decreased glomular filtration rate (Lee *et al.* 1995). Increased mean arterial pressure (MAP) and decreased renal and intestinal blood flow were observed in cats following isovolemic ET with a high O_2 affinity (P50 = 17 mm Hg) bovine hemoglobin intramolecularly cross-linked with diaspirin between the β subunits at lysine 82, and also with a low O_2 affinity (P50 = 34 mm Hg) ββ cross-linked human hemoglobin (Ulatowski *et al.* 1995). Similar increases in systemic arterial pressure and vascular resistance have been observed upon use of human hemoglobin cross-linked with diaspirin between the α subunits at lysine 99 (αα–Hb) in swine (Hess, Macdonald and Brinkley 1993) and in rats (Hamilton *et al.* 1992, Schultz *et al.* 1993, Keipert *et al.* 1993, Motterlini 1996, Vandegriff *et al.* 1996, Migita *et al.* 1997). Cell-free αα-Hb solution has been shown to augment sympathetic coronary vasoconstriction in isolated rabbit heart (Macdonald and Motterlini 1994), and similarly, genetically engineered recombinant human hemoglobin inhibits endothelium-dependent vasorelaxation in isolated rabbit aortic ring preparations (Rioux, Drapeau and Marceau 1995). Pyridoxalated hemoglobin polyoxyethylene conjugate, a surface modified cell-free HBOC, has also been shown in increase arterial blood pressure in both conscious and anesthetized rats (Kida *et al.* 1995).

The physiological consequences of an increase in mean arterial pressure with an associated increase in systemic vascular resistance due to vasoconstriction upon administration of cell-free HBOCs remain controversial. Some evidence suggests that in certain clinical circumstances, the vasopressor properties of cell-free hemoglobins may lead to increased tissue oxygenation, which may be beneficial in the treatment of hemorrhagic or septic shock (Doyle *et al.* 1996, Gulati *et al.* 1996, Greenburg and Kim 1995). Conversely, other evidence indicates peripheral vasoconstriction results in decreased functional capillary density causing decreased tissue oxygenation (Pohl and Lamontagne 1991, Tsai, Kerger and Intaglietta 1995, Vandegriff and Winslow 1995, Tsai, Kerger and Intaglietta 1996, Rohlfs *et al.* 1996). This may lead to a somewhat contradictory situation in which administration of a cell-free HBOC for the purpose of improving tissue oxygenation may in fact have the opposite effect. Resolution of this issue requires an understanding of the mechanisms behind physiological control of vascular tone in order to understand the vasopressor effect of cell-free HBOCs.

14.1.2 Endothelium-derived relaxing factor: nitric oxide

Control of systemic blood pressure and resistance to blood flow is achieved by a dynamic constriction and relaxation of smooth muscle tissue which surrounds all blood vessels except capillaries. Vascular smooth muscle tension is continually adjusted by a complex system that acts to cause either vasoconstriction or vasodilation depending on metabolic need. Research performed over the last decade has established nitric oxide (NO) as an endothelium-derived relaxing factor that can cause vasodilation. Among the findings was the demonstration that molecules that act as NO donors (*e.g.*, nitroprusside, nitroglycerin) lead to vasorelaxation through activation of guanylate cyclase (GC), whereas molecules that either inhibit the biosynthesis of NO (*e.g.*, N^G-monomethyl-L-arginine) or remove NO (*e.g.*, hemoglobin) cause vasoconstriction (Arnold *et al.* 1977, Katsuki *et al.* 1977, Martin, Smith and White 1986, Palmer, Ferrige and Moncada 1987, Ignarro *et al.* 1987, Ignarro, Byrns, and Wood 1988, Furchgott 1988, Moncada, Palmer and Higgs 1991). NO is synthesized from L-arginine in endothelial cells which lie between the intravascular space and the surrounding smooth muscle (Palmer, Ashton and Moncada 1988). Free NO rapidly diffuses out of and away from the endothelial cell in all directions. NO that diffuses into adjacent smooth muscle cells is able to bind to the heme group of GC causing a conformational change that activates the enzyme to produce cGMP. Elevated levels of cGMP cause smooth muscle relaxation by stimulation of intracellular binding of free calcium (For a review, see Ignarro 1990).

Despite the wide variation that exists in the physical properties (O_2 affinity, molecular mass, solution properties) of different cell-free HBOCs, it appears that the vasopressor response is a feature common to nearly all of these red cell substitutes. This suggests a common mechanism for HBOC-induced vasoconstriction based on a common physical property. It is well established that human deoxyhemoglobin reversibly binds NO very rapidly and with extremely high affinity (Cassoly and Gibson 1975, Moore and Gibson 1976). Additionally, it has been shown that NO will react directly and irreversibly with oxyhemoglobin at least as rapidly as NO binds to deoxy hemoglobin (Doyle and Hoekstra 1981, Eich *et al.* 1996). Either or both of these reactions might occur with cell-free HBOCs and may be responsible for reducing NO concentrations *in vivo.*

14.1.3 Nitric oxide scavenging by hemoglobin-based oxygen carriers

The identification of nitric oxide as an important messenger in endothelium-dependent vasorelaxation coupled with the known reactivity of hemoglobin toward NO has led to the suggestion that the vasoconstriction observed upon use of cell-free HBOCs is primarily due to NO scavenging. Recent evidence in support of this conclusion comes from experiments using site-directed mutagenesis of recombinant human hemoglobin (Lemon *et al.* 1996). Recombinant hemoglobins were designed and isolated in which specific residues within the binding pocket were mutated to amino acids with large hydrophobic side chains (*e.g.*, phenylalanine). The intent was to reduce the rate of NO reaction with these mutant hemoglobins by sterically restricting ligand access to the heme pocket. The bimolecular rates of NO-induced oxidation for the resulting mutant oxyhemoglobins were up to 20-fold lower than the rate observed for wild-type oxyhemoglobin. Administration of these recombinant hemoglobins elicited a diminished pressor response in rats relative to the increase in MAP observed with recombinant human hemoglobin (rHb 1.1) containing the hemoglobin Presbyterian mutant (β108 Asn $\rightarrow$ Lys). There was a direct correlation between the amount of increase in MAP observed *in vivo* and the bimolecular rate of NO-induced oxidation. The more rapid the rate of NO-induced oxidation observed *in vitro*, the larger the increase in MAP observed *in vivo.* These results are the first to show that modulating the reactivity of a cell-free HBOC toward NO may alter the vasopressor effect.

The results of Lemon *et al.* (1996) are especially significant in view of the circular logic that has evolved in the literature regarding the relationship between vasoactivity and the reaction of NO with cell-free hemoglobin. Researchers attempting to identify the endothelium-derived relaxing factor have used the observation that cell-free hemoglobin has the ability to either inhibit vasodilation or promote vasoconstriction as evidence to support the conclusion that the endothelium-derived relaxing factor is NO (Martin *et al.* 1985, Furchgott 1988, Ignarro, Byrns and Wood 1988). Similarly, researchers in the field of red cell substitutes often conclude that increases in MAP upon administration of a cell-free HBOC are due to NO scavenging based on the high reactivity and affinity toward NO displayed by native human hemoglobin (Schultz *et al.* 1993, Greenburg and Kim 1995, Rioux, Drapeau and Marceau 1995, Ulatowski *et al.* 1995, Gulati *et al.* 1996).

In the face of this evidence, it is tempting to conclude that NO scavenging is the principal, if not sole mechanism for cell-free HBOC-induced vasoconstriction. However, it is well established that multiple factors contribute to the physiological control of vascular smooth muscle tone. Cell-free HBOCs may influence these other factors, and vasoconstriction may result from a combination of mechanisms that may or may not include NO scavenging. For example, experimental evidence has existed for quite some time that vascular smooth muscle tension responds to arteriolar O_2 levels. Decreases in vascular tone in response to decreases in O_2 tension have been demonstrated in isolated coronary blood vessels (Gellai, Norton and Detar 1973). Conversely, other experimental evidence has shown that increases in O_2 tension cause arteriolar constriction, perhaps through inhibition of the synthesis of endothelium-derived vasodilator prostaglandins (Messina *et al.* 1994). In the case of red cell substitutes, low O_2 affinity cell-free HBOCs may deliver an excessive amount of O_2 to the arterioles: under circumstances of high O_2 levels in the microcirculation, metabolic autoregulatory processes may lead to vasoconstriction and decreased functional capillary density resulting in impaired tissue oxygenation (Tsai, Kerger and Intaglietta 1995, Vandegriff and Winslow 1996, Tsai, Kerger and Intaglietta 1996).

Recently, it has been suggested that *S*-nitrosolyated hemoglobin and low molecular weight *S*-nitrosothiols (RSNOs) may play an important role in the regulation of vascular smooth muscle tone (Li *et al.* 1996, Stamler and Slivka 1996). RSNOs, in which the NO group is formally a nitrosium ion (NO^+), appear to exhibit vasorelaxant properties that are similar to the neutral NO radical. Experimental evidence indicates that low molecular weight *S*-nitrosothiols are able to modify human hemoglobin by a transnitrosation reaction with the highly reactive sulfhydryl group of Cysβ93. It is possible that NO is carried through the circulation in this form and is then liberated to another thiol bearing species *via* another transnitrosation reaction at a site where it is needed. An attractive feature of this model is that it may explain why the Cysβ93 residue of hemoglobin is so highly conserved throughout nature. Another attractive feature is the fact that RSNOs do not react at the heme groups of either deoxy- or oxyhemoglobin, which are the sites where NO scavenging reactions are believed to take place. However, it remains to be seen how an *S*-nitrosothiol might activate GC at physiologically relevant rates, since current models of GC activation rely specifically on NO radical binding to the heme group of GC (Moncada, Palmer and Higgs 1991, Arnelle and Stamler 1995). This would indicate that the free radical form of NO, rather than the nitrosium ion form is required. There are no published examples of *S*-nitrosylation of a cell-free HBOC. Any effect this class of red cell substitute may have on *S*-nitrosothiols or how this may relate to vasopressor properties is unknown.

Because the vasopressor properties of most cell-free HBOCs are similar, it has been difficult to directly assess the extent to which NO scavenging contributes to vasoactivity observed upon administration of these solutions. To address this, we have studied two cell-free HBOCs that exhibit different vasopressor responses: (1) αα–Hb which is observed to cause an increase in MAP, and (2) PEG-Hb which is observed to cause no significant increase in MAP (Migita *et al.* 1997). This allows a direct test of the hypothesis that the difference in MAP response may be due to differences in reactivity between these hemoglobins and NO. The balance of this chapter further investigates the relationship between the reactivity of NO with the heme of cell-free HBOCs *in vitro* and the *in vivo* change in MAP observed upon isovolemic ET with solutions of these HBOCs.

14.2 Experimental Design

14.2.1 Materials and sample preparation

Human hemoglobin cross-linked with bis-(3,5-dibromosalicyl) fumarate between α chains at α-lysine 99 (αα–Hb) was a gift from the U.S. Army. The αα–Hb was dissolved in Ringer's lactate to a concentration of 7.9 g/dl to produce a stock solution that is both iso-ionic and iso-oncotic with blood. Bovine hemoglobin conjugated to unbranched methoxypolyethylene glycol (PEG-Hb) was a gift of Enzon, Inc. PEG-Hb exhibits a molecular weight of 125 ± 15 kD (Nucci, Shorr and Abuchowski 1996) and was dissolved in isotonic Ringer's lactate to produce a stock solution at a concentration of 5.5 g/dl. Stock NO solutions (1.97 mM) were prepared by equilibration of anaerobic buffer under 1 atm of NO gas. Nitrosylhemoglobin samples were prepared by equilibration of anaerobic deoxyhemoglobin under 1 atm of NO gas.

14.2.2 Kinetic measurements

NO bimolecular association kinetics were measured using a flash photolysis apparatus equipped with a Lumonics XeCl Excimer (508 nm) pumped dye laser. The laser produces a light pulse 4 nanoseconds in duration that averages 3 mJ per pulse at 540 nm. The observation light was provided by a xenon arc lamp, and both the photolysis and observation beams were focused on the front face of a 2-mm pathlength cuvette containing the Hb-NO sample. NO recombination kinetic transients were monitored in the Soret region at the wavelength of maximal absorbance change (435 nm). Substantially less than 1% photolysis was produced by 100% laser light intensity due to the extremely low quantum yield of Hb-NO complexes (Saffran and Gibson 1977), and thus 1000 transients were signal averaged for each sample to improve the signal-to-noise ratio and produce the resulting NO recombination time courses. The time courses were fitted to a single exponential expression using an iterative linear least squares algorithm to obtain the observed rate constants. Under these conditions, the reaction is pseudo first order and the bimolecular rate constants were obtained by dividing the observed rate constants by the NO concentration ($k' = k_{obs}/[NO]$).

NO unimolecular dissociation kinetics were measured by ligand displacement reactions. Approximately 1 mg of solid sodium dithionite was added to a 1-cm path length cuvette that was sealed with a rubber septum. The cuvette was flushed with N_2 and then completely filled, such that there was no gas space, with anaerobic 0.1 M bis-Tris propane, 0.1 M NaCl, pH 7.4 buffer that had been equilibrated previously with 1 atm carbon monoxide gas ([CO] = 1 mM). The NO displacement reaction was initiated by introducing a few μl of stock nitrosylhemoglobin solution prepared as described above. The excess dithionite reacts with free NO dissolved in solution but does not react with NO bound to hemoglobin (Moore and Gibson 1976). As the NO dissociates, it is destroyed by the dithionite, and CO binds to the heme. Kinetic transients were monitored as the conversion of Hb-NO to Hb-CO with a Milton Roy 3000 diode array spectrophotometer, and kinetic time courses were fitted to a biexponential expression using an iterative linear least squares algorithm to obtain the observed rate constants. Under these conditions, the observed rate constants are nearly identical to the actual dissociation rate constants ($k_{obs} = k$, Olson 1981). Overall dissociation equilibrium constants were calculated as the ratio of the weighted mean of the dissociation rate constants for each hemoglobin to the corresponding association rate constant ($K_d = k / k'$).

The kinetics of NO-induced oxidation of oxyhemoglobin were measured by conventional rapid mixing techniques using an Applied Photophysics stopped-flow spectrophotometer. Solutions of air-equilibrated hemoglobin were mixed against anaerobic solutions of NO, and the conversion of oxyhemoglobin to methemoglobin was monitored by the absorbance change at 419 nm. The value of the bimolecular rate constant for this reaction is reported to be extremely large (Doyle and Hoekstra 1981, Eich *et al.* 1996), so the concentration of NO after mixing was kept low (2 μM) in order to minimize loss of the reaction time course in the mixing time of the stopped-flow apparatus. Under these conditions, the rate of the autoxidation reaction of NO with dissolved O_2 is negligible compared to the rate of reaction with oxyhemoglobin (Kharitonov, Sundquist and Sharma 1994). The concentration of oxyhemoglobin after mixing was at least a factor of 5 less than that of NO in order to use a pseudo first order approximation. The low oxyhemoglobin concentrations resulted in small absorbance changes, and several kinetic transients were signal averaged for each kinetic time course in order to improve the signal-to-noise ratio. The time courses were fitted to a single exponential expression using an iterative linear least squares algorithm to obtain the observed rate constants. The bimolecular rate constants were obtained by dividing the observed rate constants by the NO concentration (k'_{ox} = k_{obs}/[NO]).

14.2.3 MAP measurements

Measurements of mean arterial pressure *in vivo* were conducted using Male Sprague-Dawley rats (250-350 g). Animals were handled according to institutional guidelines and the National Research Council guide for the care and use of laboratory animals. Animals were instrumented as described by Migita *et al.* (1997). One day prior to the exchange-transfusion experiment, specially designed catheters were surgically implanted in the femoral artery of one leg and the femoral vein of the other leg. The catheters were passed subcutaneously to the tail and were held in place by a plastic sheath assembly. On the day after surgery, conscious rats were placed in a plastic restrainer, and an isovolemic exchange transfusion to 50% of total blood volume (TBV = 0.065 × g body mass) was performed with a stock solution of cell-free hemoglobin. Fluids were exchanged using a peristaltic pump at a rate of 0.5 ml/min with completion of the ET taking approximately 30 minutes. Mean arterial pressure was monitored continuously throughout the experiment by a pressure transducer (UFI model 1050 BPR) connected to the arterial line. Signals from the pressure transducer were digitized and amplified (BioPac Systems Model MP100) and stored as MAP as a function of time on a personal computer for analysis.

14.3 Results

14.3.1 Mean arterial pressure response to 50% isovolemic exchange transfusion

Figure 14.1 shows the effect of a 50% isovolemic ET with either αα–Hb or PEG-Hb on MAP (Migita *et al.* 1997). The data represent the average values for MAP at each time point for groups of rats that received either αα–Hb (n = 6) or PEG-Hb (n = 5). The ET begins at time = 0 minutes in Figure 14.1 for each group and ends after 30 minutes. Animals that received αα–Hb show a significant ($p < 0.05$) increase in MAP within seconds of the start of the ET from the pre-exchange baseline value (111 ± 3 mm Hg). The maximal MAP (137 ± 6 mm Hg) is achieved approximately 8 minutes after the start of the ET. The elevated blood pressure observed with the αα–Hb group persists throughout the ET procedure. This persistence of elevated MAP is consistent with other reports on the effect of MAP in rats following either isovolemic ET or bolus administration of αα cross-linked human hemoglobin. The elevated MAP values persist for at least 2 hours after introduction of this cell-free HBOC (Keipert *et al.* 1993, Hamilton *et al.* 1992, Schultz *et al.* 1993, Motterlini 1996, Vandegriff *et al.* 1996, Migita *et al.* 1997). The MAP response in the PEG-Hb group to 50% isovolemic ET is markedly different to the response observed in the αα–Hb group. No significant increase in MAP above the baseline value (107 ± 4 mm Hg) is observed for this group at anytime during ET or within 2 hours after ET (Migita *et al.* 1997). A small, insignificant increase in MAP (maximal value = 114 ± 4 mm Hg) is observed approximately 12 minutes after the start of ET, and this trend returns to baseline by the end of the ET. The stark contrast between the vasopressor response observed with αα–Hb and the lack of one observed with PEG-Hb implies that differences in one or more physical properties of these cell-free HBOCs must exist in order to account for the differences observed in the 50% isovolemic ET experiment.

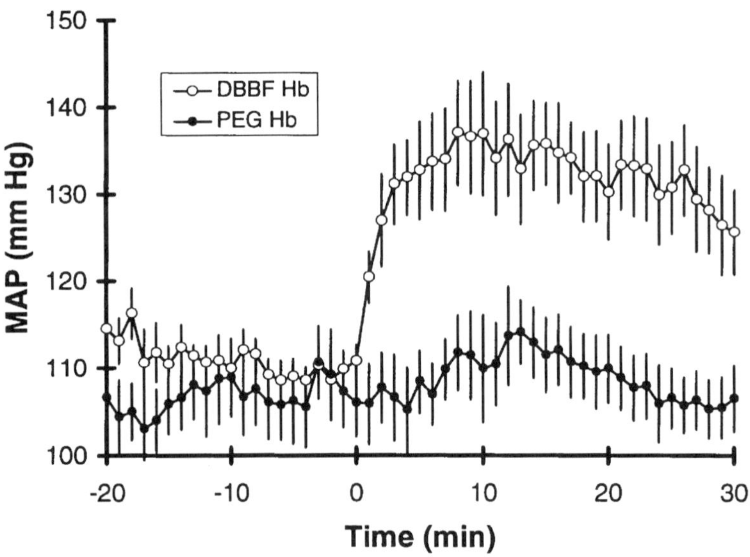

Figure 14.1. Mean arterial pressure response to 50% isovolemic exchange transfusion. The average value of MAP is plotted *versus* time for αα–Hb (n = 6, *open circles*) and PEG-Hb (n = 5, *black circles*). The *error bars* represent the standard error of the mean at each time point. The *x-axis* is scaled such that the ET begins at time = 0 minutes and ends at time = 30 minutes. (Adapted from Migita *et al.* 1997).

The blood pressure begins to rise within seconds of the start of ET with αα–Hb. This implies that very little of this material (< 10 mg) is required to elicit the vasopressor response, and the rate of the reaction(s) that cause the response is very rapid. This would tend to rule out any mechanism for vasoconstriction that involves either augmentation or suppression of expression of macromolecule biosynthesis (*e.g.*, proteins or hormones). However, it does not rule out NO scavenging, or release of stored prostaglandins as the mechanism, since those reactions are extremely rapid. The time period between the start of the ET and the first appearance of increased MAP is approximately the same as the circulation time within the rat. In humans, the circulation time has been estimated at 5-10 seconds at sea level (Monge *et al.* 1955).

14.3.2 Nitric oxide reaction kinetics

The evidence that has accumulated over the last decade implicating NO in an important role in the control of vascular smooth muscle tone suggests that the different pressor responses exhibited by these two cell-free HBOCs (Figure 14.1 and Migita *et al.* 1997) may be the result of differences in reactivity toward NO. The lack of an increase in MAP in response to ET with PEG-Hb may be due to a decreased reactivity toward NO relative to αα–Hb, analogous to the results of Lemon *et al.* (1996). In order to test this hypothesis, the reaction of NO with these hemoglobins was studied *in vitro*. Kinetic and equilibrium binding constants were determined for the reaction between NO and the reduced, unliganded form of these hemoglobins. The reaction between NO and the oxygenated forms of these hemoglobins was also studied. This often overlooked reaction is at least as important as NO binding to deoxy-HBOC, since cell-free HBOCs are expected to be significantly saturated with O_2 *in vivo*, and the rate of this reaction with native human hemoglobin is at least as rapid as the rate of NO binding to deoxyhemoglobin (Doyle and Hoekstra 1981, Eich *et al.* 1996).

14.3.2.1 Bimolecular association rates

Overall bimolecular association rate constants for the binding of NO to αα–Hb and PEG-Hb were investigated by laser flash photolysis, a technique which takes advantage of the photosensitivity of the bond between ferrous heme protein and ligand (Saffran and Gibson 1977). Flash photolysis has an advantage over conventional rapid mixing techniques in that one can monitor very rapid reactions that would otherwise be lost in the mixing time of a stopped-flow apparatus. The measurement consists of exposing a sample of ligand bound heme protein to a brief pulse of light that photolyses a fraction of ligands off the heme. Of this population of photolysed ligands, a fraction immediately rebinds to the heme from within the protein (geminate recombination, Carver *et al.* 1990), and a fraction escapes from the heme pocket all the way out of the protein and into the solvent. Time courses for geminate processes are independent of ligand concentration whereas the observed rate of bimolecular recombination from the surrounding solvent depends on ligand concentration. Bimolecular recombination of the ligand from solvent to the heme occurs as the system relaxes back to equilibrium. Experiments are monitored by absorbance change before, during and after the flash pulse.

Figure 14.2 shows ligand recombination time courses for photolysis of the nitrosyl complexes of αα–Hb and PEG-Hb each in the presence of 1.97 mM NO (1 atm). As a control, a sample of human hemoglobin A_0 was prepared along with the other samples in a manner identical to sample preparation used for αα–Hb and PEG-Hb (HbA_0-NO time course omitted for clarity). The *x-axis* is scaled such that the laser pulse begins at time = 50 μs. Due to the extremely small quantum yield of nitrosylhemoglobin complexes (Saffran and Gibson 1977), very small absorbance changes are obtained, and the signal-to-noise ratio for an individual flash is very poor. The time courses in Figure 14.2 are plotted as the normalized absorbance change *versus* time and are the result of signal averaging of 1000 flash pulses for each sample.

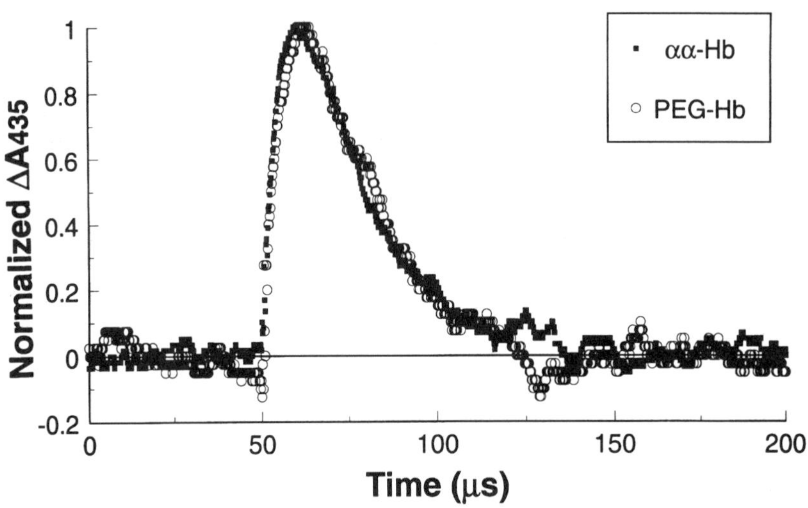

Figure 14.2. Nitric oxide recombination to hemoglobin following laser photolysis. Normalized Δ absorbance values collected at 435 nm with the laser photolysis apparatus are plotted *versus* time for αα–Hb (*black squares*) and PEG-Hb (*open circles*). The time courses represent the average of 1000 flashes for each sample. The *x-axis* is scaled such that the laser pulse begins at time = 50 μseconds. Each sample contains [Hb] = 100 μM (heme) and [NO] = 1.97 mM (1 atm) in 0.1 M bis-Tris propane, 0.1 M NaCl, pH 7.4, 23°C.

It is immediately apparent from Figure 14.2 that the bimolecular recombination time courses for NO binding to αα–Hb and PEG-Hb are identical within experimental error. The recombination time courses subsequent to the laser pulse for all three hemoglobins are best described by a single exponential function, and each time course exhibits a half-time of 10 μs ($k_{obs} =$ 69,000 s^{-1}). Since the concentration of free NO (1.97 mM) is in vast excess of photolysed hemes (< 1 μM), a pseudo first order approximation is made for the recombination reaction. The overall bimolecular association rate constants for these reactions are obtained by dividing the fitted value of the observed rate constant by the concentration of NO (Table 14.1). All three hemoglobins studied (αα–Hb, PEG-Hb, HbA_0) exhibited values for the association rate constant that are, within experimental error, the same as the value previously reported for NO binding to native human hemoglobin (Table 14.1 and Cassoly and Gibson 1975).

Table 14.1 Rate and equilibrium binding constants for nitric oxide reactions with hemoglobin.

Hemoglobin	k' (μ$M^{-1}s^{-1}$)	k (× $10^{-5}s^{-1}$)	K_d (pM)	k'_{ox} (μ$M^{-1}s^{-1}$)
HbA_0	32 ± 4	4.7 ± 1	1.5	30 ± 9
αα-Hb	37 ± 4	23 ± 2	6.2	31 ± 12
PEG-Hb	34 ± 3	14 ± 1	4.2	30 ± 10

The rate constants represent the mean of at least three separate determinations. The bimolecular association rate constants (k') were measured by flash photolysis of nitrosylhemoglobin samples in the presence of 1 atm NO gas. Dissociation rate constants (k) were determined by ligand displacement with CO in the presence of excess dithionite and represent the weighted mean of the observed rate constants obtained from biexponential fits of the time courses (see text). The errors in the rate constants were determined as the standard deviation of the mean. Equilibrium binding constants (K_d) were calculated as the ratio of the dissociation rate constant to the association rate constant ($K_d = k/k'$). The bimolecular rate constants for NO oxidation of the different oxyhemoglobins (k'_{ox}) were determined by the stopped-flow rapid mixing technique.

14.3.2.2 Unimolecular dissociation rates

The dissociation of NO from αα–Hb and PEG-Hb was studied by CO replacement in the presence of excess sodium dithionite (Figure 14.3). The time courses for the conversion of nitrosylhemoglobin to carbonylhemoglobin display distinctly biphasic kinetic behavior for each HBOC and were fitted to a double exponential expression to obtain observed rate constants. The αα–Hb-NO displacement time course exhibits an observed rate constant of 6.2 × 10^{-4} s^{-1} for the rapid kinetic phase which accounts for 30% of the total absorbance change. The slower kinetic phase displays a fitted observed rate constant of 0.5 × 10^{-4} s^{-1} and accounts for the remaining 70% of the total absorbance change. In the PEG-Hb measurements, the rapid kinetic phase fitted to an observed rate constant of 2.1 × 10^{-4} s^{-1} (60%) with a value of 0.5 × 10^{-4} s^{-1} obtained for the slower kinetic phase (40%). The time courses for the dissociation of NO from purified human HbA_0 (measured as a control) yielded values of 9.2 $\times$ 10^{-4} s^{-1} for the rapid kinetic phase observed rate constant (40% of the total absorbance change) and 0.2 $\times$ 10^{-4} s^{-1} for the slower kinetic phase (60%). These results are consistent with previously reported time courses for the NO dissociation reaction (Salhany, Ogawa and Shulman 1975, Moore and Gibson 1976, Sharma and Ranney 1978).

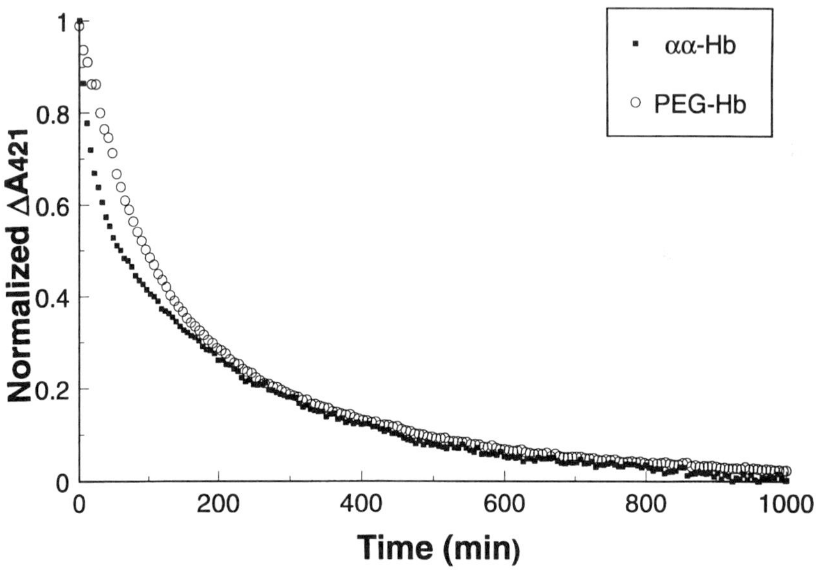

Figure 14.3. Normalized time courses for the displacement of NO by CO in the presence of excess dithoinite. The *black squares* represent the time course for αα–Hb, and the *open circles* represent the time course for Peg Hb. The reactions were carried out at 23°C in the presence of 1 mM CO. The buffer conditions were 0.1 M bis-Tris propane, 0.1 M NaCl, pH 7.4.

It should be noted that the amplitudes for the rapid and slow kinetic phases for a given Hb-NO dissociation time course are not equal, indicating that the observed biphasic kinetic behavior cannot be due simply to differences between the α and β chains. Moore and Gibson (1976) reported that for native nitrosylhemoglobin dissolved in borate buffer at pH 9.1, the replacement of NO by CO is best described by a single exponential function with an observed rate constant of 0.14 $\times$ 10^{-4} s^{-1}. As the pH was lowered, the time course of the reaction began to deviate from monophasic behavior with the appearance of a rapid kinetic phase, interpreted as being due to dissociation of NO from the low-affinity (T) state quaternary conformation of hemoglobin. The amplitude of the rapid kinetic phase increased as the pH decreased, while the observed rate constant for the slower kinetic phase remained nearly unchanged from the value obtained at pH 9.1.

The kinetic heterogeneity observed for HbA_0, αα–Hb and PEG-Hb suggests cooperative dissociation of NO and the existence of significant levels of both high affinity (R) and low affinity (T) quaternary structures of fully liganded nitrosylhemoglobin at neutral pH. Significant levels of fully liganded T-state native human nitrosylhemoglobin have been identified by nuclear magnetic resonance and ultraviolet circular dichroism spectroscopy under suitable solution conditions (Salhany, Ogawa and Shulman 1975). As NO dissociates from hemoglobin in the presence of CO, a solution of nitrosylhemoglobin that is partially in the high-affinity (R) state and partially in the low-affinity (T) state is converted to carbonomoxyhemoglobin which is entirely in the high-affinity (R) state. For human HbA_0 and αα–Hb, most of the absorbance change is associated with the slower kinetic phase implying that, under these conditions, the majority of the fully liganded nitrosylhemoglobin molecules are in the R-state conformation. However, in the case of the PEG-Hb, the rapid kinetic phase accounts for approximately 60% of the total absorbance change, with the slower kinetic phase accounting for about 40% of the total reaction. This suggests that the majority of fully saturated PEG-Hb-NO molecules are in the T-state conformation under these reaction conditions (0.1 M bis-Tris propane, 0.1 M NaCl, pH 7.4). Addition of the allosteric effector inositol hexaphosphate (IHP) has been shown to convert a solution of fully liganded human Hb-NO completely to the low-affinity (T) state (Salhany, Ogawa and Shulman 1975). In contrast, PEG-Hb is produced from bovine hemoglobin which has a quaternary conformation that is very sensitive to the presence of chloride ion as an allosteric effector (Fronticelli, Bucci and Orth 1984). It is possible that the 0.1 M NaCl present in the buffer used for these NO displacement reactions shifts the PEG-Hb-NO conformational equilibrium, such that the T-state is favored in a manner similar to the effect IHP has on human Hb-NO.

14.3.2.3 Equilibrium constants for NO binding to HBOCs

Due to the extremely high affinity of hemoglobin binding to NO, it is generally not possible to determine the values of overall dissociation equilibrium constants by titration methods. In such cases, the equilibrium dissociation constants are calculated as the ratio of the unimolecular dissociation rate constant to the bimolecular association rate constant ($K_d = k/k'$). The biphasic kinetic behavior displayed by the nitrosylhemoglobin displacement reactions means that each time course yields two observed dissociation rate constants since the solution contains significant populations of both R- and T-state nitrosylhemoglobins. The overall equilibrium dissociation constants were estimated by taking the average values for the observed dissociation rate constant, weighted by the relative contributions to the total absorbance change, and dividing by the values obtained for the bimolecular association rate constants (Table 14.1). The values of the equilibrium constants calculated in this manner show that αα–Hb binds NO more weakly than PEG-Hb (6.2 *versus* 4.2 *p*M and both of these HBOCs display a weaker NO binding than human HbA_0 (Table 14.1). Despite the observation that αα–Hb elicits a vasopressor response *in vivo* in contrast to PEG-Hb (Figure 14.1), αα–Hb binds NO more weakly than PEG-Hb.

14.3.2.4 Reaction rates of nitric oxide-induced oxidation of oxyhemoglobin

Overall bimolecular rate constants for the reaction of NO with the oxygenated forms of αα–Hb and PEG-Hb were measured by conventional rapid mixing techniques. This irreversible reaction proceeds by direct bimolecular combination of NO with O_2 bound to hemoglobin and is not an O_2 displacement reaction (Doyle and Hoekstra 1981). Oxyhemoglobin acts as a superoxide donor in this reaction, and the immediate products are peroxynitrite anion ($OONO^-$) and methemoglobin. Peroxynitrite anion is also the product of the direct reaction of NO with superoxide. The conjugate acid, peroxynitrous acid (HOONO, pK_a = 6.8), can isomerize to form nitrate, undergo homolytic cleavage to form hydroxyl and nitrite free radicals ($HO^•$ and $^•NO_2$), or isomerize to an oxidation-reduction active peroxynitrous acid species (Pryor and Squadrito 1995). Regardless of the chemical mechanism, peroxynitrite has been implicated as a possible harmful intermediate in the alteration of vascular tone and endothelial injury (Beckman *et al.* 1990) and in cardiac tissue damage during reoxygenation following hypoxia (Matheis *et al.* 1992). Thus, in addition to a possible role in NO scavenging, the products of the reaction of oxygenated cell-free HBOCs with NO may be harmful.

Figure 14.4 shows time courses for the reaction of 2 μM NO with 0.4 μM of αα–Hb and PEG-Hb. As was observed for the NO bimolecular recombination reaction (Figure 14.2), there is no difference in the reaction kinetics between αα–Hb and PEG-Hb within experimental noise limits. The reaction time courses following mixing are best described by a single exponential function, and each exhibit a half-time of 12 ms (k_{obs} = 60 s^{-1}). The rate of NO combination with oxyhemoglobin is extremely rapid, and the ability to monitor rapid reactions in the stopped-flow apparatus is limited by the mixing time of the device. NO concentrations were kept at a low value to minimize the fraction of the reaction time course lost during mixing. As a consequence, the concentration of oxyhemoglobin after mixing was kept low (0.4 μM) so that a pseudo first order approximation could be used. The use of low oxyhemoglobin concentrations gave small absorbance changes for each mixing event, and an average of 10 kinetic transients were collected and signal averaged to produce each time course. Due to all of these factors, the measurement of this reaction tests the limits of the rapid mixing technique, and the resulting rate constants are associated with somewhat large standard deviation (Table 14.1). Nevertheless, the values of the rates determined for the NO-induced oxidation reaction are consistent with those obtained for the bimolecular association reaction with the deoxyhemoglobins.

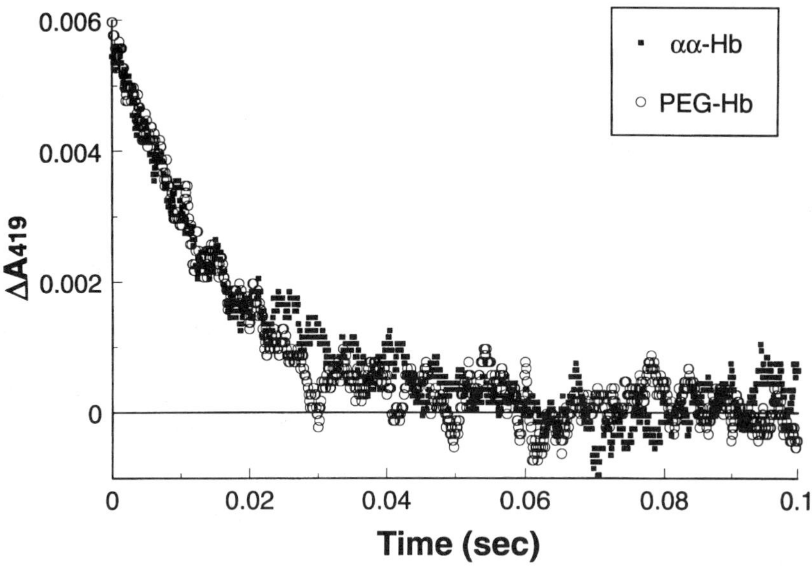

Figure 14.4. Nitric oxide oxidation of oxyhemoglobin. The Δ absorbance values at 419 nm collected with the stopped-flow rapid mixing apparatus are plotted *versus* time for αα–Hb *(black squares)* and PEG-Hb (*open circles*). The time courses represent the average of 10 mixing events for each sample. The conditions for each reaction after mixing are [Hb] = 0.4 μM (heme) and [NO] = 2 μM in 0.1 M bis-Tris propane, 0.1 M NaCl, pH 7.4, 23°C.

The overall bimolecular association rate constants for these reactions are obtained by dividing the fitted value of the observed rate constant by the concentration of NO ($k'_{ox} = k_{obs}$/[NO], Table 14.1). Both the αα–Hb and PEG-Hb experiments yielded k'_{ox} values of 30 ± 10 $\mu M^{-1}s^{-1}$. As a control, a sample of human hemoglobin A_0 was prepared along with the other samples in a manner identical to sample preparation used for αα–Hb and PEG-Hb, and a value of 30 ± 9 $\mu M^{-1}s^{-1}$ was obtained for the reaction of human oxyhemoglobin with NO.

In their recent study of the mechanism of NO-induced oxidation of hemoglobin, Eich *et al.* (1996) reported bimolecular rate constant values in the range 30-50 $\mu M^{-1}s^{-1}$ for the reaction of NO with wild-type human oxyhemoglobin, which are slightly larger than the values obtained in this study. We cannot account for the minor discrepancy in these two studies at this time. However, it is apparent that under identical reaction conditions, the rates of reaction between NOand the oxygenated forms of αα–Hb and PEG-Hb are identical.

14.4 Discussion

A series of experimental findings obtained over the years has led researchers in the field of red cell substitutes to draw the conclusion that the vasopressor response usually observed upon administration of cell-free HBOCs is due to NO scavenging by hemoglobin. NO is well established as an endothelium-derived relaxing factor (EDRF) that is believed to work by activating GC within smooth muscle cells upon binding to the heme group of this enzyme. Physiologic control of vascular smooth muscle tone is achieved by a dynamic balance of factors that cause vasoconstriction and vasorelaxation. Reduction in concentration or complete removal of EDRF *in vivo* is expected to result in an increase in vascular smooth muscle tension since a factor believed to counterbalance vasoconstrictive processes is lost. The reactions between hemoglobin and the neutral free radical form of NO that activates GC are extremely rapid and essentially irreversible. NO binds to the deoxy-form of hemoglobin with *p*M affinity, and NO reacts irreversibly with oxyhemoglobin. Both of these reactions occur with bimolecular rate constants in excess of 3×10^7 $M^{-1}s^{-1}$ at 37°C. Thus it is easy to conclude that cell-free HBOCs cause vasoconstriction by rapid removal of this EDRF.

Until recently, no direct tests of the hypothesis that the vasopressor response observed upon administration of the cell-free HBOC *in vivo* is related to the reactivity of the hemoglobin with NO measured *in vitro* have been presented. There are two reasons why such experimental evidence has proven elusive. First, a cell-free HBOC that exhibits the appropriate vasopressor response must be studied. Demonstration that reduced reactivity toward NO results in a decreased vasopressor response requires a cell-free HBOC that exhibits little or no vasoactivity. Virtually all HBOCs studied and reported on to date have been observed to cause an increase in MAP *in vivo*. Second, a hemoglobin that exhibits reduced reactivity with NO relative to native human hemoglobin must be studied. Such a hemoglobin is extremely rare due to the nature of NO binding to heme proteins.

The mechanism for diatomic ligand binding to hemoglobin is best described as a process consisting of at least two distinct steps (Rohlfs, Olson and Gibson 1988, Carver *et al.* 1990). Ligand in solution must first diffuse into and through the protein matrix that surrounds the heme active site. In a second step, ligand binds to the iron atom of the heme from within the heme pocket. In the case of NO, binding from within the heme pocket occurs on a *pico*second time scale. This process occurs so rapidly that the rate limiting step in the overall bimolecular association of NO to hemoglobin is diffusion into and throughout the surrounding protein matrix. The magnitude of the difference between the rate of binding from within the pocket and the rate of diffusion into and throughout the protein is so great that the overall bimolecular association rate constant is essentially equal to the rate of ligand diffusion into and throughout the protein. This is in contrast to what is observed for CO (where the rate limiting step is binding from within the heme pocket) and O_2 (where both steps contribute approximately equally to the overall binding process) and explains why there is no difference in the bimolecular association rates for NO binding to high-affinity (R) and low-affinity (T) state hemoglobin (Cassoly and Gibson 1975). The rate of the reaction of NO with O_2 bound to hemoglobin from within the active site must also be extremely rapid since the overall bimolecular rates for this NO-induced oxidation reaction are the same as the rate of NO binding to deoxyhemoglobin (Table 14.1, Doyle and Hoekstra 1981, Eich *et al.* 1996).

Based on these findings, it appears that in order to modulate the reactivity of a heme protein with NO, the kinetic barrier for ligand diffusion into and throughout the protein to the binding site must be increased. This was achieved for myoglobin and hemoglobin (Eich *et al.* 1996, Lemon *et al.* 1996) by decreasing the volume of the distal pocket through the use of site-directed mutagenesis. The bimolecular rates determined for NO-induced oxidation of the mutant oxyhemoglobins were up to 20-fold lower than the rate observed for wild-type oxyhemoglobin, and mutant oxyhemoglobins that exhibited reduced rates of reaction with NO also exhibited decreased vasopressor responses relative to recombinant human hemoglobin containing the β108 Asn → Lys (Hb Presbyterian) mutant. Thus it would appear that a causal relationship exists between NO reactivity and the vasopressor response, and by modulating the reactivity of a cell-free HBOC toward NO, one can reduce the increases in MAP observed upon use of the hemoglobin *in vivo*.

We have found that bovine hemoglobin conjugated to methoxypolyethylene glycol, PEG-Hb, exhibits no significant increase in MAP during isovolemic 50% ET in rat, in contrast to the significant and persistent increase in MAP that is observed when the same experiment is performed using αα–Hb (Figure 14.1 and Migita *et al.* 1997). If this difference in vasopressor response is due to differences in reactivity toward NO, then the reactivity of PEG-Hb toward NO is expected to be reduced relative to αα–Hb due to, for example, a possible increase in the kinetic barrier to NO diffusion presented by the polyethylene glycol chains. The results of this study show that this cannot be the case (Table 14.1, Figures 14.2, 14.3, and 14.4). NO reaction rates with the deoxy- and-oxy- forms of PEG-Hb, αα–Hb, and human HbA_0 are all the same. The dissociation rate constants are the only measurable difference in NO binding parameters between αα–Hb and PEG-Hb. NO appears to dissociate more rapidly from αα–Hb than from PEG-Hb. When the association and dissociation rate constants are used to calculate the equilibrium dissociation constants, the cell-free HBOC that is observed to cause an increase in MAP (αα–Hb) exhibits approximately a factor of two weaker NO binding than the cell-free HBOC that does not exhibit a vasopressor response

(PEG-Hb), exactly the opposite of what would be expected based on the hypothesis that increases in MAP are due to NO binding.

In the context of this study alone, there appears to be no relationship between NO reactivity and the vasopressor response. However, the differences observed upon 50% ET with solutions of these cell-free HBOCs must arise from differences in one or more physical properties exhibited by these solutions. PEG-Hb and αα-Hb display different O_2 binding parameters (Migita *et al.* 1997) and different solution properties including viscosity and colloid osmotic pressure (Vandegriff, Rohlfs and Winslow 1997).

It has been suggested that while cell-free HBOCs do carry O_2 *in vivo*, the presence of a low O_2 affinity cell-free HBOC may not necessarily lead to a corresponding high level of O_2 delivery to the tissues (Tsai, Kerger and Intaglietta 1995). Cell-free HBOCs may overcome a diffusive limitation to O_2 delivery (Page *et al.* 1996) resulting in abnormally high O_2 levels in the regulatory arterioles. This has the potential to produce an autoregulatory response in which vasoconstriction causes increased vascular resistance and reduced flow (Vandegriff and Winslow 1995, Tsai, Kerger and Intaglietta 1996, Winslow and Vandegriff 1997). In this model, the shape and position of the O_2 equilibrium curve, in addition to the total O_2 carrying capacity, are crucial in determining the amount of O_2 delivered to the regulatory regions of the microcirculation. The differences observed in vasoactivity between αα-Hb and PEG-Hb are consistent with this model since O_2 equilibrium binding studies indicate a significantly lower O_2 affinity and higher cooperativity for αα-Hb relative to PEG-Hb (Migita *et al.* 1997).

It has become increasingly apparent over the last few years that mechanical forces associated with blood flow play important roles in the control of vascular tone (Davies 1995). The endothelium is exposed to hemodynamic shear stress which works to regulate blood flow. When flow increases, shear stress increases, causing arteries to dilate by endothelial-dependent, nervous-system-independent, relaxation of the smooth muscle cells. For a Newtonian fluid, shear stress is directly proportional to viscosity. In the case of blood, or mixtures of blood and cell-free HBOC solutions which are non-Newtonian, shear stress increases with increasing viscosity. The effects of solution viscosity on O_2 delivery have been observed by comparing tissue oxygenation following hemodilution with either colloids or with crystalloids (Tsai, Kerger and Intaglietta 1995). Again, the difference in MAP response observed between αα-Hb and PEG-Hb is consistent with this model of shear stress-mediated vasoregulation. PEG-Hb exhibits significantly higher viscosity than αα-Hb solutions when measured at the same hemoglobin concentration and shear rate (McCarthy *et al.*, unpublished).

Because of its size and solution properties, PEG-Hb occupies a much greater molecular volume in solution than does αα-Hb (Vandegriff,

Rohlfs and Winslow 1997). This may be important if the mechanism for HBOC-induced increases in MAP requires movement of the hemoglobin from the circulation to the extravascular space. It is possible that NO scavenging occurs at levels significant enough to cause vasoconstriction only when hemoglobin enters the interstitial space between endothelial cells and smooth muscle cells. If this is the case, then PEG-Hb may not cause vasoconstriction due to its molecular size which may prevent passage of PEG-Hb through endothelial cell junctions. Both fluorescently labeled αα-Hb and PEG-Hb have been shown to extravasate within minutes in the intestine of anesthetized rats despite observations that suggest that this type of junction is too small to permit passage of PEG-Hb (Baldwin 1997). This suggests that the difference in MAP response between αα-Hb and PEG-Hb is probably not due to differences in the tendency of these hemoglobins to diffuse out of the lumen. However, the issue of extravasation may be irrelevant since the endothelial cell can be considered as a point source of NO. Once synthesized, NO diffuses in all directions. Even in the absence of extravasation, intravascular NO scavenging reactions can still act as a NO sink that will reduce the effective concentration of NO in and around smooth muscle cells (Lancaster 1994).

In conclusion, it must be remembered that physiological control of vascular smooth muscle tone relies on many factors, any or all of which may be affected by the presence of a cell-free HBOC. This study has addressed only one such factor: the ability of a cell-free HBOC to react with NO at the heme ligand binding site. The full physiological relevance of NO scavenging reactions will only be discovered through continued investigations of the mechanisms involved in regulating blood pressure.

14.5 Acknowledgments

We would like to acknowledge the contributions of Professor Doug Magde and Michael D. Magde Jr. in the preparation of this chapter. This work was supported in part by a grant from the United States Public Health Service National Heart, Lung and Blood Institute of the National Institutes of Health (No. HL48018).

14.6 References

Arnelle, D.R., and J.S. Stamler. NO^+, NO, and NO^- donations by *S*-nitrosothiols: Implications for regulation of physiological functions by *S*-nitrosylation and acceleration of disulfide formation. *Arch. Biochem. Biophys.* 318: 279-285, 1995.

Arnold, W.P., C.K. Mittal, S. Katsuki, and F. Murad. Nitric oxide activates guanylate cyclase and increases guanosine 3',5'-cyclic monophosphate levels in various tissue preparations. *Proc. Natl. Acad. Sci. USA* 74: 3203-3207, 1977.

Beckman, J.S., T.W. Beckman, J. Chen, P.A. Marshall, and B.A. Freeman. Apparent hydroxyl radical production by peroxynitrite: implications for endothelial injury from nitric oxide. *Proc. Natl. Acad. Sci.* USA 87: 1620-1624, 1990.

Baldwin, A. Blood substitutes and the intestinal microcirculation: Extravasation and ultrastructural alterations. In *Advances in Blood Substitutes: Industrial Opportunities and Medical Challenges* (R.M. Winslow, K.D. Vandegriff and M. Intaglietta, Eds.) Boston: Birkhäuser, 1997.

Carver, T.E., R.J. Rohlfs, J.S. Olson, Q.H. Gibson, R.S. Blackmore, B.A. Springer, and S.G. Sligar. Analysis of the kinetic barriers for ligand binding to sperm whale myoglobin using site-directed mutagenesis and laser photolysis techniques. *J. Biol. Chem.* 265: 20007-20020, 1990.

Cassoly, R., and Q.H. Gibson. Conformation, co-operativity and ligand binding in human hemoglobin. *J. Mol. Biol.* 91: 301-313, 1975.

Davies, P.F. Flow-mediated endothelial mechanotransduction. *Physiol. Rev.* 75: 519-560, 1995.

Doyle, M.P., N. Fink, G.J. Rosenthal, and R. Gorczynski. Efficacy of recombinant human hemoglobin to restore oxygen consumption following hemorrhage. *Artif. Cells, Blood Substitutes, Immobil. Biotech.* 24: 330, 1996.

Doyle, M.P. and J.W. Hoekstra. Oxidation of nitrogen oxides by bound dioxygen in hemoproteins. *J. Inorg. Biochem.* 14: 351-358, 1981.

Eich, R.F., T. Li, D.D. Lemon, D.H. Doherty, S.R. Curry, J.F. Aitken, A.J. Mathews, K.A. Johnson, R.D. Smith, G.N. Phillips Jr., and J.S. Olson. Mechanism of NO-induced oxidation of myoglobin and hemoglobin. *Biochemistry* 35: 6976-6983, 1996.

Fronticelli C., E. Bucci, and C. Orth. Solvent regulation of oxygen affinity in hemoglobin. Sensitivity of bovine hemoglobin to chloride ions. *J. Biol. Chem.* 259: 10841-10844, 1984.

Furchgott, R.F. Studies on the relaxation of rabbit aorta by sodium nitrite: the basis for the proposal that the acid-activatable factor from bovine retractor penis is inorganic nitrite and the endothelium-derived relaxing factor is nitric oxide. In *Mechanisms of Vasodilation* (P.M. Vanhoutte, ed.) New York: Raven, 1988, pp. 401-414.

Gellai, M., J.M. Norton, and R. Detar. Evidence for control of coronary vascular tone by oxygen. *Circ. Res.* 32, 279-289, 1973.

Greenburg, A.G., and H.W. Kim. Nitrosyl hemoglobin formation after intravenous administration of a hemoglobin-based oxygen carrier in endotoxemic rats. *Artif. Cells, Blood Substitutes, Immobil. Biotech.* 23: 271-276, 1995.

Gulati, A., A.P. Sen, A. Kumar, and M.G. Tyagi. Increase in endothelin and removal of nitric oxide (NO) contribute toward the efficacy of diaspirin crosslinked hemoglobin in hemorrhaged rats. *Artif. Cells, Blood Substitutes, Immobil. Biotech.* 24: 345, 1996.

Hamilton, I., S.C. Schultz, F. Cole, K. Burhop, and D. Malcolm. Characterization of diaspirin cross-linked hemoglobin's pressor response. *Crit. Care Med.* 20: S106, 1992.

Hess, J.R., V.W. Macdonald, and W.W. Brinkley. Systemic and pulmonary hypertension after resuscitation with cell-free hemoglobin. *J. Appl. Physiol.* 74: 1769-1778, 1993.

Ignarro, L.J. Biosynthesis and metabolism of endothelium-derived nitric oxide. *Ann. Rev.Pharmacol. Toxicol.* 30: 535-560, 1990.

Ignarro, L.J., G.M. Buga, K.S. Wood, R.E. Byrns, and G. Chaudhuri. Endothelium-derived relaxing factor produced and released from artery and vein is nitric oxide. *Proc. Natl. Acad. Sci. USA* 84: 9265-9269, 1987.

Ignarro, L.J., R.E. Byrns, and K.S. Wood. Biochemical and pharmacological properties of endothelium-derived relaxing factor and its similarity to nitric oxide radical. In *Mechanisms of Vasodilation* (P.M. Vanhoutte, ed.) New York: Raven, 1988, pp. 427-435.

Jia, L., C. Bonaventura, J. Bonaventura, and J.S. Stamler. *S*-nitrosohaemoglobin: a dynamic activity of blood involved in vascular control. *Nature* 380: 221-226, 1996.

Jones, R.T., C.G. Head, T.S. Fujita, D.T.-B. Shih, J. Wodzinska, and R. Kluger. Modification of human hemoglobin with methyl acyl phosphates derived from dicarboxylic acids. Systematic relationships between cross-linked structure and oxygen-binding properties. *Biochemistry* 32: 215-223, 1993.

Katsuki, S., W. Arnold, C. Mittal, and F. Murad. Stimulation of guanylate cyclase by sodium nitroprusside, nitroglycerin and nitric oxide in various tissue preparations and comparison to the effects of sodium azide and hydroxylamine. *J. Cyclic Nucleotide Res.* 3: 23-35, 1977.

Keipert. P.E., A. Gonzales, C.L. Gomez, V.W. Macdonald, J.R. Hess, and R.M. Winslow. Acute changes in systemic blood pressure and urine output of conscious rats following exchange transfusion with diaspirin-crosslinked hemoglobin solution. *Transfusion* 33: 701-708, 1993.

Kharitonov, V.G., A.R. Sundquist, and V.S. Sharma. Kinetics of nitric oxide autoxidation in aqueous solution. *J. Biol. Chem.* 269: 5881-5883, 1994.

Kida, Y., M. Maeda, S. Iwata, Y. Iwashita, K. Goto, and K. Nishi. Effects of pyridoxalated hemoglobin polyoxyethylene conjugate and other hemoglobin-related substances on arterial blood pressure in anesthetized and conscious rats. *Artif. Organs* 19: 117-128, 1995.

Lancaster, J.R. Jr. Simulation of the diffusion and reaction of endogenously produced nitric oxide. *Proc. Natl. Acad. Sci. USA* 91: 8137-8141, 1994.

Lee, R., K. Neya, T.A. Svizzero, and G.J. Vlahakes. Limitations of the efficacy of hemoglobin-based oxygen-carrying solutions. *J. Appl. Physiol.* 79: 236-242, 1995.

Lemon, D.D., D.H. Doherty, S.R. Curry, A.J. Mathews, M.P. Doyle, T.J. Fattor, and J.S. Olson. Control of the nitric oxide-scavenging activity of hemoglobin. *Artif. Cells, Blood Substitutes, Immobil. Biotech.* 24: 378, 1996.

Lieberthal, W., E.F. Wolf, E.W. Merrill, N.G. Levinsky, and C.R. Valeri. Hemodynamic effects of different preparations of stroma free hemolysates in the isolated perfused rat kidney. *Life Sciences* 41: 2525-2533, 1987.

Macdonald V.W., and R. Motterlini. Vasoconstrictor effects in isolated rabbit heart perfused with bis(3,5- dibromosalicyl)fumarate cross-linked hemoglobin (αα Hb). *Artif. Cells, Blood Substitutes, Immobil. Biotech.* 22: 565-575, 1994.

Martin, W., J.A. Smith, and D.G. White. The mechanism by which hemoglobin inhibits the relaxation of rabbit aorta induced by nitrovasodilators, nitric oxide, or bovine retractor penis inhibitory factor. *Br. J. Pharmacol.* 89: 563-571, 1986.

Martin, W., G.M. Villani, D. Jothianandan, and R.F. Furchgott. Selective blockade of endothelium-dependent and glyceryl trinitrate-induced relaxation by hemoglobin and by methylene blue in the rabbit aorta. *J. Pharmacol. Exp. Ther.* 232: 708-16, 1985.

Matheis, G., M.P. Sherman, G.D. Buckberg, D.M. Haybron, H.H. Young, and L.J. Ignarro. Role of L-arginine nitric oxide pathway in myocardial reoxygenation injury. *Am. J. Physiol.* 262: H616-H620, 1992.

Messina, E.J., D. Sun, A. Koller, M.S. Wolin, and G. Kelly. Increases in oxygen tension evoke arteriolar constriction by inhibiting endothelial prostaglandin syntheses. *Microvasc. Res.* 48: 151-160, 1994.

Migita, R., A. Gonzales, M.L. Gonzales, K.D. Vandegriff, and R.M. Winslow. Blood volume and cardiac index in rats after 50% exchange transfusion with hemoglobin-based oxygen carriers. *Am. J. Physiol.* in press, 1997.

Moncada, S., R.M.J. Palmer, and E.A. Higgs. Nitric oxide: physiology, pathophysiology, and pharmacology. *Pharmacol. Rev.* 43: 109-142, 1991.

Monge, C., C.A. Cazorla, G. Whittembury, Y. Sakata, and C. Rizo-Patron. A description of the circulatory dynamics in the heart and lungs of people at sea level and at high altitude by means of the dye dilution technique. *Acta Physiol. Latinoam.* 5: 189-210, 1955.

Moore, E.G., and Q.H. Gibson. Cooperativity in the dissociation of nitric oxide from hemoglobin. *J. Biol. Chem.* 251: 2788-2794, 1976.

Motterlini, R. Interaction of hemoglobin with nitric oxide and carbon monoxide: physiological implications. In *Blood Substitutes: New Challenges* (R.M. Winslow, K.D. Vandegriff and M. Intaglietta, eds.) Boston: Birkhäuser, 1996 pp. 74-98.

Nucci, M.L., R.G.L. Shorr, and A. Abuchowski. PEG- Hemoglobin. Oxygen carrying blood substitute. *Drugs Fut.* 21: 29-32, 1996.

Olson, J.S. Stopped-flow, rapid mixing measurements of ligand binding to hemoglobin and red cells. *Meth. Enzymol.* 76: 631-651, 1981.

Page, T.C., McKay, C.B., Light, W.R., and Hellums, J.D. Experimental simulation of oxygen transport in microvessels. In *Blood Substitutes: New Challenges* (R.M. Winslow, K.D. Vandegriff and M. Intaglietta, eds.) Boston: Birkhäuser, 1996 pp. 132-145.

Palmer, R.M.J., A.G. Ferrige, S. Moncada. Nitric oxide release accounts for the biological activity of endothelium-derived relaxing factor. *Nature* 327: 524-526, 1987.

Palmer, R.M.J., D.S. Ashton, S. Moncada. Vascular endothelial cells synthesize nitric oxide from L-arginine. *Nature* 333: 664-666, 1988.

Pohl U., and D. Lamontagne. Impaired tissue perfusion after inhibition of endothelium-derived nitric oxide. *Basic Res. Cardiol.* 86 Suppl 2: 97-105, 1991.

Pryor, W.A. and G.L. Squadrito. The chemistry of peroxynitrite: a product from the reaction of nitric oxide with superoxide. *Am. J. Physiol.* 268: L699-722, 1995.

Rioux F., G. Drapeau , and F. Marceau. Recombinant human hemoglobin (rHb1.1) selectively inhibits vasorelaxation elicited by nitric oxide donors in rabbit isolated aortic rings. *J. Cardiovasc. Pharmacol.* 25: 587-594, 1995.

Rohlfs, R.J., A. Gonzales, D. Baker, M. McCarthy, M.D. Magde Jr., K.D. Vandegriff, J.G. Adamson, and R.M. Winslow. Effect of altering O_2 binding properties of cell-free hemoglobin on pCO_2 and lactate levels during exponential hemorrhage following 50% exchange transfusion. *Artif. Cells, Blood Substitutes, Immobil. Biotech.* 24: 413, 1996.

Rohlfs, R.J., J.S. Olson, and Q.H. Gibson. A comparison of the geminate recombination kinetics of several monomeric heme proteins. *J. Biol. Chem.* 263: 1803-1813, 1988.

Saffran, W.A., and Q.H. Gibson. Photodissociation of ligands from heme and heme proteins. Effect of temperature and organic phosphate. *J. Biol. Chem.* 261: 7955-7958, 1977.

Salhany, J.M., S. Ogawa, and R.G. Shulman. Correlation between quaternary structure and ligand dissociation kinetics for fully liganded hemoglobin. *Biochemistry* 14: 2180-2190, 1975.

Schultz S.C., B. Grady, F. Cole, I. Hamilton, K. Burhop, and D.S. Malcolm. A role for endothelin and nitric oxide in the pressor response to diaspirin cross-linked hemoglobin. *J. Lab. Clin. Med.* 122: 301-308, 1993.

Sharma, V.S., and H.M. Ranney. The dissociation of NO from nitrosylhemoglobin. *J. Biol. Chem.* 253: 6467-6472, 1978.

Stamler, J.S., and A. Slivka. Biological chemistry of thiols in the vasculature and in vascular-related disease. *Nutr. Rev.* 54: 1-30, 1996.

Tsai, A.G., H. Kerger, and M. Intaglietta. Microcirculatory consequences of blood substitution with αα-hemoglobin In *Blood Substitutes: Physiological Basis of Efficacy* (R.M. Winslow, K.D. Vandegriff and M. Intaglietta, eds.) Boston: Birkhäuser, 1995, pp. 155-174.

Tsai, A.G., H. Kerger, and M. Intaglietta. Microvascular oxygen distribution: effects due to free hemoglobin in plasma In *Blood Substitutes: New Challenges* (R.M. Winslow, K.D. Vandegriff and M. Intaglietta, eds.) Boston: Birkhäuser, 1996, pp. 124-131.

Ulatowski, J.A, R.C. Koehler, T. Nishikawa, R.J. Traystman, A. Razynska, H. Kwansa, B. Urbaitis, and E. Bucci. Role of nitric oxide scavenging in peripheral vasoconstrictor response to beta-beta cross-linked hemoglobin. *Artif. Cells, Blood Substitutes, Immobil. Biotech.* 23: 236-269, 1995.

Vandegriff, K.D. and R.M. Winslow. A theoretical analysis of oxygen transport: a new strategy for the design of hemoglobin-based blood substitutes. In *Blood Substitutes: Physiological Basis of Efficacy* (R.M. Winslow, K.D. Vandegriff, and M. Intaglietta, eds.) Boston: Birkhäuser, 1995, pp. 143-154.

Vandegriff, K.D., R.J. Rohlfs, A. Gonzales, M.L. Gonzales, M. McCarthy, M.D. Magde Jr., G. Adamson, and R.M. Winslow. Effect of altering O_2 binding properties of cell free hemoglobins on mean arterial pressure following 50% exchange transfusion. *Artif. Cells, Blood Substitutes, Immobil. Biotech.* 24: 447, 1996.

Vandegriff, K.D., R.J. Rohlfs, and R.M. Winslow. Colloid osmotic effect of hemoglobin-based oxygen carriers. In *Advances in Blood Substitutes: Industrial Opportunities and Medical Challenges* (R.M. Winslow, K.D. Vandegriff and M. Intaglietta, eds.) Boston: Birkhäuser, 1997.

Winslow, R.M. *Hemoglobin-based Red Cell Substitutes.* Baltimore: Johns Hopkins University Press, 1992.

Winslow, R.M., and Vandegriff, K.D. Hemoglobin oxygen affinity and the design of red cell substitutes. In *Advances in Blood Substitutes: Industrial Opportunities and Medical Challenges* (R.M. Winslow, K.D. Vandegriff and M. Intaglietta, Eds.) Boston: Birkhäuser, 1997.

Wojciechowski, P. Controlling the molecular weight of an oligomerized HBOC. *Artif. Cells, Blood Substitutes, Immobil. Biotech.* 24: 461, 1996.

14.7 Discussion

Torchilin: May I ask you about the molecular weight of the polyethylene glycol which has been used in this experiment and molecular ratio of PEG to hemoglobin in the complex?

Rohlfs: If I understand your question, you want the overall molecular weight of the conjugated hemoglobin?

Torchilin: No, no, just of a single chain because what you showed is that you have several chains of PEG conjugated with a hemoglobin.

Rohlfs: Right, 5000 molecular weight PEG chains.

Torchilin: Why in this case, does it gives the size of 280 Ångstroms, because if you are using 5000 Dalton molecular weight PEG, it gives about 90 Ångstroms altogether.

Rohlfs: I should have explained that more thoroughly when that slide came up. Those values came from some oncotic pressure measurements that Dr. Vandegriff will talk about on Wednesday, and that diameter came from a radius of gyration calculated from the concentration dependence of the osmotic pressure.

Torchilin: Because this radius can really exist only under the condition of polymeric brush in which all PEG chains are so densely located to each other that they protrude into the solution. This is not usually the case. They still keep some flexibility and if so, they have a much thinner layer because they have normal tendencies as a flexible polymer to a point.

Rohlfs: Yes, I hope I didn't give the wrong impression with my cartoon drawing, but these PEG groups do not stick out like I showed in the cartoon.

Torchilin: What is known, so I do have several minor questions, and I will commence if you don't mind. The first time when PEG was used to modify proteins was with enzymes was quite long ago, in the early 1970s when Abuchowski and his group did it. What was known about it was that usually low molecular weight substrates were always converted with the same kinetic parameters, like for PEG-free enzymes. At that time, it was quite a solid conclusion, which has been supported now in experiments for years, that PEG does not change diffusion coefficients for small molecules, and these should not be a mechanism of any changes unless PEG modification somehow modifies that binding site which also might happen.

Rohlfs: No, I think you're exactly right.

Torchilin: And, I think this might be a very good explanation to what you know because this is a random modification. All reactive groups might be touched by PEG. It's very interesting to know what was the chemistry of modification. And it might just somehow modify the binding site or just the absorption site for NO•, and this is why you can see such a difference.

Rohlfs: We actually thought that might be the case when we started this study, but I think we've shown that it has no effect as all these other studies have shown, that small molecule diffusion up to the active site is unaffected.

Torchilin: And, just one small question which I did not understand, when you said that kinetic barriers are the same for reaction association and disassociation, what did you mean? Did you mean energy of activation, because if you are talking about energy of activation, you need Arrhenius slopes. Because, if at a given temperature, you do have the same constants, it still doesn't mean that the energy barrier is the same. It depends upon the slope of Arrhenius curves.

Rohlfs: That's very true, and I'm sorry if I caused confusion in this. What I meant to suggest was that for the two different reactions, NO binding to deoxyhemoglobin and NO reacting with oxyhemoglobin, it is likely that those kinetic barriers are the same.

Torchilin: At the given temperature.

Rohlfs: Yes, at the temperature of our experiment, which was 23°C.

Keipert: One quick question and then a more complex one. Was this hemoglobin that you Pegylated yourself, or was this the Enzon product?

Rohlfs: This was a gift from Enzon.

Keipert: And, is that correct, that it has a P50 of 10 torr?

Rohlfs: Right, that's what we find.

Keipert: The other thing. You're looking at *in vitro* comparisons here of nitric oxide binding in a test tube, and I'm personally not that surprised that they are very similar. I mean, I think many people have always felt that this is an intrinsic binding property to the heme. And, then at the end, you talk about some differences in these solutions that may explain the physiological differences you see in the 50% exchange, and you invoke things like colloidal oncotic pressure and P50, etc., but there seems to me that there's one dramatic difference that you haven't eluded to yet or talked about, and that's the drastic difference in intravascular retention time between these two products.

Rohlfs: Right.

Keipert: You've got an αα-hemoglobin that clearly has been shown to extravasate; it's cleared very quickly; it'll get into the interstitial space between the vascular smooth muscle wall and the endothelial cell and, presumably, that's where the nitric oxide binding will cause vasoconstriction, and the pegylated hemoglobin has probably the longest blood half-life because the pegylation keeps it intravascular.

Rohlfs: I can give you a short answer and a long answer. The short answer is that Dr. Baldwin will talk about this either tomorrow or Wednesday. The long answer is that, as Joe Bonaventura pointed out and as Lancaster has pointed out, even if it does not extravasate, it is still going to act as an NO sink in the vascular space, and this will effectively reduce the NO concentration throughout the system. I also want to point out that blood does not cause vasoconstriction, and how does one explain why NO is not being scavenged by blood. I would suggest to you that the kinetic barrier presented by the RBC membrane is not sufficient to slow down NO binding if this were, in fact, the mechanism.

Keipert: I thought red cells were a sink for nitric oxide binding for whatever does diffuse into the vascular space.

Rohlfs: Well then, if that's the case, then it still doesn't explain why alpha-alpha hemoglobin shows vasoconstriction and PEG hemoglobin doesn't. Whether they are scavenging nitric oxide or not, you cannot invoke a difference in vasoactivity based on a difference in NO reactivity at the heme as an explanation for it.

Keipert: I agree that for the hemoglobin that's inside the vasculature, they may both be a sink to equal degrees, but if one of them gets on the other side of that cell and the other one doesn't, that could cause a difference.

Rohlfs: Yes, and then again, I'll say even if it doesn't extravasate, it still will act as a sink from within the vasculature which will effectively lower the NO concentration.

Winslow: Let me interject something, Ron, if you don't mind. Peter, the paper that Ron mentioned by Migita *et al.*, in press in the *J. Appl. Physiol.,* shows that the short-term half-life for these two hemoglobins is exactly the same; that is, if you look at the half-life over 25 minutes, the curves are superimposable, and so I don't think that you can explain this on the basis of a rapid elimination into some other space as a difference between the two hemoglobins.

Bonaventura: Nice talk. Thanks a lot. You talked about the reaction of oxyhemoglobin and nitric oxide. What are the products?

Rohlfs: The products are methemoglobin and peroxynitrite anion, initially.

Bonaventura: And there are no intermediates that you can think of?

Rohlfs: Well, not that I'm aware of. This is all based on what I've read in the literature.

Bonaventura: And so, the stoichiometry?

Rohlfs: Is 1:1.

Bonaventura: Have you measured it?

Rohlfs: I have not quantified the amount of peroxynitrite produced. We can quantify the amount of methemoglobin produced by the absorbance change, and that's 1:1.

Bonaventura: So you have no data to suggest that it's not 1:1.

Rohlfs: That's correct.

Gonzales: If you actually look at the MAP graph, PEG hemoglobin does increase a little bit. There is some vasoactivity.

Rohlfs: It's not statistically significant over baseline.

Gonzales: Well, I guess my point is that I just think it's fair to say that there could be possible vasoconstriction going on there.

Rohlfs: Yes, I agree. It is possible, and I tried to touch on this in the last slide. It is possible that the PEG hemoglobin is scavenging NO, but some other property of that molecule can either attenuate or mask that effect.

Gonzales: Just to throw in a variable, the αα-hemoglobin is at 8 g/dl, whereas the PEG hemoglobin is at 5.5 g/dl.

Winslow: May I ask one final question, Ron, or maybe Joe Bonaventura might comment on this. We're left at the end of this story without an explanation for why one hemoglobin is vasoactive and the other one isn't. We seem to be ruling out possibilities here. I wonder if somebody who understands eNOS might comment on the possibility that if we have a hemoglobin that unloads oxygen very readily if, in fact, we may be suppressing eNOS activity enough to cause this degree of vasoactivity in this kind of a time span.

Rohlfs: I'd look to Vijay to comment on that one.

Sharma: Interesting data. You see, the second order rate constant for the reaction of NO with oxyhemoglobin is 2×10^7, and this is if we assume it is simply the rate for oxygen diffusing into the heme pocket. Then the rate constant for the reaction of NO with oxygen, you can assume somewhere around 10^{10} on the basis of geminate recombination of NO with heme proteins. This is the same rate constant that you have for the reaction of NO with O_2^-. So what it seems is that oxygen is sitting there more or less like O_2^-. This may not be the case if oxygen affinity is high in a hemoglobin variant. In other words, how much dissociated oxygen comes out O_2^-. It will depend on how much oxygen affinity that protein has for oxygen. High affinity proteins are less likely to leave O_2^- than low affinity mutants, and that is where the probable explanation of the question you asked.

Index

A

B

C

D

Q

R

Y

Z

Permissions

[1] Figure 4.2, page 50 is reprinted from *J. Natl. Canc. Inst.* 81, pp. 570-576, © Bethesda: U.S. National Cancer Institute 1989.

[2] Table 11.1, page 218 is reprinted from *Biophys. Chem.* (in press), © Amsterdam: Elsevier Science 1997.

[3] Table 11.2, page 224 is adapted from *J. Appl. Physiol.* (in press), © Bethesda: American Physiological Society 1997.

[4] Figure 11.1, page 217 is reprinted from *Biophys. Chem.* (in press), © Amsterdam: Elsevier Science 1997.

[5] Figure 11.2, page 218 is reprinted from *Biophys. Chem.* (in press), © Amsterdam: Elsevier Science 1997.

[6] Figure 11.3, page 219 is reprinted from *Biophys. Chem.* (in press), © Amsterdam: Elsevier Science 1997.

[7] Figure 11.4, page 222 is reprinted from *Biophys. Chem.* (in press), © Amsterdam: Elsevier Science 1997.

[8] Figure 11.5, page 222 is reprinted from *Biophys. Chem.* (in press), © Amsterdam: Elsevier Science 1997.

[9] Figure 11.6, page 223 is reprinted from *Biophys. Chem.* (in press), © Amsterdam: Elsevier Science 1997.

[10] Figure 13.1, page 256 is adapted from *J. Liposome Res.* 4, pp. 725-739, © Amsterdam: Elsevier Science 1994.

[11] Figure 13.3, page 258 is reprinted from *Biochim. Biophys. Acta* 1195, pp. 11-20, © Amsterdam: Elsevier Science 1994a.

[12] Figure 13.4, page 260 is adapted from *Biochim. Biophys. Acta* 1279, pp. 75-83, © Amsterdam: Elsevier Science 1996.

[13] Figure 13.5, page 262 is reprinted from *Adv. Drug Delivery Rev.* 16, pp. 157-182, © Amsterdam: Elsevier Science 1995a.

[14] Figure 13.10, page 273 is reprinted from *Biochim. Biophys. Acta* 1195, pp. 181-184, © Amsterdam: Elsevier Science 1994b.